# Taking SIDES

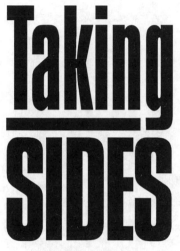

## Clashing Views on Controversial Issues in Health and Society

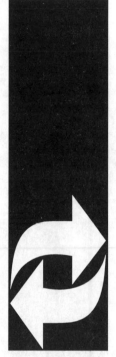

**Fourth Edition**

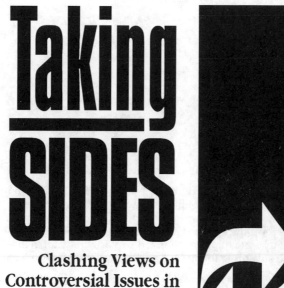

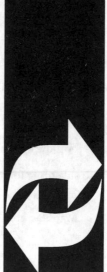

# Taking SIDES

### Clashing Views on Controversial Issues in Health and Society

**Fourth Edition**

**Edited, Selected, and with Introductions by**

## Eileen L. Daniel

*State University of New York College at Brockport*

Dushkin/McGraw-Hill
A Division of The McGraw-Hill Companies

*To Ann*

**Photo Acknowledgments**

© 1999 by PhotoDisc, Inc.

**Cover Art Acknowledgment**

Charles Vitelli

**Library of Congress Cataloging-in-Publication Data**

Main entry under title:
    Taking sides: clashing views on controversial issues in health and society/edited, selected,
and with introductions by Eileen L. Daniel.—4th ed.
    Includes bibliographical references and index.
    1. Health. 2. Medical care—United States. 3. Medical ethics. 4. Social medicine—United
States. I. Daniel, Eileen L., *comp.*

362.1

0-07-303191-7

ISSN: 1094-7531

 Printed on Recycled Paper

# PREFACE

This book contains 42 selections arranged in 21 pro and con pairs. Each pair addresses a controversial issue in health and society, expressed in terms of a question in order to draw the lines of debate more clearly.

Most of the questions that are included here relate to health topics of modern concern, such as AIDS, abortion, environmental health, and drug use and abuse. The authors of the selections take strong stands on specific issues and provide support for their positions. Although we may not agree with a particular point of view, each author clearly defines his or her stand on the issues.

This book is divided into six parts, each containing related issues. Each part opener provides a brief overview of the issues and offers several related sites on the World Wide Web, including Web addresses. Each issue is preceded by an *introduction*, which sets the stage for the debate, gives historical background on the subject, and provides a context for the controversy. Each issue concludes with a *postscript*, which offers a summary of the debate and some concluding observations and suggests further readings on the subject. The postscript also raises further points, since most of the issues have more than two sides. At the back of the book is a listing of all the *contributors to this volume*, which gives information on the physicians, professors, journalists, and scientists whose views are debated here.

*Taking Sides: Clashing Views on Controversial Issues in Health and Society* is a tool to encourage critical thought on important health issues. Readers should not feel confined to the views expressed in the selections. Some readers may see important points on both sides of an issue and may construct for themselves a new and creative approach, which may incorporate the best of both sides or provide an entirely new vantage point for understanding.

**Changes to this edition**    The fourth edition of *Taking Sides: Clashing Views on Controversial Issues in Health and Society* includes some important changes from the third edition. Eight completely new issues have been added: *Should Human Cloning Ever Be Permitted?* (Issue 5); *Is Stress Responsible for Disease?* (Issue 6); *Does Tobacco Advertising Influence Teens to Smoke?* (Issue 8); *Should Confidentiality Remain a Priority for People With AIDS?* (Issue 13); *Should Partial-Birth Abortion Be Banned?* (Issue 14); *Will Most Postmenopausal Women Benefit from Estrogen Replacement Therapy?* (Issue 15); *Should a Low-Fat, High-Carbohydrate Diet Be Recommended for Everyone?* (Issue 19); and *Should All Children Be Immunized Against Childhood Diseases?* (Issue 20). In addition, for four of the issues, I have retained the question from the third edition but have replaced one of the selections in order to bring the debate up-to-date or to focus more clearly on the controversy: Issue 1 on managed care, Issue 3 on limiting health care for the elderly, Issue 18 on global warming, and Issue 21 on homeopathic remedies. In all, there are 20 new readings. The issue introductions and postscripts have all been revised and updated.

**A word to the instructor**　An *Instructor's Manual With Test Questions* (both multiple-choice and essay) is available through the publisher for instructors using *Taking Sides* in the classroom. Also available is a general guidebook, *Using Taking Sides in the Classroom,* which discusses teaching techniques and methods for integrating the pro-con approach of *Taking Sides* into any classroom setting. An online version of *Using Taking Sides in the Classroom* and a correspondence service for Taking Sides adopters can be found at http://www.dushkin.com/usingts/. For students, we offer a field guide to analyzing argumentative essays, *Analyzing Controversy: An Introductory Guide,* with exercises and techniques to help them to decipher genuine controversies.

*Taking Sides: Clashing Views on Controversial Issues in Health and Society* is only one title in the Taking Sides series. If you are interested in seeing the table of contents for any of the other titles, please visit the Taking Sides Web site at http://www.dushkin.com/takingsides/.

**Acknowledgments**　Special thanks again to John, Diana, and Jordan. Also, thanks to my colleagues at the State University of New York College at Brockport for all their helpful contributions. Finally, I appreciate the assistance of the staff at Dushkin/McGraw-Hill.

Eileen L. Daniel
State University of New York
College at Brockport

# CONTENTS IN BRIEF

# CONTENTS

Surgeon David Jacobsen makes the claim that health maintenance organizations (HMOs) offer quality care and that high-quality medical care at an affordable price is not only possible under managed care; it is a reality. Pediatrician and author Ronald J. Glasser argues that managed care companies care more for profits than for people.

Marcia Angell, executive editor of *The New England Journal of Medicine*, asserts that physician-assisted suicide should be permitted under some circumstances and that not all of the pain of the dying can be controlled. Physician Kathleen M. Foley argues that doctors do not know enough about their patients, themselves, or suffering to provide assistance with dying as a medical treatment for the relief of suffering.

Hastings Center director Daniel Callahan contends that medical care for
elderly people who have lived their natural life expectancy should consist
only of pain relief rather than expensive health care services that serve only
to forestall death. Patricia Lanoie Blanchette, a physician and a professor of
medicine and public health, argues that health care should not be rationed
by age and that age bias should be recognized and confronted.

Josh Sugarmann, executive director of the Violence Policy Center, argues
that guns increase the costs of hospitalization, rehabilitation, and lost wages,
making them a serious public health issue. Attorney Don B. Kates, professor of
genetics Henry E. Schaffer, and William C. Waters IV, a physician, counter that
most gun-related violence is caused by aberrants, not ordinary gun owners.

Attorney John A. Robertson contends there are many benefits to cloning and
that a ban on privately funded cloning research is unjustified. Attorney and
medical ethicist George J. Annas argues that cloning devalues people by
depriving them of their uniqueness.

The editors of the *Harvard Health Letter* maintain that there is evidence that individuals who are chronically stressed possess an increased risk of cancer and heart disease. Writer Christopher Caldwell argues that no one, including doctors, can come to an agreement on what stress is, so stress can not be blamed as the cause of disease.

Herbert Benson, an associate professor of medicine at Harvard Medical School, and journalist Marg Stark contend that faith and spirituality will enhance and prolong life. William B. Lindley, associate editor of *Truth Seeker*, counters that there is no scientific way to determine that spirituality can heal.

Professor of business Richard W. Pollay states that teens are influenced to smoke by advertising that appeals to them. He argues that the advertisements portray smokers as independent and successful in the quest for social approval. Editor and journalist Jacob Sullum argues that there is no evidence that advertising encourages people, particularly teens, to smoke.

Writer Dave Shiflett contends that for years the antidrinking establishment has insisted that even moderate drinking is bad for health despite the fact that science indicates otherwise. Physicians Meir J. Stampfer and Eric B. Rimm and professor Diana Chapman Walsh argue that encouraging the use of alcohol, even in moderation, could lead to an increase in its consumption, with potentially dangerous results.

Eric A. Voth, medical director of Chemical Dependency Services at St. Francis Hospital in Topeka, Kansas, argues that marijuana produces many adverse effects and that its effectiveness as a medicine is supported only by anecdotes. Ethan A. Nadelmann, director of the Lindesmith Center, a New York drug policy research institute, asserts that government officials continue to promote the myth that marijuana is harmful and leads to the use of hard drugs.

Reporter Jennifer Washburn challenges two studies that claim silicone gel implants do no harm and finds that over 10 percent of the women who received implants are ill. Journalist Michael Fumento argues that special interests and the press have conspired to ban implants despite the fact that no scientific study has linked them to cancer or other diseases.

Health and medical reporters Leslie Laurence and Beth Weinhouse assert that women have been excluded from most research on new drugs and medical treatments. Physician Andrew G. Kadar argues that women actually receive more medical care and benefit more from medical research than men do.

Journalist Gabriel Rotello contends that there are good reasons to exempt AIDS from the traditional public health tracking of infectious diseases. Disease intervention specialist William B. Kaliher argues that treating the disease as a public health issue rather than as a political issue can help reduce the number of AIDS cases.

Professor and neurosurgeon Robert J. White states that Congress should completely ban late-term, partial-birth abortion. John M. Swomley, a professor emeritus of social ethics, maintains that the increased medical risk caused by banning late-term, partial-birth abortion is reason enough for Congress to allow the practice.

Health columnist Michael Castleman asserts that unless a woman has a history of breast cancer, the benefits of postmenopausal hormone replacement therapy far outweigh the risks. Writer Julie Felner interviews physician Dr. Susan Love, who states that she is alarmed that many physicians prescribe hormone replacement therapy for all menopausal patients indefinitely.

Journalists Dennis Bernstein and Thea Kelley maintain that disabling, sometimes life-threatening medical problems related to environmental and chemical exposure are currently affecting thousands of soldiers who fought in the
Persian Gulf War. Michael Fumento, a science and economics reporter, argues
that medical experts have not found any evidence to support the existence of
a syndrome related to the war.

Martha Honey, a research fellow at the Institute for Policy Studies, asserts that
pesticides in the food chain are building up in animals and humans and are
disrupting the immune system, causing cancers, and creating birth defects.
Bruce Ames, a professor of biochemistry and molecular biology, argues that
any risks from pesticides in foods are minimal and that fears are greatly
exaggerated.

Journalist Ross Gelbspan contends that we need to act now to prevent future
catastrophic climatic changes that may result from global warming. Chemists
Arthur B. Robinson and Zachary W. Robinson argue that even though carbon
dioxide levels have increased during the past 20 years, global temperatures
have decreased.

# INTRODUCTION

## Dimensions and Approaches to the Study of Health and Society

Eileen L. Daniel

### WHAT IS HEALTH?

Traditionally, being healthy meant being absent of illness. If someone did not have a disease, then he or she was considered healthy. The overall health of a nation or specific population was determined by numbers measuring illness, disease, and death rates. Today this rather negative view of assessing individual health and health in general is changing. A healthy person is one who is not only free from disease but also fully well.

Being well, or wellness, involves the interrelationship of many dimensions of health: physical, emotional, social, mental, and spiritual. This multifaceted view of health reflects a holistic approach, which includes individuals taking responsibility for their own well-being.

Our health and longevity are affected by the many choices we make every day. Medical reports tell us that if we abstain from smoking, drugs, excessive alcohol consumption, fat, and cholesterol, and if we get regular exercise, our rate of disease and disability will significantly decrease. These reports, although not totally conclusive, have encouraged many people to make positive lifestyle changes. Millions of people have quit smoking, alcohol consumption is down, and more and more individuals are exercising regularly and eating low-fat diets. These changes are encouraging, but the many people who have been unable or unwilling to make them are left feeling worried and/or guilty over continuing their negative health behaviors.

Additionally, experts disagree about the exact nature of positive health behaviors, and this causes confusion. For example, some scientists maintain that overweight Americans should make efforts to lose weight, even if it takes many tries. Others assert that losing weight and gaining it back repeatedly is worse for one's health than remaining overweight. Another debatable issue is whether or not people should consume moderate amounts of alcohol to help prevent heart disease. Many studies have shown it to be beneficial, while others indicate that alcohol may increase the risk of breast cancer.

Health status is also affected by society and government. Societal pressures have helped pass smoking restrictions in public places, mandatory safety belt legislation, and laws permitting condom distribution in public schools. The government plays a role in the health of individuals as well, although it has failed to provide minimal health care for many low-income Americans.

Unfortunately, there are no absolute answers to many questions regarding health and wellness issues. Moral questions, controversial concerns, and individual perceptions of health matters all can create opposing views. As you evaluate the issues in this book, you should keep an open mind toward both sides. You might not change your mind regarding partial-birth abortion or the limitation of health care for the elderly, but you will still be able to learn from the opposing viewpoint.

## HEALTH AND SOCIETY

The issues in this book are divided into six parts. The first deals with health care and society. Part 1 begins with a debate on whether or not managed health care offers consumers an improvement over traditional care. In the United States approximately 35 to 40 million Americans have no health insurance. Furthermore, there has been a resurgence in diseases such as tuberculosis and antibiotic-resistant strains of bacterial infections, which threaten thousands of Americans and strain the current system. Those enrolled in government programs such as Medicaid often find few, if any, physicians who will accept them as patients because reimbursements are low and the paperwork is cumbersome. On the other hand, Americans continue to live longer and longer, and for most of us, the health care available is among the best in the world.

Issue 2 deals with whether or not physicians should intervene to hasten death for hopelessly ill persons. Many Americans agree that we cannot and should not prolong the lives of terminally ill patients, although others believe that physicians should not hasten the process of dying but rather should offer these individuals relief from pain and quality of life management strategies. A related debate is presented in Issue 3, which questions the wisdom of using expensive life-prolonging treatments on elderly patients. The fourth controversy in this section is about the epidemic of homicide and the potential benefits of more stringent gun control. Doctors and public health officials claim that homicides involving guns are increasing, which is driving health care costs up and diminishing quality of life. They maintain that gun control would help reduce the shootings and deaths. Opponents of gun control argue that under such a policy only criminals—not law-abiding citizens—would have access to guns. They also contend that doctors should leave the gun control issue to criminologists. Issue 5 asks, Should human cloning ever be permitted? Cloning technology offers the *potential* to asexually produce a human child. While there are pros and cons to the ability to clone cells, ethical and moral questions also arise.

## MIND/BODY RELATIONSHIP

Part 2 discusses two important issues related to the relationship between mind and body. Is stress responsible for disease, and can spirituality overcome disease? Over the past 10 years, both laypeople and the medical profession have placed an emphasis on the prevention of illness as a way to improve health. Not smoking, for instance, certainly reduces the risk of developing lung cancer. Unfortunately, the current U.S. health care system places an emphasis on treatment rather than on prevention, even though prevention is less expensive, less painful, and more humane. Stress management programs have arisen to prevent stress-related illness, which many believe is responsible for the majority of doctor visits. Does stress cause disease, and will managing stress actually prevent disease? Issue 7 discusses the role of spirituality in the prevention of disease. Many studies have found that religion and spirituality play a role in recovery from sickness. Should health providers encourage their patients to seek spirituality?

## SUBSTANCE USE AND ABUSE

Part 3 introduces current issues related to drug use and abuse in the United States. Millions of Americans use and abuse drugs that alter their minds and affect their bodies. These drugs range from illegal substances, such as crack cocaine and marijuana, to the widely used legal drugs, such as alcohol and tobacco. Use of these substances can lead to physical and psychological addiction and the related problems of family dysfunction, reduced worker productivity, and crime. Because of drug-related crime, many experts have argued for the legalization of drugs, particularly marijuana. The argument is that if currently illegal drugs were legalized, the enormous profits from illegal drug sales would no longer exist, which would reduce criminal behavior in this area and free law enforcement officials to focus on other crime areas.

The American drug crisis is often related to changes in or a breakdown of traditional values. The collapse of strong family and religious influences may affect drug usage, especially among young people. It has been argued, however, that some people, regardless of societal or familial influences, will use drugs based on need. For example, some people have testified that cancer patients can benefit from marijuana because it reduces the severity of the effects of chemotherapy. Although there is a movement to legalize this drug for its medicinal purposes, many experts want marijuana to remain illegal (see Issue 10). Alcohol and its role in the prevention of heart disease are also discussed in this section. Alcohol is a factor in car crashes, violence, and health problems. Heavy drinkers are at risk for cirrhosis, cancer, hypertension, malnutrition, and other illnesses. Although these risks are well known, some experts maintain that moderate drinking can actually improve health by reducing stress and heart attacks. They believe that moderate drinking should be promoted as a means of reducing heart disease.

Also in this section is a debate on the role of advertising and smoking. Almost all smokers began smoking as teenagers. Many factors, including peer pressure, influence teens to smoke. Is exposure to cigarette ads one of those major factors?

## SEXUALITY AND GENDER ISSUES

For years, women in North America have had the option of augmenting the size of their breasts by having silicone implants placed under their skin. Some women have the operation to reconstruct their breasts following a mastectomy, but most opt for the surgery for cosmetic reasons. Recently, some women with breast implants have claimed that the silicone has caused health problems ranging from headaches to autoimmune diseases. Several successful lawsuits were based on the premise that silicone caused these health problems. Jennifer Washburn holds this opinion, but Michael Fumento argues that there is no conclusive evidence that silicone causes disease.

The second issue discussed in this section is whether or not our health care system favors men at the expense of women. Although they live longer than men, many women claim that they have been excluded from drug tests and other medical research and receive inferior care when they see doctors. Opponents of this view maintain that women see their doctors more frequently than men, are hospitalized more often, and continue to outlive men by several years.

As the AIDS epidemic continues, should physicians take a traditional public health approach in combatting the disease? If so, partners of afflicted people would likely be tracked and encouraged to seek treatment. On the other hand, tracking might discourage individuals from getting tested for AIDS in the first place. The issue of confidentiality for people with AIDS is presented in Issue 13.

The abortion issue continues to cause major controversy. More restrictions have been placed on the right to abortion as a result of the political power wielded by the pro-life faction. Pro-choice followers, however, argue that making abortion illegal again will force many women to obtain dangerous "back-alley" abortions. Complicating the issue has been the recent killings and shootings of doctors and other personnel in abortion and women's health clinics and the recent debates over late-term, or partial-birth, abortion, which is the focus of Issue 14.

Routinely prescribing estrogen replacement hormones for postmenopausal women is the final issue discussed in this section. Many doctors are against the routine use of these drugs, while others argue that they should always be prescribed unless there is a specific reason not to.

## ENVIRONMENTAL ISSUES

Debate continues over the two fundamental issues surrounding the environment: human needs and the future of the environment. The debate becomes more heated as the environmental issues move closer to human concerns, such as health, economic interests, and politics. In Issue 16, for example, the debate focuses on whether or not troops stationed overseas during the Persian Gulf War were exposed to harmful environmental or chemical substances that caused their present health problems. Issue 17 discusses the safety of pesticide usage on fruits and vegetables. The Alar (a chemical growth regulator for apples) scare convinced many Americans that the apple supply was not safe and that an apple a day could cause cancer. At the same time, nutritionists as well as the Department of Agriculture were urging people to eat more fruits and vegetables to help *prevent* cancer.

The question of whether or not environmental changes are having a serious impact on the average global temperature is debated in Issue 18. Global warming has many implications, including political, health, economic, and environmental. Due to increased levels of greenhouse gases in the atmosphere, global temperatures appear to be rising. Rising temperatures could cause major catastrophes such as loss of plant and animal species, a reduction of the food supply, drought, disease, and flooding of low-lying coastal areas.

## CONSUMER HEALTH AND NUTRITION DECISIONS

Part 6 introduces questions about particular issues related to choices about health care services: (1) Should a low-fat, high-carbohydrate diet be recommended for everyone? (2) Should all children be immunized against childhood diseases? and (3) Are homeopathic remedies legitimate?

Losing weight and maintaining a healthy lifestyle are major concerns for many people nowadays. Much of the effort to lose weight has focused on reducing fat intake. Indeed, many experts agree that a low-fat, high-carbohydrate diet lowers serum cholesterol levels and risk of heart disease and, therefore, improves one's overall health. However, opponents of this view maintain that a low-fat, high-carbohydrate diet does not reduce the risk of heart disease or cancer and that it actually contributes to obesity. Issue 19 explores this debate.

At the turn of the twentieth century, millions of American children developed childhood diseases such as tetanus, polio, measles, and pertussis (whooping cough). Many of these children died or became permanently disabled because of these illnesses. Today vaccines can prevent all of these conditions; however, not all children receive their recommended immunizations. Some do not get vaccinated until the schools require them, and others are allowed exemptions. More and more, parents are requesting exemptions for some or all vaccinations based on fears over their safety and their effectiveness. The pertussis vaccination seems to generate the biggest fears. Reports of serious injury to children following the pertussis vaccination (usually given in a combination of diphtheria, pertussis, and tetanus, or DPT) have convinced many parents to forgo immunization. As a result, the incidence rates of measles and pertussis have been climbing after decades of decline. Is it safer to be vaccinated than to risk getting pertussis? Most medical societies and physicians believe so, but Richard Moskowitz argues that many vaccines are neither safe nor effective.

Current views of homeopathy and the use of homeopathic remedies are discussed in Issue 21. Due to demand by the public, homeopathy is achieving new legitimacy, despite the efforts of traditional medicine to discredit the practice. As more consumers turn their backs on traditional medicine, the use of homeopathic remedies has increased. Is homeopathy an effective treatment?

Will the many debates presented in this book ever be resolved? Some issues may resolve themselves because of the availability of resources. For instance, funding for health care for the elderly may become restricted in the United States, as it is in the United Kingdom, simply because there are increasingly limited resources to go around. As health costs continue to rise, an overhaul of the health care system to provide managed care for all while keeping costs down seems inevitable. Other controversies may require the test of time for resolution. Several more years may be required before it can be determined whether or not global warming is really a serious environmental hazard. The debates over the effectiveness of stress management, the health effects of moderate use of alcohol, and the benefits of estrogen replacement therapy may also require years of additional research.

Other controversies may never resolve themselves. There may never be a consensus over the abortion issue, gun control, tracking people with AIDS, or physician-assisted suicide. This book will introduce you to many ongoing controversies on a variety of sensitive and complex health-related topics. In order to have a good grasp of one's own viewpoint, it is necessary to be familiar with and understand the points made by the opposition.

# On the Internet . . .

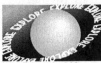
http://www.dushkin.com

## National Committee for Quality Assurance
The National Committee for Quality Assurance's Web page features an HMO accreditation status list that is updated monthly. It also provides accreditation summary reports on a number of HMO plans and other consumer information on managed care plans.
*http://www.ncqa.org*

## Euthanasia World Directory
This site is about euthanasia and contains a newsletter and a main page featuring Dr. Jack Kevorkian. There is also a discussion on the book *Final Exit* and numerous citations about different laws regarding assisted suicide.
*http://www.efn.org/~ergo/*

## Huffington Center on Aging
The Huffington Center on Aging, Baylor College of Medicine's home page offers links to related sites on aging and Alzheimer's disease. *http://www.hcoa.org*

## GunCite
This Web site is dedicated to a comprehensive discussion of gun control and Second Amendment issues. It includes analyses of firearms statistics, research, and gun control policies. *http://www.guncite.com*

## The Human Cloning Page
This page lists links related to human cloning, morals, ethics, and how cloning is done, as well as providing background about cloning sheep and other mammals.
*http://users.andara.com/~bpaul/humanclone.html*

# PART 1

## Health and Society

*The United States currently faces many health challenges, including an aging population and providing quality health services in a managed care environment. Society must confront the financial cost of providing health care to the elderly. At the same time, millions of Americans have enrolled in health maintenance organizations, which attempt to control health care costs through managing care. Although many people are happy with managed care, others claim it restricts access to the health care they need. To further complicate health issues, public policy and medical ethics have not always kept pace with rapidly growing technology and scientific advances. This section discusses some of the major controversies concerning the role of society in health concerns.*

■ Will Managed Care Improve Health Care in the United States?

■ Should Doctors Ever Help Terminally Ill Patients to Commit Suicide?

■ Should Health Care for the Elderly Be Limited?

■ Is Gun Control a Public Health Issue?

■ Should Human Cloning Ever Be Permitted?

# ISSUE 1

## Will Managed Care Improve Health Care in the United States?

**YES: David Jacobsen,** from "Cost-Conscious Care," *Reason* (June 1996)

**NO: Ronald J. Glasser,** from "The Doctor Is Not In: On the Managed Failure of Managed Health Care," *Harper's Magazine* (March 1998)

### ISSUE SUMMARY

**YES:** Surgeon David Jacobsen makes the claim that health maintenance organizations (HMOs) offer quality care and that high-quality medical care at an affordable price is not only possible under managed care; it is a reality.

**NO:** Pediatrician and author Ronald J. Glasser argues that managed care companies care more for profits than for people.

Many Americans have perceived serious wrongs with the current health care system. In general, these concerns are (1) increasing health care access to the uninsured, (2) gaining the ability to keep one's health insurance when one changes or loses a job, and (3) controlling the escalating costs of health care.

Health care in the United States is handled by various unrelated agencies and organizations and through a number of programs, including private insurance, government-supported Medicaid for the needy, and Medicare for the elderly. Currently there are between 35 and 40 million people—about 16 percent of the population—who do not have any health insurance and who do not qualify for government-sponsored programs. These people must often do without any medical care or suffer financial catastrophe if illness occurs. A *New York Times* article in 1992 claimed that 50 percent of personal bankruptcies in the United States have been attributed to medical costs.

In addition to the number of uninsured people, America's health care is the most expensive in the world. The United States spends more on health care than any other nation, about $2,600 per capita. The share of the national output of wealth, the gross domestic product (GDP), expended by the United States on health is 14 percent and rising. Yet the United States has a lower life expectancy, higher infant mortality, and a higher percentage of low birth weight infants than Canada, Japan, or most western European nations. Ironically, the United States is the only industrialized nation other than South Africa that does not provide government-sponsored health care to all its citizens.

One solution to America's health care problems has been the shift to managing care through various plans, such as health maintenance organizations (HMOs). HMOs are organizations that provide health care in return for pre-fixed payments. Most HMOs provide care through a network of doctors and hospitals that their members must use in order to be covered. Currently, more than 50 million workers—70 percent of the nation's eligible employees—now have health care through some type of managed care. The rise in managed care is related to employer efforts to reduce health care benefit costs. There are cost savings, but consumer groups and physicians worry that managed care will move medical decisions from doctors to accountants. Proponents of the managed care industry argue that health care will actually improve under its care. They claim that it makes good financial sense for managed care providers to intervene before patients get sicker. Unfortunately, seriously ill patients, who are the most expensive to treat, may lose out under managed care.

The underlying principle of managed health care is to maintain the health of a community by offering early detection tests and preventive care, such as cholesterol screenings, vaccinations, physical exams, and smoking cessation programs. These services are usually provided at a modest fee or co-payment. In exchange for these reduced fees, the consumer agrees to see a limited group of doctors and providers selected by the managed care plan. The plan keeps rates down by limiting the patient's access to costly specialists and procedures, using less expensive and lesser-trained providers, and reducing hospital stays. Some health care workers have complained that pressure has been put on them to discharge patients as quickly as possible. Managed care plans have also increasingly demanded that certain medical procedures that were once done only in a hospital now be done in a less costly outpatient setting.

Does managed care compromise quality? Studies comparing traditional fee-for-service and managed care have found that the quality of care is similar. Consumer satisfaction surveys do not necessarily agree. Managed care patients are less likely to be satisfied with their care than those in a traditional practice. The more seriously ill they are, the more dissatisfaction they report. A recent survey by the Harvard School of Public Health found that managed care patients reported longer waits to see a specialist. They were also more likely to report incorrect care by their primary care physicians. Most experts believe there is a wide range in quality among managed care plans. In cities where managed care is relatively new, managed care plans tend to offer the lowest possible premiums in order to attract new subscribers. Quality is often sacrificed. In communities where managed care has been well established, the quality tends to be higher.

In the following selections, David Jacobsen argues that HMOs offer quality care that is comparable with the traditional fee-for-service. Ronald J. Glasser argues that managed care companies are more concerned with profits than with patients.

# YES
David Jacobsen

# COST-CONSCIOUS CARE

"Torture by HMO" is the title of a March 18 [1996] column by Bob Herbert in *The New York Times*. Herbert tells the story of a North Carolina family with a baby suffering from leukemia. Their health maintenance organization insisted that the child undergo treatment in another state, at great cost and inconvenience. Herbert condemns the HMO's "inflexible and thoroughly inhumane" policies, adding that "humanitarian concerns are not what corporate care is about. In the competition with profits, patients must always lose."

This portrait of HMOs as soulless money-making machines has become increasingly popular in recent years, as skyrocketing health care costs have driven a shift from fee-for-service medicine to managed care. Critics such as Harvard Medical School professor David Himmelstein contend that HMOs reward doctors for providing less care, trapping them in a conflict between their incomes and their patients' welfare, and impose "gag clauses" that forbid them to discuss this conflict with patients. "The bottom line is superseding the Hippocratic oath," write Jeff Cohen and Norman Solomon in their syndicated column. "Cost-cutting edicts from HMO managements put doctors in a box.... Faced with directives to help maximize profits, many physicians are under constant pressure to shift their allegiance from patients to company stockholders."

From my perspective as both a physician and a patient in the same HMO, these charges do not ring true. I do not doubt that HMOs, like any other business, sometimes serve their customers poorly. But there is no reason to believe that managed care systematically undermines patient welfare because of the imperative to cut costs. To the contrary, I have found that efficiency is perfectly compatible with compassionate, effective health care. (Since this article was written, I have myself become a cancer patient. Thus far, my care has been unsurpassed. I have the option of being treated outside my HMO, but would not think of going anywhere else. I expect from my plan the same level of care as a patient that I have provided as a physician.)

My plan delivers care at several neighborhood health centers. Each member chooses a "home" center and a primary care physician at that center. Surgical, pediatric, obstetrical, and mental health services, as well as radiology, laboratory, pharmacy, and physical therapy, are all provided under one roof. While our "staff model" HMO does not offer as extensive a choice of physicians as many "network" HMOs, our arrangement does offer economies of scale and strict control of physician quality. Surveys consistently show that patients rate quality of care above greater choice of providers.

I am paid a straight salary and modest bonuses tied to both the plan's profitability and a patient satisfaction index. Frequent advisory audits help me and my patients sort out health care they *need* from health care they *want*. My goal is healthy, satisfied patients and a financially sound business. Every day, I put my professional reputation on the line. So does my HMO. Our challenge is to cut costs without cutting quality. Fortunately, there are many ways to do this.

* * *

Changing the venue of medical care from hospital to out-patient center, office, or home is the most important factor driving health care costs down and quality up. Hospitals are very expensive pieces of architecture. They are also complex places and therefore potentially hazardous to your health. Despite rigorous safeguards, medication and treatment errors can and do occur. As many as 15 percent of hospitalized patients go home with a hospital-acquired infection, often caused by antibiotic-resistant organisms. Furthermore, most patients do not wish to be in a hospital. In the last three years, my HMO has reduced hospital use by 25 percent.

Inguinal hernia repair is one of the most frequently performed operations.

Just a few years ago, the cost of this operation included a preoperative night in the hospital, one to two hours in the operating room under general anesthesia, and up to five postoperative days in the hospital. The patient had to take four to six weeks off work, and the recurrence rate was 10 percent. In 1996, at my HMO, this operation requires 40 minutes of surgery in a free-standing, outpatient surgical center under local anesthesia using a $100 plastic-mesh plug. Patients have less discomfort, return to unrestricted work in one week, and enjoy a recurrence rate of less than 1 per 1,000. This approach to hernia repair has been technically feasible for several years but was usually employed sporadically, at the discretion of the surgeon or the patient. In the era of cost containment, it has rapidly become the standard in the profession, regardless of reimbursement mode.

Thanks to the innovation of laparoscopic surgery, 80 percent of my patients who need their gallbladder removed can undergo the operation as outpatients and return to work in a week. The original inspiration for this procedure was the development of miniature video cameras, and the early reports were dismissed as mere technical wizardry. But as it became clear that laparoscopic gallbladder removal was not only safe but much less expensive than conventional surgery, surgeons quickly adopted the procedure as the standard approach, and patients demanded it.

* * *

The challenge of providing better care at lower cost has spurred not only the development of new procedures but the resurrection of old ones. Pilonidal abscess, a chronic and painful anorectal condition, used to be treated with radical surgery in the hospital. Recovery was frequently prolonged and painful. I now treat this problem with a 20-minute office procedure. Patients can return to work in two days, and the recurrence rate is less than 2 percent. This procedure was first described 15 years ago but languished until managed care created the incentive to implement it on a wider scale.

Open-heart surgery is expensive. Traditionally, the payer is billed separately by the hospital, the surgeon, and the anesthesiologist. My HMO recently negotiated a contract in which we pay a flat fee per operation that is about half our previous cost. As for concerns that surgeons might offer less surgery for less money, our studies show no change in mortality or morbidity since this contract went into effect. Beyond the question of ethics, no reputable provider group would risk a lucrative contract with a large HMO by delivering less than first-class care. Based on this experience, we are exploring package pricing for other high-cost procedures, such as organ transplantations.

Childhood asthma is a distressing and sometimes frightening problem for parents and children. Our studies showed that repeated visits to the emergency room were not only unnerving for families but accounted for a substantial portion of the cost of treating asthma. Through an aggressive program of family education, we are teaching our patients how to handle most asthma attacks at home, even how to give adrenaline injections. A nurse practitioner is available by telephone 24 hours a day to advise families whether a visit to the hospital may be necessary. Emergency room visits are down 40 percent in the last two years. So far, we have noted no adverse effects on patient care, and the response from families has been almost entirely positive.

Treatment of minor lacerations used to involve a trip to the hospital emergency room and frequently entailed a long wait. On nights and weekends our health centers are now staffed with specially trained physician assistants who repair 90 percent of all minor lacerations. In the first year this program has saved more than $100,000 in hospital emergency room charges while taking care of our patients better and more quickly.

For many of our patients with chronic wounds, such as bedsores and diabetic ulcers, treatment has often involved lengthy stays in rehabilitation hospitals or prolonged, expensive home visits by nurses. Under our wound-care program, most patients with chronic wounds can be treated directly at our health centers under the supervision of a physician. In most cases, patients and their families can be trained to do the daily wound care at home. In the first year, this program saved more than $70,000 in outside utilization costs.

Patients needing hip replacement surgery are often elderly and suffering from other medical problems. We now begin physical therapy evaluation in the patient's home *prior* to surgery. By knowing the level of family support and the location of stairs and bathrooms, we can much better prepare the patient for recuperation and rehabilitation. The new approach has cut the average hospital stay in half, eliminated the need for intermediate rehab hospital care in many cases, and accelerated recuperation.

For the past three years, my HMO has followed a policy of early discharge after childbirth. The childbirth program includes comprehensive prenatal education, post-partum home visits, and individual screening. A 16-year-old first-time mother with no family support and no telephone at home is not sent home in 24 hours. But 70 percent of women with uncomplicated vaginal deliveries are discharged in 24 to 36 hours. And despite the recent brouhaha over "drive-thru" deliveries, a recent survey documents that 90 percent of our patients are satisfied with their care—the same percentage as before the early discharge policy was adopted. There is no evidence that the health of mother or infant has been compromised. Most mothers and their babies belong at home with an attentive family, rather than in a potentially dangerous hospital.

Unnecessary diagnostic tests are probably the most familiar example of American medicine's spendthrift ways. Our computers are now set up so that every time a physician orders a laboratory test or X-ray procedure, a window on the screen displays the cost. Before managed care we neither knew nor asked. Preliminary analysis shows that this minor innovation has significantly reduced the ordering of routine laboratory and X-ray tests, especially among medical residents (physicians in training).

* * *

Much criticism of HMO care focuses not on common procedures such as these but on rare, emotionally charged illnesses. The cover story in the January 22 [1996] issue of Time, for example, chronicles the experience of a woman with advanced breast cancer whose HMO refused to pay for bone marrow transplantation. In such desperate cases, everyone understandably feels that something ought to be done. But the truth is that bone marrow transplantation for advanced breast cancer is a dangerous and expensive treatment of no proven benefit. This kind of case must be handled on an individual basis with consummate compassion and understanding, but it should not divert our attention from the myriad ways in which good medical care can be delivered for less money.

The significance of the potential conflict between physician income and patient welfare has also been exaggerated. First of all, it is offensive to me and the overwhelming majority of my colleagues to suggest that we would pad our bank accounts by obstructing or denying necessary medical care to our patients. I hew to an ethical standard of care, and so does my HMO. I am first and foremost the advocate of my patients, but always within the constraints of appropriate care and limited resources. More care is not always better care, and wishing that medicine could be exempt from the laws of economics does not make it so.

While there are various arrangements by which physicians are compensated under managed care, the incentives are to provide neither too little care nor too much care but optimal care. Under managed care, the worst course I could follow is to provide less than optimal care. Delay in diagnosis or treatment would only invite more expensive diagnosis and treatment down the line (and probably a lawsuit as well). Denying needed care is not only bad ethics; it is bad business.

As for the highly publicized "gag clauses," which have been outlawed in Massachusetts and a number of other states, my HMO does not have one. HMOs are entitled to insist on the confidentiality of proprietary information, but my HMO and most others encourage physicians to discuss financial incentives, covered benefits, and care options with patients. Many physicians are understandably dispirited by what they view as the demise of traditional health care and by projections of a 150,000-physician glut by the year 2000. But grievances and frustrations should be discussed with management and peers. Discussing them with patients can only erode an already embattled doctor–patient relationship.

\* \* \*

Despite the charges of conflict and carnage, the evidence suggests that most physicians and patients are adjusting remarkably well to the managed care revolution and that the quality of care remains high. Studies have consistently shown that HMO patients are at least as satisfied with their care as patients receiving traditional fee-for-service care. A recent survey by CareData Reports, a New York health care information firm, revealed that, among members of 33 HMOs nationwide, nearly 80 percent were satisfied with their care. (The lowest ratings were not for quality of care but for administration and communication.) A 1994 study of 25,000 employees conducted by Xerox showed that HMO patients were significantly more satisfied with their overall care than were fee-for-service patients. In a 1994 Federal Employee Health Benefits Program survey of 90,000 federal employees, 86 percent of HMO members said they were satisfied with their plans, compared with 82 percent in fee-for-service plans. Interestingly, a 1994 survey by Towers Perrin revealed that patient satisfaction with HMO care rose with years of membership.

The results of research using objective measures have been similar. A 1996 study by KPMG Peat Marwick found that, in cities where most health care was provided by HMOs, costs were 11 percent lower, hospital stays 6 percent shorter, and death rates 5 percent lower than in cities where most care was provided under fee-for-service arrangements. A study recently published in the *Journal of the American Medical Association* looked at costs and outcomes of treatment for several chronic illnesses. Compared with fee-for-service specialists, HMO primary care physicians used 40 percent fewer hospital days and 12 percent less drugs. At four- and seven-year follow-ups, patient outcomes were the same.

A 1995 North Carolina study looked at the cost and outcome of treatment for lower-back pain. Costs for a single episode ranged from $169 in an HMO to $545 at a fee-for-service chiropractor, while outcomes were identical. As David Nash, an HMO expert at Jefferson Medical College in Philadelphia, told the *Chicago Sun-Times* last year [1995], "Overwhelmingly, the published evidence supports the notion that quality of care in the managed care arena equals, if not surpasses, the care in the private, fee-for-service sector."

The shift to managed care unquestionably imposes greater responsibility on patients. More information is becoming available to enable them to compare costs and benefits and make intelligent choices. We ought to disabuse ourselves of the notion that we can have a perfect health care system in which no one is ever misdiagnosed, mismanaged, or missed altogether. But high-quality medical care at an affordable price is not only possible under managed care; it is a reality.

# NO
### Ronald J. Glasser

# THE DOCTOR IS NOT IN

We are born, we live, and then we die, but these days we do so with less and less help from a medical profession paid to discount our suffering and ignore our pain. Proofs of the bitter joke implicit in the phrase "managed care" show up in every morning's newspaper, in casual conversations with relatives or friends recently returned from a hospital or from what was once thought of as a doctor's office instead of an insurance company's waiting room, and in a country generously supplied with competent and compassionate doctors, 160.3 million of us now find ourselves held captive to corporate health-care systems that earn $952 billion a year but can't afford the luxury of a conscience or a heart.

Childless women in every city in America dread the simplest fertility workups because they know that the evaluation probably will serve as evidence denying them future payments for diseases of the vagina, uterus, or ovaries; the rest of us have had our co-payments increased, our use of prescription drugs curtailed or replaced by corporate-sanctioned medications, stays in the hospital reduced or eliminated, "pre-authorizations" required for necessary and routine tests. The broad removal of health-care benefits takes place at all points of the country's medical-industrial complex, and in line with the tone and temper of the times more than 2,300 Massachusetts physicians in December of last year signed a despairing manifesto in the *Journal of the American Medical Association:*

> The time we are allowed to spend with the sick shrinks under the pressure to increase throughput, as though we were dealing with industrial commodities rather than afflicted human beings.... Physicians and nurses are being prodded by threats and bribes to abdicate allegiance to patients, and to shun the sickest, who may be unprofitable. Some of us risk being fired or "delisted" for giving, or even discussing, expensive services, and many are offered bonuses for minimizing care.

Such forced denial of care occurs at a time when new medical and surgical technologies allow physicians to treat and often cure any number of conditions that only a few years ago barely could be diagnosed; organs now can be digitally reconstructed in three dimensions to locate previously inoperable tumors; heart attacks can be stopped with injections of a compound known as tPA; blind people may wake up and see with implanted plastic lenses; one-and-a-half-pound premature babies, once given up for lost, routinely are nursed to health; a new generation of medical research brings us genetically engineered tests and one nearly miraculous drug after the next. At the same moment, presumably well-insured women diagnosed with disseminated breast cancer must hire lawyers to have their health plans pay for life-saving bone-marrow transplants and managed-care companies can deny powered wheelchairs to handicapped children who pass a "utilization review" showing them able to stagger twenty-five feet with the help of a walker.

But although a good many of us suspect that somehow we are being swindled, and those of us who have fallen seriously ill know for a fact that the purveyors of managed care often wish we would go away or die—as quietly and quickly as possible—we're reluctant to draw the commercial moral of the tale. The system wasn't meant to care for sick people; it was meant to make and manage money.

\* \* \*

The theory of "managed care" first attracted attention in the 1940s in the coal regions of Kentucky and West Virginia. Labor unions hired doctors, constructed clinics and hospitals, and supplied prepaid medical services at a fixed monthly rate to their members and their families. The fixed rate per patient was unrelated to the patient's use of the service. By the 1950s, a few large companies had taken a similarly paternalistic stance and were offering contract health care to their own employees. The arrangement was not designed to profit anyone other than those who received care, which was why it worked.

But in the 1970s, the government and large corporate employers began to seek ways to reduce health-care costs, and the concept of contract medicine was injected with the virus of the profit motive. Cadres of systems managers, some of whom had planned the failed technowar in Vietnam, brought forth new corporate structures meant to introduce market forces into the industry and named by the several acronyms (HMO, PPO, POS, etc.) for preferred or managed medicine.[1] Not only were a lot of people going to get well, but some of them were going to get rich. First promoted by what is known as InterStudy (a health-policy think tank organized in 1972), the proposition relied on the idea that an HMO could make money if it provided medical care only to people who enjoyed the prior benefits of perfect health and a full-time job. Thus the practice known as "cherry picking," which virtually removed the burden of insuring people who were seriously ill. You simply cannot be employed full time if you suffer from the effects of a crippling disability or disease.

The full story of how and why, over the short span of twenty years, the concept of the HMO came to dominate nearly every phase of American medicine (directing the distribution of every operation, wheelchair, test, and pill) would embrace all the arts of financial chicanery made popular in the 1980s with appropriate reference to junk-bond financing, the prosperity of the drug companies, the general acceptance of the 401-K plan, the demographics of the baby boom, and probably a list of every fund-raiser attended by Presidents Ronald Reagan and George Bush. Here was but one scheme in an era of schemes, the HMO as a brilliant means of redistributing income from individual physicians to corporate executives and shareholders. The short-term profits were extraordinary: PacifiCare, for example, swelled from a $168,911 enterprise in 1986 to a $10 billion behemoth by 1997.

For corporations and small businesses burdened with rising medical costs, the HMO appeared as a gift from heaven. As recently as 1980 company health plans enrolled only a small percentage of the eligible employees; last year the plans enrolled 85 percent, up from 48 percent in 1993. The percentage of doctors practicing outside the HMOs meanwhile has dwindled to the present 19.9 percent.[2]

But the spectacular success of managed care proved to be the cause of its equally spectacular failures. Cherry picking is another name for a Ponzi scheme, and sooner or later it falls apart. Even a company blessed with tens of thousands of healthy subscribers eventually finds itself obliged to pay for the occasional premature birth at $1,500 a day, or the occasional employee who develops a brain tumor or whose wife is diagnosed with ovarian cancer. There are car accidents and near drownings. There are the late complications of diabetes, the forty-year-old struck down with a heart attack, the previously undiagnosed melanoma, the complications of hypertension. The odd executive may need a hip replacement because of an old football injury, or a chief financial officer a heart transplant after what should have been a routine viral illness. If the HMO acquires 400,000 or half a million new members (as it must if its stock price is to keep rising), the costs

mount at an exponential rate. Now there may be as many as 20,000 claims a month —a metastasis of paperwork, a hemorrhage of cash. The co-payments coming in from new enrollees can no longer keep up with the money going out. New restrictions must be implemented, new administrators hired to guarantee compliance, more controls, more advertisements to attract new members. The whole operation begins to unravel.[3]

When a company finds itself hard-pressed for profit, then behind the closed doors of the executive suite what has been left unsaid becomes the loud and forthright voice of reason: *Yes, we are a company that cares about the well-being of the American people, but the free market is the free market, and so . . .* And so, among the middle managers and accountants of the nation's health plans the talk these days turns to ways of lowering what Wall Street calls an HMO's "medical-loss ratio"—i.e., that percentage of yearly revenues allotted to patient care. The term, in and of itself, repudiates every principle that undergirds the profession of medicine and flatly contradicts the Hippocratic oath, which pledges a physician's first responsibility to the care of his or her patient. But banks don't accept payment in oaths, as was made plain by an analyst from Nutmeg Securities, Ira Zuckerman, who reminded his prospective investors last November that the attractiveness of managed-care companies as investments changes when health plans sign up members who will actually have to see a doctor. The rule of thumb holds that a managed-care business is in trouble if more than 65 percent of its enrollees submit a significant claim in any one-year period. Little wonder then that rehabilitation for stroke victims or occupational therapy for spinal-cord injuries no longer make the list of benefits. Managed-care companies actually seek to *hide* their competencies; no HMO wishes to advertise its successes with cystic fibrosis or multiple sclerosis, or, say, the skill of its subspecialists who treat AIDS. Were a company to become known for treating complicated or expensive diseases, it would run the real risk of attracting the attention of the very sick. The blurring of priorities becomes embarrassingly obvious in the newspaper ads that promote the virtues of the country's prepaid health plans. As, for instance, last December in the Minneapolis *Star Tribune:*

> We offer an extensive and unique program of reporting quality, accessibility and satisfaction data to consumers at the clinic and physician level—through the internet and other mechanisms.
>
> We developed a doctor-led organization, called the Institute for Clinical Systems Integration, that develops nationally recognized medical best practices using the best medical minds in our community.
>
> We have received numerous national awards for our community health improvement initiatives.
>
> We created the nation's first comprehensive program to encourage reading and brain stimulation for infants and young children.

In less than five years, managed care has managed to eliminate from the public-policy debate any and all words that describe suffering and disease, and together with the good news about "reporting quality," and "satisfaction data," the industry defends itself against past, present, and future criticism by explaining the symptoms that afflict the country's health-care system with at least five warm and welcome fairy tales that

the public apparently still chooses to believe:

**All doctors are rich and omnipotent:** The stereotyped image of the aloof and wealthy physician driving a Mercedes or wandering over a golf course allows the proponents of managed care to imply, usually with a good deal of success, that any doctor who speaks ill of corporatized medicine is, by definition, a greedy and callous fellow who thinks only about his fees.

As a percentage of all medical costs, the money allotted to physicians' services has remained constant over the last thirty years. Between 1993 and 1995, what the American Medical Association calls "median physician net income (after expenses, before taxes)" declined, in real terms, by 1.4 percent. Surgeons and radiologists, among them the most highly paid practitioners in any of the medical professions, earned, on average in 1995, roughly $250,000. The sums dwindle into pittances when compared with the earnings of the executives of publicly traded managed-care companies, which, on average in 1996, approached the handsome sum of $10 million. What inflates the price of medicine in the United States is the cost of corporate vice presidents, not the cost of doctors.

Which possibly explains why the number of practicing physicians in the United States has increased by no more than 20 percent in the last six years, while since 1983 the number of health-care managers has increased by 683 percent. The comparative percentages speak to the loss of authority on the part of doctors who no longer have much to say about the schedules they keep, the fees they charge, the treatments and protocols they prescribe. As often as not, they possess as little power of decision as the custodians of a hospital's linen supply.

**The operation is unnecessary:** The rich doctor requires the unnecessary operation (as well as the superfluous test, the costly prescription, the frivolous C-section or coronary bypass) not for any sound medical reason but in order to become even more rich. Thus the nation's hospitals and operating rooms supposedly overflow with patients who have no cause for serious complaint, healthy, happy people, who, were it not for the avarice of their physicians, would be baking pies or running relay races.

Once again, actual practice contradicts the heartwarming cant. The numbers of C-sections performed in the country have more to do with the availability of fetal-monitoring equipment and the fear of malpractice suits than with the will to profit on the part of the attending obstetrician. Recent reviews of coronary-bypass operations have shown that the number of inappropriate procedures varies from 0 percent to 2.4 percent, while the number deemed "equivocal" never has exceeded 7 percent. The number of inappropriate coronary angiographies in a 1994 study conducted in New York State was 5 percent. In 1992, a Medicare pre-authorization program was discontinued when, following a review of Medicare requests for coronary-bypass procedures in the state of Texas, a negligible number were found to be inappropriate.

Health-care executives like to say that doctors get away with performing needless operations because their monopoly of the standard surgical repertoire excuses them from having to explain or justify their actions. The canard ignores the fierce but societally beneficial struggle between different medical specialties, a struggle that constantly forces the argument about what is necessary and what is not. Internists develop drugs to reduce the need for the cardiovascular surgeons' bypass procedure; neonatalists use chemicals to get premature infants off respirators quicker and keep them out of the hands of pulmonologists; infectious-disease specialists develop oral regimens and home antibiotic therapies as alternatives to orthopedic surgery or in-hospital IV medications.

**The doctor is a mechanical device:** The systems planners at the Pentagon construed the Vietnam War as a manufacturing problem—victory a product, death a means of production, soldiers listed in the inventories like truck tires or boxes of ammunition. A similar habit of mind inclines our health-care managers to classify doctors as interchangeable pieces of hospital equipment. As with light bulbs and bottles of saline solution, so also with heart specialists and neurosurgeons. Every doctor serves as well as every other doctor. The proposition is patently false, but it allows the HMOs to limit their patients' choice of physician. Like nineteenth-century coal miners obliged to buy their necessities from a company store, subscribers to late-twentieth-century health plans must go to the doctors named on a company list. A number of HMOs improve the policy with a further refinement of cost-saving simplification. Not content with the assignment of absolute equality to doctors in all degrees of specialty, they suggest that the only physician whom any patient ever needs to see is the primary-care physician—i.e., the doctor who knows a little of this and a little of that, who is so well rounded that he points in no direction at all, a compliant soul content to follow a memo or a guideline because he isn't sure when an MRI is really appropriate or whether, in the attempt to rule out Lyme disease, it is best to do the expensive Western Blot test or the cheaper ELISA essay.

**The patient loves going to the hospital:**  As corollary to the story of the rich doctor, the health-care companies tell the story of the patient as spendthrift fool, who, if left to his or her own devices, will bankrupt the country with an "infinite demand" for heart transplants, kidney dialysis, and liposuction. But as with the health-care industry's other probings of imaginary symptoms, the diagnosis has been proven false. Most people check into hospitals only when they have no choice in the matter, and the nonexistent phenomenon of infinite demand doesn't lead to the unproven result of infinite cost. New medical treatments and surgical procedures, no matter how expensive when first introduced, retain their original costly forms for astonishingly short periods. Less expensive and less complicated therapies invariably replace the early experiments.

The evolving art of kidney dialysis offers the textbook case in point. Long before the advent of managed care, kidney specialists looking for an alternative to hemodialysis—with its inconvenience, risks of infection, clotting, and blood loss, as well as its complicated machinery—pursued the development of the less demanding peritoneal dialysis. So also with balloon angioplasty, which today has become the preferred alternative to the expensive coronary bypass. So also with every other specialty that anybody but an insurance agent cares to name.

An axiom of economics holds that nothing can be rationed that is itself not scarce, and, absent evidence of infinite demand and infinite cost, you can't ration health care when there are more than enough doctors, hospitals, and high-tech equipment distributed through the country to do everything and anything that needs to be done. American health care is an unsaturated demand market, and in such markets "rationing" is simply a code word for not spending the money to take care of the poor, the uninsured, the underinsured, and the high-risk patient.

**Sickness is the patient's fault, and death is a preventable disease:**  Because we live in a society that equates youth and wellness with intelligence and superior moral character, the health-care industry can pretend that it really isn't supposed to do anything at all. If the patient hadn't been so careless—if he or she had given up smoking and drinking, read the complete works of Andrew Weil, cut down on the day's fat intake, checked the blood pressure, ridden the stationary bicycle, ingested the correct amounts of garlic and zinc, gotten in touch with the inner child —then the patient wouldn't be making so many awful noises, wouldn't be conspiring to harm the "medical-loss ratio," wouldn't be bothering doctors (busy and important people, albeit overpaid) with the miserable proofs of their weakness and stupidity.

No health plan advertises the fact that a good many patients admitted to the hospital with a diagnosis of a myocardial infarct have few or none of the so-called risk factors for a heart attack: they are not smokers; they are not overweight; they are not hypertensive; they exercised; they have normal cholesterol. No plan sends out notices or memos that one in twenty-five births will have a congenital defect, or that a third of patients with diabetes run the risk of going blind.

In truth, it is a dangerous world out there. Slip through the ice, get hit on the freeway, wake up with blood in your urine, have trouble breathing, stumble about after a splitting headache, lose the ability to feel, have trouble remembering things, experience ringing in your ears, find mucus in your stools, start gasping at night, and garlic pills will be of little help. But wellness is the panacea of the 1990s, and the health plans promote the wonders of aerobic exercise and fat-free diets in order to obscure the real purpose of medicine, which is the treatment of illness and the relief of suffering. To the extent that the plans can shift the burden of health care to the private sectors of personal hygiene and morality, they excuse themselves from the tedious and increasingly expensive chores of providing a public service or addressing the common good.

*  *  *

For the last twenty years the theory and practice of managed care has enjoyed the protection of the political and financial interests—insurance companies, the pharmaceutical industry, large business corporations, suppliers of hospital equipment, members of Congress—eager to keep the Ponzi scheme profitably in place. Assured of the approval of the best people that money can buy, the HMOs have gone calmly about the business of eliminating one treatment after another and adding one doctor after the next to their rosters. For the time being they probably can count on their formularies of false diagnosis to preserve the illusions of compassion and competence. But every month another 315,000 Americans reach the age of fifty, a figure that will

rise over the next fifteen years. Of the money spent on medical care during the course of an average American's lifetime, the bulk of it is spent during the last two or three years of that life, and by the year 2010, people over the age of sixty-five will constitute the most rapidly multiplying sector of the population. They will want, expect, and need medical care, but who will pay the bill? The government has been steadily depleting the funds intended to meet the future costs of Social Security and Medicare, and the working children of what promises to be the most long-lived generation in the country's history can't be counted on to come up with either the money or the will to support a pyramid scheme.

Because Americans as they grow older tend to become more political, the demographics also imply the likelihood of active protests on the part of large numbers of people (surprisingly vigorous, remarkably well informed) bent on redressing what they will come to perceive, not without reason, as a balance of wrongs. The reaction already has begun. A few months ago the Massachusetts physicians published their manifesto, and the American College of Rheumatology recently recommended that chronic arthritis patients should be seen at least once by a rheumatologist both for confirmation of the diagnosis and the development of an adequate treatment plan. The American College of cardiology has compiled its own guidelines for heart disease and posted them on the Internet in the hope that Americans might learn from a computer what they never will learn from a doctor sworn to silence by an HMO.

All the symptoms of protest confirm the same diagnosis—a health-care industry sickened with the virus of "medical-loss ratio" and unlikely to recover until cured of its addiction to the profit motive. A physician is not by nature a commodities broker, a clinic is not a meatpacking plant, and unless the health-care industry quits caring for money instead of people, its chronic pathology almost certainly will be referred to the consulting rooms of government. Not that the politicians will want to take the case, but let enough people make strong enough complaint, and the therapeutics committees in the country's legislatures might be forced to write a new and not so mean-spirited set of guidelines.

## NOTES

1. Alan Enthoven, who served as a systems analyst under Defense Secretary Robert McNamara during the Vietnam War, devised the theory of managed competition and still serves as its principal apologist, both in his capacity as chairman of California's Managed Health Care Improvement Task Force and as a professor of health-care economics at Stanford University.

2. The wealthier American zip codes continue to support a troupe of expensive physicians whose skills (at unclogging beefeater hearts or smoothing the wrinkles in a woman's neck) are so renowned, or whose clients are so prosperous, that they do not accept any form of insurance. Such practices are, in effect, boutiques, and the practitioner is able to lavish time and attention on his patients, who may in turn congratulate themselves on the quality of the care they have received.

3. Last fall, Oxford Health Plans, Inc., a "model" HMO that aggressively marketed its friendliness toward consumers, reported losses of $125 million, citing higher medical costs than expected. Not surprisingly, the stock price of Oxford lost 80 percent of its value over the span of four months. Shortly thereafter, investors accused Oxford executives of withholding information about the company's balance sheet while they sold large blocks of shares. The Securities and Exchange Commission and the New York Attorney General's Office are investigating the complaint.

# POSTSCRIPT

## Will Managed Care Improve Health Care in the United States?

Should managed care scare the typical health care consumer? Will our access to necessary care be denied in favor of the bottom line? Many experts think that is the case since managed care plans reward physicians for providing less care. In some plans, gag orders have been imposed on member doctors. The doctors are forbidden, or "gagged," from disclosing expensive treatment options not covered by the plan. As more and more workers are enrolled in managed care programs by their employers, can we assume that companies can make better health care choices than their employees would individually? On the other hand, can we as a nation cope with rising health costs, especially as our population ages?

An overview of managed care is provided in "Managed-Care Plan Performance Since 1980: A Literature Analysis," *Journal of the American Medical Association* (May 18, 1994) and "Managed Care: Do Health-Care Firms Sacrifice Quality to Cut Costs?" *CQ Researcher* (April 12, 1996).

Although there are dissatisfied consumers, several articles claim that the quality of care through managed care is comparable to fee-for-service care. These include "Managed Care Can Help Curb Medicare Costs," *USA Today* (February 8, 1995); "Managed Care Means Shared Responsibilities," *St.Louis Post-Dispatch* (January 29, 1996); and "Learning to Accentuate the Positive in Managed Care," *The New England Journal of Medicine* (February 13, 1997).

Many articles, books, and reports, however, claim that patients suffer under managed care. These include "Bedside Mania: Medicine Turned Upside Down," *The American Prospect* (March/April 1997); "The Sick Business: Why For-Profit Medicine Couldn't Care Less," *The New Republic* (December 29, 1997); "Why HMOs Are the Opposite of Free Markets," *Human Events* (January 30, 1998); "Should We Accept Mediocrity?" *The New England Journal of Medicine* (April 9, 1998); and "Health Care Update," *American Enterprise* (March/April 1998).

If managed care is not the solution for reforming medical services in the United States, are there alternatives? The Canadian system has often been considered the solution to rising health care costs in the United States. The Canadian medicare program, however, has been under attack for not providing necessary services for its patients, especially in regard to making referrals to specialists. For information on the Canadian system, read "Bitter Medicine: Canada Is Taking an Ax to Its Popular Health Care System," *In These Times* (January 20, 1997).

# ISSUE 2

## Should Doctors Ever Help Terminally Ill Patients to Commit Suicide?

**YES: Marcia Angell,** from "The Supreme Court and Physician-Assisted Suicide: The Ultimate Right," *The New England Journal of Medicine* (January 2, 1997)

**NO: Kathleen M. Foley,** from "Competent Care for the Dying Instead of Physician-Assisted Suicide," *The New England Journal of Medicine* (January 2, 1997)

### ISSUE SUMMARY

**YES:** Marcia Angell, executive editor of *The New England Journal of Medicine,* asserts that physician-assisted suicide should be permitted under some circumstances and that not all of the pain of the dying can be controlled.

**NO:** Physician Kathleen M. Foley argues that doctors do not know enough about their patients, themselves, or suffering to provide assistance with dying as a medical treatment for the relief of suffering.

Should doctors ever help their patients die? Whereas doctors should provide every support possible to their dying patients, do they have the right or obligation to actually hasten the process of death even if a patient requests it? This topic has been the subject of numerous debates over the past decade.

Some of the practices that were controversial a short time ago in the care of terminally ill patients have become accepted and routine. Many doctors now believe that it is ethical to use "do-not-resuscitate" orders on dying patients, while others feel that it is also acceptable to withhold food and water from patients who are hopelessly ill and dying. The word *euthanasia,* which comes from Greek roots—the prefix *eu,* meaning good, fortunate, or easy, and the word *thanatos,* meaning death—describes a good or easy death. Withdrawing care or treatment (referred to as *passive euthanasia*) may be acceptable to many doctors, but *active euthanasia,* or playing an active role in a patient's death, may not. One form of active euthanasia, physician-assisted suicide, has been the subject of numerous debates in recent years.

In early 1988 the *Journal of the American Medical Association* published a short article entitled "It's Over, Debbie" (January 8, 1988), which was written by an anonymous physician who described administering a lethal dose of morphine to a young woman with terminal cancer. The doctor claimed her suffering was extreme and that there was absolutely no hope of recovery.

The morphine was requested by the patient, who said, "Let's get this over with." The patient died within minutes of receiving the drug, while the doctor looked on. This article generated a great deal of criticism because the doctor had met the patient for the first time that evening and had not consulted with colleagues or family members before making his decision. The doctor did, however, believe he was correctly responding to the patient's request.

Soon after this incident, Dr. Jack Kevorkian assisted in the suicide of an Oregon woman who suffered from Alzheimer's disease. Dr. Kevorkian supplied the woman with a device that he developed—a "suicide machine"—that allowed her to give herself a lethal dose of drugs. Intense criticism followed regarding the ability of Dr. Kevorkian to diagnose the patient's illness (which was not immediately terminal) and whether or not the patient was able to make an informed decision to end her life.

In March 1991 Dr. Timothy E. Quill published an editorial in *The New England Journal of Medicine* that described an assisted suicide. A woman, Quill's patient for eight years, was suffering from leukemia. She had decided not to undergo chemotherapy, which would have offered her only a 25 percent chance of long-term survival with considerable side effects. In addition to refusing treatment, the patient requested that Quill help her commit suicide. She later killed herself with sleeping pills that Quill had prescribed. Quill is an outspoken advocate of physician-assisted suicide under certain conditions.

Other physicians believe that many hopelessly ill patients contemplate taking their own lives because their doctors do not help them manage their pain. Pain is one of the principal reasons the sick ask their doctors to help them to die. Many doctors believe that the best antidote to the appeal of doctor-assisted suicide would be better treatment of pain. In "The Quality of Mercy: Effective Pain Treatments Already Exist. Why Aren't Doctors Using Them?" *U.S. News and World Report* (March 17, 1997), the authors claim that health providers are unwilling to treat pain adequately out of fear of litigation, fear their patients will become addicted, or because they lack adequate knowledge about pain management.

The debate over aided suicide has reached a new plateau. In June 1997 the Supreme Court justices unanimously rejected a plea to declare physician-assisted suicide a constitutional right. The justices did leave the way open for states to legalize the practice. Although most states make aided suicide a crime, legislators in nine states want to repeal the laws. In Oregon voters narrowly approved the legalization of assisted suicide in 1994; a bill to repeal the legislation was rejected in November 1997.

In the following articles, Dr. Marcia Angell supports a patient's right to assisted suicide and cites personal reasons for her decision. Dr. Kathleen M. Foley argues that physicians should provide competent care for the dying, including adequate pain management, and should not offer physician-assisted suicide.

# YES

Marcia Angell

## THE SUPREME COURT AND PHYSICIAN-ASSISTED SUICIDE— THE ULTIMATE RIGHT

The U.S. Supreme Court will decide later this year whether to let stand decisions by two appeals courts permitting doctors to help terminally ill patients commit suicide.[1] The Ninth and Second Circuit Courts of Appeals last spring held that state laws in Washington and New York that ban assistance in suicide were unconstitutional as applied to doctors and their dying patients.[2,3] If the Supreme Court lets the decisions stand, physicians in 12 states, which include about half the population of the United States, would be allowed to provide the means for terminally ill patients to take their own lives, and the remaining states would rapidly follow suit. Not since *Roe* v. *Wade* has a Supreme Court decision been so fateful.

The decision will culminate several years of intense national debate, fueled by a number of highly publicized events. Perhaps most important among them is Dr. Jack Kevorkian's defiant assistance in some 44 suicides since 1990, to the dismay of many in the medical and legal establishments, but with substantial public support, as evidenced by the fact that three juries refused to convict him even in the face of a Michigan statute enacted for that purpose. Also since 1990, voters in three states have considered ballot initiatives that would legalize some form of physician-assisted dying, and in 1994 Oregon became the first state to approve such a measure.[4] (The Oregon law was stayed pending a court challenge.) Several surveys indicate that roughly two thirds of the American public now support physician-assisted suicide,[5,6] as do more than half the doctors in the United States,[6,7] despite the fact that influential physicians' organizations are opposed. It seems clear that many Americans are now so concerned about the possibility of a lingering, high-technology death that they are receptive to the idea of doctors' being allowed to help them die.

In this editorial I will explain why I believe the appeals courts were right and why I hope the Supreme Court will uphold their decisions. I am aware that this is a highly contentious issue, with good people and strong arguments on both sides. The American Medical Association (AMA) filed an amicus brief opposing the legalization of physician-assisted suicide,[8] and the Massachusetts Medical Society, which owns the *Journal* was a signatory to it. But here I speak for myself not the *Journal* or the Massachusetts Medical Society. The legal aspects of the case have been well discussed elsewhere, to me most compellingly in Ronald Dworkin's essay in the *New York Review of Books*.[9] I will focus primarily on the medical and ethical aspects.

I begin with the generally accepted premise that one of the most important ethical principles in medicine is respect for each patient's autonomy, and that when this principle conflicts with others, it should almost always take precedence. This premise is incorporated into our laws governing medical practice and research, including the requirement of informed consent to any treatment. In medicine, patients exercise their self-determination most dramatically when they ask that life-sustaining treatment be withdrawn. Although others may sometimes consider the request ill-founded, we are bound to honor it if the patient is mentally competent—that is, if the patient can understand the nature of the decision and its consequences.

A second starting point is the recognition that death is not fair and is often cruel. Some people die quickly, and others die slowly but peacefully. Some find personal or religious meaning in the process, as well as an opportunity for a final reconciliation with loved ones. But others, especially those with cancer, AIDS, or progressive neurologic disorders, may die by inches and in great anguish, despite every effort of their doctors and nurses. Although nearly all pain can be relieved, some cannot, and other symptoms, such as dyspnea, nausea, and weakness, are even more difficult to control. In addition, dying sometimes holds great indignities and existential suffering. Patients who happen to require some treatment to sustain their lives, such as assisted ventilation or dialysis, can hasten death by having the life-sustaining treatment withdrawn, but those who are not receiving life-sustaining treatment may desperately need help they cannot now get.

If the decisions of the appeals courts are upheld, states will not be able to prohibit doctors from helping such patients to die by prescribing a lethal dose of a drug and advising them on its use for suicide. State laws barring euthanasia (the administration of a lethal drug by a doctor) and assisted suicide for patients who are not terminally ill would not be affected. Furthermore, doctors would not be *required* to assist in suicide; they would simply have that option. Both appeals courts based their decisions on constitutional questions. This is important, because it shifted the focus of the debate from what the majority would approve through the political process, as exemplified by the Oregon initiative, to a matter of fundamental rights, which are largely immune from the political process. Indeed, the Ninth Circuit Court drew an explicit analogy between suicide and abortion, saying that both were personal choices protected by the Constitution and that forbidding doctors to assist would in effect nullify these rights. Although states could regulate assisted suicide, as they do abortion, they would not be permitted to regulate it out of existence.

It is hard to quarrel with the desire of a greatly suffering, dying patient for a quicker, more humane death or to disagree that it may be merciful to help bring that about. In those circumstances, loved ones are often relieved when death finally comes, as are the attending doctors and nurses. As the Second Circuit Court said, the state has no interest in prolonging such a life. Why, then, do so many people oppose legalizing physician-assisted suicide in these cases? There are a number of arguments against it, some stronger than others, but I believe none of them can offset the overriding duties of doctors to relieve suffering and to respect their patients' autonomy. Below I list several of the more important arguments against physician-assisted suicide and discuss why I believe they are in the last analysis unpersuasive.

*Assisted suicide is a form of killing, which is always wrong. In contrast, withdrawing life-sustaining treatment simply allows the disease to take its course.* There are three methods of hastening the death of a dying patient: withdrawing life-sustaining treatment, assisting suicide, and euthanasia. The right to stop treatment has been recognized repeatedly since the 1976 case of Karen Ann Quinlan[10] and was affirmed by the U.S. Supreme Court in the 1990 *Cruzan* decision[11] and the U.S. Congress in its 1990 Patient Self-Determination Act.[12] Although the legal underpinning is the right to be free of unwanted bodily invasion, the purpose of hastening death was explicitly acknowledged. In contrast, assisted suicide and euthanasia have not been accepted; euthanasia is illegal in all states, and assisted suicide is illegal in most of them.

Why the distinctions? Most would say they turn on the doctor's role: whether it is passive or active. When life-sustaining treatment is withdrawn, the doctor's role is considered passive and the cause of death is the underlying disease, despite the fact that switching off the ventilator of a patient dependent on it looks anything but passive and would be considered homicide if done without the consent of the patient or a proxy. In contrast, euthanasia by the injection of a lethal drug is active and directly causes the patient's death. Assisting suicide by supplying the necessary drugs is considered somewhere in between, more active than switching off a ventilator but less active than injecting drugs, hence morally and legally more ambiguous.

I believe, however, that these distinctions are too doctor-centered and not sufficiently patient-centered. We should ask ourselves not so much whether the doctor's role is passive or active but whether the *patient's* role is passive or active. From that perspective, the three methods of hastening death line up quite differently. When life-sustaining treatment is withdrawn from an incompetent patient at the request of a proxy or when euthanasia is performed, the patient may be utterly passive. Indeed, either act can be performed even if the patient is unaware of the decision. In sharp contrast, assisted suicide, by definition, cannot occur without the patient's knowledge and participation. Therefore, it must be active—that is to say, voluntary. That is a crucial distinction, because it provides an inherent safeguard against abuse that is not present with the other two methods of hastening death. If the loaded term "kill" is to be used, it is not the doctor who kills, but the patient. Primarily because euthanasia can be performed without the patient's participation, I oppose its legalization in this country.

*Assisted suicide is not necessary. All suffering can be relieved if care givers are sufficiently skillful and compassionate, as illustrated by the hospice movement.* I have no doubt that if expert palliative care were available to everyone who needed it, there would be few requests for assisted suicide. Even under the best of circumstances, however, there will always be a few patients whose suffering simply cannot be adequately alleviated. And there will be some who would prefer suicide to any other measures available, including the withdrawal of life-sustaining treatment or the use of heavy sedation. Surely, every effort should be made to improve palliative care, as I argued 15 years ago,[13] but when those efforts are unavailing and suffering patients desperately long to end their lives, physician-assisted suicide should be allowed. The argument that permitting it would divert us from redoubling our commitment to comfort care asks these patients to pay the penalty for our failings. It is also illogical. Good comfort care and the availability of physician-assisted suicide are no more mutually exclusive than good cardiologic care and the availability of heart transplantation.

*Permitting assisted suicide would put us on a moral "slippery slope." Although in itself assisted suicide might be acceptable, it would lead inexorably to involuntary euthanasia.* It is impossible to avoid slippery slopes in medicine (or in any aspect of life). The issue is how and where to find a purchase. For example, we accept the right of proxies to terminate life-sustaining treatment, despite the obvious potential for abuse, because the reasons for doing so outweigh the risks. We hope our procedures will safeguard patients. In the case of assisted suicide, its voluntary nature is the best protection against sliding down a slippery slope, but we also need to ensure that the request is thoughtful and freely made. Although it

is possible that we may someday decide to legalize voluntary euthanasia under certain circumstances or assisted suicide for patients who are not terminally ill, legalizing assisted suicide for the dying does not in itself make these other decisions inevitable. Interestingly, recent reports from the Netherlands, where both euthanasia and physician-assisted suicide are permitted, indicate that fears about a slippery slope there have not been borne out.[14-16]

*Assisted suicide would be a threat to the economically and socially vulnerable. The poor disabled, and elderly might be coerced to request it.* Admittedly, overburdened families or cost-conscious doctors might pressure vulnerable patients to request suicide, but similar wrongdoing is at least as likely in the case of withdrawing life-sustaining treatment, since that decision can be made by proxy. Yet, there is no evidence of widespread abuse. The Ninth Circuit Court recalled that it was feared *Roe* v. *Wade* would lead to coercion of poor and uneducated women to request abortions, but that did not happen. The concern that coercion is more likely in this era of managed care, although understandable, would hold suffering patients hostage to the deficiencies of our health care system. Unfortunately, no human endeavor is immune to abuses. The question is not whether a perfect system can be devised, but whether abuses are likely to be sufficiently rare to be offset by the benefits to patients who otherwise would be condemned to face the end of their lives in protracted agony.

*Depressed patients would seek physician-assisted suicide rather than help for their depression. Even in the terminally ill, a request for assisted suicide might signify treatable depression, not irreversible suffering.* Patients suffering greatly at the end of life may also be depressed, but the depression does not necessarily explain their decision to commit suicide or make it irrational. Nor is it simple to diagnose depression in terminally ill patients. Sadness is to be expected, and some of the vegetative symptoms of depression are similar to the symptoms of terminal illness. The success of antidepressant treatment in these circumstances is also not ensured. Although there are anecdotes about patients who changed their minds about suicide after treatment,[17] we do not have good studies of how often that happens or the relation to antidepressant treatment. Dying patients who request assisted suicide and seem depressed should certainly be strongly encouraged to accept psychiatric treatment, but I do not believe that competent patients should be *required* to accept it as a condition of receiving assistance with suicide. On the other hand, doctors would not be required to comply with all requests; they would be expected to use their judgment, just as they do in so many other types of life-and-death decisions in medical practice.

*Doctors should never participate in taking life. If there is to be assisted suicide, doctor must not be involved.* Although most doctors favor permitting assisted suicide under certain circumstances, many who favor it believe that doctors should not provide the assistance.[6,7] To them, doctors should be unambiguously committed to life (although most doctors who hold this view would readily honor a patient's decision to have life-sustaining treatment withdrawn). The AMA, too, seems to object to physician-assisted suicide primarily because it violates the profession's mission. Like others, I find that position too abstract.[18] The highest ethical imperative of doctors should

be to provide care in whatever way best serves patients' interests, in accord with each patient's wishes, not with a theoretical commitment to preserve life no matter what the cost in suffering.[19] If a patient requests help with suicide and the doctor believes the request is appropriate, requiring someone else to provide the assistance would be a form of abandonment. Doctors who are opposed in principle need not assist, but they should make their patients aware of their position early in the relationship so that a patient who chooses to select another doctor can do so. The greatest harm we can do is to consign a desperate patient to unbearable suffering —or force the patient to seek out a stranger like Dr. Kevorkian. Contrary to the frequent assertion that permitting physician-assisted suicide would lead patients to distrust their doctors, I believe distrust is more likely to arise from uncertainty about whether a doctor will honor a patient's wishes.

*Physician-assisted suicide may occasionally be warranted, but it should remain illegal. If doctors risk prosecution, they will think twice before assisting with suicide.* This argument wrongly shifts the focus from the patient to the doctor. Instead of reflecting the condition and wishes of patients, assisted suicide would reflect the courage and compassion of their doctors. Thus, patients with doctors like Timothy Quill, who described in a 1991 *Journal* article how he helped a patient take her life,[20] would get the help they need and want, but similar patients with less steadfast doctors would not. That makes no sense.

*People do not need assistance to commit suicide. With enough determination, they can do it themselves.* This is perhaps the cruelest of the arguments against physician-assisted suicide. Many patients at the end of life are, in fact, physically unable to commit suicide on their own. Others lack the resources to do so. It has sometimes been suggested that they can simply stop eating and drinking and kill themselves that way. Although this method has been described as peaceful under certain conditions,[21] no one should count on that. The fact is that this argument leaves most patients to their suffering. Some, usually men, manage to commit suicide using violent methods. Percy Bridgman, a Nobel laureate in physics who in 1961 shot himself rather than die of metastatic cancer, said in his suicide note, "It is not decent for Society to make a man do this to himself."[22]

My father, who knew nothing of Percy Bridgman, committed suicide under similar circumstances. He was 81 and had metastatic prostate cancer. The night before he was scheduled to be admitted to the hospital, he shot himself. Like Bridgman, he thought it might be his last chance. At the time, he was not in extreme pain, nor was he close to death (his life expectancy was probably longer than six months). But he was suffering nonetheless—from nausea and the side effects of antiemetic agents, weakness, incontinence, and hopelessness. Was he depressed? He would probably have freely admitted that he was, but he would have thought it beside the point. In any case, he was an intensely private man who would have refused psychiatric care. Was he overly concerned with maintaining control of the circumstances of his life and death? Many people would say so, but that was the way he was. It is the job of medicine to deal with patients as they are, not as we would like them to be.

I tell my father's story here because it makes an abstract issue very concrete. If physician-assisted suicide had been available, I have no doubt my father would have chosen it. He was protective of his family, and if he had felt he had the choice, he would have spared my mother the shock of finding his body. He did not tell her what he planned to do, because he knew she would stop him. I also believe my father would have waited if physician-assisted suicide had been available. If patients have access to drugs they can take when they choose, they will not feel they must commit suicide early, while they are still able to do it on their own. They would probably live longer and certainly more peacefully, and they might not even use the drugs.

Long before my father's death, I believed that physician-assisted suicide ought to be permissible under some circumstances, but his death strengthened my conviction that it is simply a part of good medical care—something to be done reluctantly and sadly, as a last resort, but done nonetheless. There should be safeguards to ensure that the decision is well considered and consistent, but they should not be so daunting or violative of privacy that they become obstacles instead of protections. In particular, they should be directed not toward reviewing the reasons for an autonomous decision, but only toward ensuring that the decision is indeed autonomous. If the Supreme Court upholds the decisions of the appeals courts, assisted suicide will not be forced on either patients or doctors, but it will be a choice for those patients who need it and those doctors willing to help. If, on the other hand, the Supreme Court overturns the lower courts' decisions, the issue will continue to be grappled with state by state, through the political process. But sooner or later, given the need and the widespread public support, physician-assisted suicide will be demanded of a compassionate profession.

## REFERENCES

1. Greenhouse L. High court to say if the dying have a right to suicide help. New York Times. October 2, 1996:A1.
2. Compassion in Dying v. Washington, 79 F.3d 790 (9th Cir. 1996).
3. Quill v. Vacco, 80 F.3d 716 (2d Cir. 1996).
4. Annas GJ. Death by prescription—the Oregon initiative. N Engl J Med 1994;331:1240-3.
5. Blendon RJ, Szalay US, Knox RA. Should physicians aid their patients in dying? The public perspective. JAMA 1992;267:2658-62.
6. Bachman JG, Alcser KH, Doukas DJ, Lichtenstein RL, Corning AD, Brody H. Attitudes of Michigan physicians and the public toward legalizing physician-assisted suicide and voluntary euthanasia. N Engl J Med 1996;334:303-9.
7. Lee MA, Nelson HD, Tilden VP, Ganzini L, Schmidt TA, Tolle SW. Legalizing assisted suicide—views of physicians in Oregon. N Engl J Med 1996;334:310-5.
8. Gianelli DM. AMA to court: no suicide aid. American Medical News. November 25, 1996:1, 27, 28.
9. Dworkin R. Sex, death, and the courts. New York Review of Books. August 8, 1996.
10. In re: Quinlan, 70 N.J. 10, 355 A.2d 647 (1976).
11. Cruzan v. Director, Missouri Department of Health, 497 U.S. 261, 110 S.Ct. 2841 (1990).
12. Omnibus Budget Reconciliation Act of 1990, P.L. 101-508, sec. 4206 and 4751, 104 Stat. 1388, 1388-115, and 1388-204 (classified respectively at 42 U.S.C. 1395cc(f) (Medicare) and 1396a(w) (Medicaid) (1994).
13. Angell M. The quality of mercy. N Engl J Med 1982;306:98-9.
14. van der Maas PJ, van der Wal G, Haverkate I, et al. Euthanasia, physician-assisted suicide, and other medical practices involving the end of life in the Netherlands, 1990–1995. N Engl J Med 1996;335:1699-705.
15. van der Wal G, van der Maas PJ, Bosma JM, et al. Evaluation of the notification procedure for physician-assisted death in the Netherlands. N Engl J Med 1996;335:1706-11.
16. Angell M. Euthanasia in the Netherlands—good news or bad? N Engl J Med 1996;335:1676-8.
17. Chochinov HM, Wilson KG, Enns M, et al.Desire for death in the terminally ill. Am J Psychiatry 1995;152:1185-91.
18. Cassel CK, Meier DE. Morals and moralism in the debate over euthanasia and assisted suicide. N Engl J Med 1990;323:750-2.
19. Angell M. Doctors and assisted suicide. Ann R Coll Physicians Surg Can 1991;24:493-4.
20. Quill TE. Death and dignity—a case of individualized decision making. N Engl J Med 1991;324:691-4.
21. Lynn J, Childress JF. Must patients always be given food and water? Hastings Cent Rep 1983;13(5):17-21.
22. Nuland SB. How we die. New York: Alfred A. Knopf, 1994:152.

# NO

## Kathleen M. Foley

## COMPETENT CARE FOR THE DYING INSTEAD OF PHYSICIAN-ASSISTED SUICIDE

While the Supreme Court is reviewing the decisions by the Second and Ninth Circuit Courts of Appeals to reverse state bans on assisted suicide, there is a unique opportunity to engage the public, health care professionals, and the government in a national discussion of how American medicine and society should address the needs of dying patients and their families. Such a discussion is critical if we are to understand the process of dying from the point of view of patients and their families and to identify existing barriers to appropriate, humane, compassionate care at the end of life. Rational discourse must replace the polarized debate over physician-assisted suicide and euthanasia. Facts, not anecdotes, are necessary to establish a common ground and frame a system of health care for the terminally ill that provides the best possible quality of living while dying.

The biased language of the appeals courts evinces little respect for the vulnerability and dependency of the dying. Judge Stephen Reinhardt, writing for the Ninth Circuit Court, applied the liberty-interest clause of the Fourteenth Amendment, advocating a constitutional right to assisted suicide. He stated, "The competent terminally ill adult, having lived nearly the full measure of his life, has a strong interest in choosing a dignified and humane death, rather than being reduced to a state of helplessness, diapered, sedated, incompetent."[1] Judge Roger J. Miner, writing for the Second Circuit Court of Appeals, applied the equal-rights clause of the Fourteenth Amendment and went on to emphasize that the state "has no interest in prolonging a life that is ending."[2] This statement is more than legal jargon. It serves as a chilling reminder of the low priority given to the dying when it comes to state resources and protection.

The appeals courts' assertion of a constitutional right to assisted suicide is narrowly restricted to the terminally ill. The courts have decided that it is the patient's condition that justifies killing and that the terminally ill are special—so special that they deserve assistance in dying. This group alone can receive

From Kathleen M. Foley, "Competent Care for the Dying Instead of Physician-Assisted Suicide," *The New England Journal of Medicine*, vol. 336, no. 1 (January 2, 1997), pp. 54–58. Copyright © 1997 by The Massachusetts Medical Society. Reprinted by permission. All rights reserved.

such assistance. The courts' response to the New York and Washington cases they reviewed is the dangerous form of affirmative action in the name of compassion. It runs the risk of further devaluing the lives of terminally ill patients and may provide the excuse for society to abrogate its responsibility for their care.

Both circuit courts went even farther in asserting that physicians are already assisting in patients' deaths when they withdraw life-sustaining treatments such as respirators or administer high doses of pain medication that hasten death. The appeals courts argued that providing a lethal prescription to allow a terminally ill patient to commit suicide is essentially the same as withdrawing life-sustaining treatment or aggressively treating pain. Judicial reasoning that eliminates the distinction between letting a person die and killing runs counter to physicians' standards of palliative care.[3] The courts' purported goal in blurring these distinctions was to bring society's legal rules more closely in line with the moral value it places on the relief of suffering.[4]

In the real world in which physicians care for dying patients, withdrawing treatment and aggressively treating pain are acts that respect patients' autonomous decisions not to be battered by medical technology and to be relieved of their suffering. The physician's intent is to provide care, not death. Physicians do struggle with doubts about their own intentions.[5] The courts' arguments fuel their ambivalence about withdrawing life-sustaining treatments or using opioid or sedative infusions to treat intractable symptoms in dying patients. Physicians are trained and socialized to preserve life. Yet saying that physicians struggle with doubts about their inten-

tions in performing these acts is not the same as saying that their intention is to kill. In palliative care, the goal is to relieve suffering, and the quality of life, not the quantity, is of utmost importance.

Whatever the courts say, specialists in palliative care do not think that they practice physician-assisted suicide or euthanasia.[6] Palliative medicine has developed guidelines for aggressive pharmacologic management of intractable symptoms in dying patients, including sedation for those near death.[3,7,8] The World Health Organization has endorsed palliative care as an integral component of a national-health care policy and has strongly recommended to its member countries that they not consider legalizing physician-assisted suicide and euthanasia until they have addressed the needs of their citizens for pain relief and palliative care.[9] The courts have disregarded this formidable recommendation and, in fact, are indirectly suggesting that the World Health Organization supports assisted suicide.

Yet the courts' support of assisted suicide reflects the requests of the physicians who initiated the suits and parallels the numerous surveys demonstrating that a large proportion of physicians support the legalization of physician-assisted suicide.[10-15] A smaller proportion of physicians are willing to provide such assistance, and an even smaller proportion are willing to inject a lethal dose of medication with the intent of killing a patient (active voluntary euthanasia). These survey data reveal a gap between the attitudes and behavior of physicians; 20 to 70 percent of physicians favor the legalization of physician-assisted suicide, but only 2 to 4 percent favor active voluntary euthanasia, and only approximately 2 to 13 percent have actually aided patients in dying, by either providing a prescription or administering a lethal injection. The limitations of these surveys, which are legion, include inconsistent definitions of physician-assisted suicide and euthanasia, lack of information about nonrespondents, and provisions for maintaining confidentiality that have led to inaccurate reporting.[13,16] Since physicians' attitudes toward alternatives to assisted suicide have not been studied, there is a void in our knowledge about the priority that physicians place on physician-assisted suicide.

The willingness of physicians to assist patients in dying appears to be determined by numerous complex factors, including religious beliefs, personal values, medical specialty, age, practice setting, and perspective on the use of financial resources.[13,16–19] Studies of patients' preferences for care at the end of life demonstrate that physicians' preferences strongly influence those of their patients.[13] Making physician-assisted suicide a medical treatment when it is so strongly dependent on these physician-related variables would result in a regulatory impossibility.[19] Physicians would have to disclose their values and attitudes to patients to avoid potential conflict.[13] A survey by Ganzini et al. demonstrated that psychiatrists' responses to requests to evaluate patients were highly determined by their attitudes.[13] In a study by Emanuel et al., depressed patients with cancer said they would view positively those physicians who acknowledged their willingness to assist in suicide. In contrast, patients with cancer who were suffering from pain would be suspicious of such physicians.[11]

In this controversy, physicians fall into one of three groups. Those who support physician-assisted suicide see it as a compassionate response to a medical need, a symbol of nonabandonment, and a means to reestablish patients' trust in doctors who have used technology excessively.[20] They argue that regulation of physician-assisted suicide is possible and, in fact, necessary to control the actions of physicians who are currently providing assistance surreptitiously.[21] The two remaining groups of physicians oppose legalization.[19,22–24] One group is morally opposed to physician-assisted suicide and emphasizes the need to preserve the professionalism of medicine and the commitment to "do no harm." These physicians view aiding a patient in dying as a form of abandonment, because a physician needs to walk the last mile with the patient, as a witness, not as an executioner. Legalization would endorse justified killing, according to these physicians, and guidelines would not be followed, even if they could be developed. Furthermore, these physicians are concerned that the conflation of assisted suicide with the withdrawal of life support or adequate treatment of pain would make it even harder for dying patients because there would be a backlash against existing policies. The other group is not ethically opposed to physician-assisted suicide and, in fact, sees it as acceptable in exceptional cases, but these physicians believe that one cannot regulate the unregulatable.[19] On this basis, the New York State Task Force on Life and the Law, a 24-member committee with broad public and professional representation, voted unanimously against the legalization of physician-assisted suicide.[24] All three groups of physicians agree that a national effort is needed to improve the care of the dying. Yet it does seem that those in favor of legalizing physician-assisted suicide are disingenuous in their use of this issue as a wedge. If this form of assistance with dying is legalized, the courts will be forced to broaden the assistance to include active voluntary euthanasia and, eventually, assistance in response to requests from proxies.

One cannot easily categorize the patients who request physician-assisted suicide or euthanasia. Some surveys of physicians have attempted to determine retrospectively the prevalence and nature of these requests.[10] Pain, AIDS, and neurodegenerative disorders are the most common conditions in patients requesting assistance in dying. There is a wide range in the age of such patients, but many are younger persons with AIDS.[10] From the limited data available, the factors most commonly involved in requests for assistance are concern about future loss of control, being or becoming a burden to others, or being unable to care for oneself and fear of severe pain.[10] A small number of recent studies have directly asked terminally ill patients with cancer or AIDS about their desire for death.[25-27] All these studies show that the desire for death is closely associated with depression and that pain and lack of social support are contributing factors.

Do we know enough, on the basis of several legal cases, to develop a public policy that will profoundly change medicine's role in society?[1,2] Approximately 2.4 million Americans die each year. We have almost no information on how they die and only general information on where they die. Sixty-one percent die in hospitals, 17 percent in nursing homes, and the remainder at home, with approximately 10 to 14 percent of those at home receiving hospice care.

The available data suggest that physicians are inadequately trained to assess and manage the multifactorial symptoms commonly associated with patients' requests for physician-assisted suicide. According to the American Medical Association's report on medical education, only 5 of 126 medical schools in the United States require a separate course in the care of the dying.[28] Of 7048 residency programs, only 26 percent offer a course on the medical and legal aspects of care at the end of life as a regular part of the curriculum. According to a survey of 1068 accredited residency programs in family medicine, internal medicine, and pediatrics and fellowship programs in geriatrics, each resident or fellow coordinates the care of 10 or fewer dying patients annually.[28] Almost 15 percent of the programs offer no formal training in terminal care. Despite the availability of hospice programs, only 17 percent of the training programs offer a hospice rotation, and the rotation is required in only half of those programs; 9 percent of the programs have residents or fellows serving as members of hospice teams. In a recent survey of 55 residency programs and over 1400 residents, conducted by the American Board of Internal Medicine, the residents were asked to rate their perception of adequate training in care at the end of life. Seventy-two percent reported that they had received adequate training in managing pain and other symptoms; 62 percent, that they had received adequate training in telling patients that they are dying; 38 percent, in describing what the process will be like; and 32 percent, in talking to patients who request assistance in dying or a hastened death (Blank L: personal communication).

The lack of training in the care of the dying is evident in practice. Several studies have concluded that poor communication between physicians and patients, physicians' lack of knowledge about national guidelines for such care, and their lack of knowledge about the control of symptoms are barriers to the provision of good care at the end of life.[23,29,30]

Yet there is now a large body of data on the components of suffering in patients with advanced terminal disease, and these data provide the basis for treatment algorithms.[3] There are three major factors in suffering: pain and other physical symptoms, psychological distress, and existential distress (described as the experience of life without meaning). It is not only the patients who suffer but also their families and the health care professionals attending them. These experiences of suffering are often closely and inextricably related. Perceived distress in any one of the three groups amplifies distress in the others.[31,32]

Pain is the most common symptom in dying patients, and according to recent data from U.S. studies, 56 percent of outpatients with cancer, 82 percent of outpatients with AIDS, 50 percent of hospitalized patients with various diagnoses, and 36 percent of nursing home residents have inadequate management of pain during the course of their terminal illness.[33-36] Members of minority groups and women, both those with cancer and those with AIDS, as well as the elderly, receive less pain treatment than other groups of patients. In a survey of 1177 physicians who had treated a total of more than 70,000 patients with cancer in the previous six months, 76 percent of the respondents cited lack of knowledge as a barrier to their ability to control pain.[37] Severe pain that is not adequately controlled interferes with the quality of life, including the activities of daily living, sleep, and social interactions.[33,38]

Other physical symptoms are also prevalent among the dying. Studies of patients with advanced cancer and of the elderly in the year before death show that they have numerous symptoms that worsen the quality of life, such as fatigue, dyspnea, delirium, nausea, and vomiting.[36,38]

Along with these physical symptoms, dying patients have a variety of well-described psychological symptoms, with a high prevalence of anxiety and depression in patients with cancer or AIDS and the elderly.[27,39] For example, more than 60 percent of patients with advanced cancer have psychiatric problems, with adjustment disorders, depression, anxiety, and delirium reported most frequently. Various factors that contribute to the prevalence and severity of psychological distress in the terminally ill have been identified.[39] The diagnosis of depression is difficult to make in medically ill patients[3,26,40]; 94 percent of the Oregon psychiatrists surveyed by Ganzini et al. were not confident that they could determine, in a single evaluation, whether a psychiatric disorder was impairing the judgment of a patient who requested assistance with suicide.[13]

Attention has recently been focused on the interaction between uncontrolled symptoms and vulnerability to suicide in patients with cancer or AIDS.[41] Data from studies of both groups of patients suggest that uncontrolled pain contributes to depression and that persistent pain interferes with patients' ability to receive support from their families and others. Patients with AIDS have a high risk of suicide that is independent of physical symptoms. Among New York City residents with AIDS, the relative risk of suicide in men between the ages of 20 and 59 years was 36 times higher than the risk among men without AIDS in the same age group and 66 times higher than the risk in the general population.[41] Patients with AIDS who committed suicide generally did so within nine months after receiving the diagnosis; 25 percent had made a previous suicide attempt, 50 percent had reported severe depression, and 40 percent had seen a psychiatrist within four days before committing suicide. As previously noted, the desire to die is most closely associated with the diagnosis of depression.[26,27] Suicide is the eighth leading cause of death in the United States, and the incidence of suicide is higher in patients with cancer or AIDS and in elderly men than in the general population. Conwell and Caine reported that depression was under-diagnosed by primary care physicians in a cohort of elderly patients who subsequently committed suicide; 75 percent of the patients had seen a primary care physician during the last month of life but had not received a diagnosis of depression.[22]

The relation between depression and the desire to hasten death may vary among subgroups of dying patients. We have no data, except for studies of a small number of patients with cancer or AIDS. The effect of treatment for depression on the desire to hasten death and on requests for assistance in doing so has not been examined in the medically ill population, except for a small study in which four of six patients who initially wished to hasten death changed their minds within two weeks.[26]

There is also the concern that certain patients, particularly members of minority groups that are estranged from the health care system, may be reluctant to receive treatment for their physical or psychological symptoms because of the fear that their physicians will, in fact, hasten death. There is now some evidence that the legalization of assisted suicide in the Northern Territory of Australia has undermined the Aborigines' trust in the medical care system[42]; this experience may serve as an example for the United States, with its multicultural population.

The multiple physical and psychological symptoms in the terminally ill and elderly are compounded by a substantial degree of existential distress. Reporting on their interviews with Washington State physicians whose patients had requested assistance in dying, Back et al. noted the physicians' lack of sophistication in assessing such nonphysical suffering.[10]

In summary, there are fundamental physician-related barriers to appropriate, humane, and compassionate care for the dying. These range from attitudinal and behavioral barriers to educational and economic barriers. Physicians do not know enough about their patients, themselves, or suffering to provide assistance with dying as a medical treatment for the relief of suffering. Physicians need to explore their own perspectives on the meaning of suffering in order to develop their own approaches to the care of the dying. They need insight into how the nature of the doctor-patient relationship influences their own decision making. If legalized, physician-assisted suicide will be a substitute for rational therapeutic, psychological, and social interventions that might otherwise enhance the qualify of life for patients who are dying. The medical profession needs to take the lead in developing guidelines for good care of dying patients. Identifying the factors related to physicians, patients, and the health care system that pose barriers to appropriate care at the end of life should be the first step in a national dialogue to educate health care professionals and the public on the topic of death and dying. Death is an issue that society as a whole faces, and it requires a compassionate response. But we should not confuse compassion with competence in the care of terminally ill patients.

## REFERENCES

1. Reinhardt, Compassion in Dying v. State of Washington, 79 F. 3d 790 9th Cir. 1996.

2. Miner, Quill v Vacco 80 F. 3d 716 2nd Cir. 1996.

3. Doyle D, Hanks GWC, MacDonald N. The Oxford textbook of palliative medicine. New York: Oxford University Press, 1993.

4. Orentlicher D. The legalization of physician-assisted suicide. N Engl J Med 1996;335:663-7.

5. Wilson WC, Smedira NG, Fink C, McDowell JA, Luce JM. Ordering and administration of sedatives and analgesics during the withholding and withdrawal of life support from critically ill patients. JAMA 1992;267:949-53.

6. Foley KM. The relationship of pain and symptom management to patient requests for physician-assisted suicide. J Pain Symptom Manage 1991;6:289-97.

7. Cherny NI, Coyle N, Foley KM. Guidelines in the care of the dying patient. Hematol Oncol Clin North Am 1996;10:261-86.

8. Cherny NI, Portenoy RK. Sedation in the management of refractory symptoms: guidelines for evaluation and treatment. J Palliat Care 1994;10(2):31-8.

9. Cancer pain relief and palliative care. Geneva: World Health Organization, 1989.

10. Back AL, Wallace JI, Starks, HE, Pearlman RA. Physician-assisted suicide and euthanasia in Washington State: patient requests and physician responses. JAMA 1996;275:919-25.

11. Emanual EJ, Fairclough DL, Daniels ER, Clarridge BR. Euthanasia and physician-assisted suicide: attitudes and experiences of oncology patients, oncologists, and the public. Lancet 1996;347:1805-10.

12. Lee MA, Nelson HD, Tilden VP, Ganzini L, Schmidt TA, Tolle SW. Legalizing assisted suicide —views of physicians in Oregon. N Engl J Med 1996;334:310-5.

13. Ganzini L, Fenn DS, Lee MA, Heintz RT, Bloom JD. Attitudes of Oregon psychiatrists toward physician-assisted suicide. Am J Psychiatry 1996; 153:1469-75.

14. Cohen JS, Fihn SD, Boyko EJ, Jonsen AR, Wood RW. Attitudes toward assisted suicide and euthanasia among physicians in Washington State. N Engl J Med 1994;331:89-94.

15. Doukas DJ, Waterhouse D, Gorenflo DW, Seid J. Attitudes and behaviors on physician-assisted death: a study of Michigan oncologists. J Clin Oncol 1995;13:1055-61.

16. Morrison E, Meier D. Physician-assisted dying. fashioning public policy with an absence of data. Generations, Winter 1994:48-53.

17. Portenoy RK, Coyle N, Kash K, et al. Determinants of the willingness to endorse assisted suicide: a survey of physicians, nurses, and social workers. Psychosomatics (in press).

18. Fins J. Physician-assisted suicide and the right to care. Cancer Control 1996;3:272-8.

19. Callahan, D, White M. The legalization of physician-assisted suicide: creating a regulatory Potemkin Village. U Richmond Law Rev 1996;30:1-83.

20. Quill TE. Death and dignity—a case of individualized decision making. N Engl J Med 1991;324:691-4.

21. Quill TE, Cassel CK, Meier DE. Care of the hopelessly ill—proposed clinical criteria for physician-assisted suicide. N Engl J Med 1992;327:1380-4.

22. Conwell Y. Caine ED. Rational suicide and the right to die—reality and myth. N Engl J Med 1991;325:1100-3.

23. Foley KM. Pain, physician assisted suicide and euthanasia. Pain Forum 1995;4:163-78.

24. When death is sought: assisted suicide and euthanasia in the medical context. New York: New York State Task Force on Life and the Law, May 1994.

25. Brown JH, Henteleff P, Barakat S, Towe CJ. Is it normal for terminally ill patients to desire death? Am J Psychiatry 1986;143:208-11.

26. Chochinov HM, Wilson KG, Enns M, et al. Desire for death in the terminally ill. Am J Psychiatry 1995;152:1185-91.

27. Breitbart W. Rosenfeld BD, Passik SD. Interest in physician-assisted suicide among ambulatory HIV-infected patients, Am J Psychiatry 1996;153:238-42.

28. Hill TP. Treating the dying patient: the challenge for medical education. Arch Intern Med 1995;155:1265-9.

29. Callahan, D. Once again reality: now where do we go? Hastings Cent Rep 1995;25(6):Suppl:S33-S36.

30. Solomon MZ, O'Donnell L, Jennings B, et al. Decisions near the end of life: professional views on life-sustaining treatments. Am J Public Health 1993;83:14–23.

31. Cherny NI, Coyle, N. Foley KM. Suffering in the advanced cancer patient: definition and taxonomy. J Palliat Care 1994;10(2):57-70.

32. Cassel EJ. The nature of suffering and the goals of medicine. N Engl J Med 1982;306:639-45.

33. Cleeland CS, Gonin R, Hatfield AK, et al. Pain and its treatment in outpatients with metastatic cancer. N Engl J Med 1994;330:592-6.

34. Breitbart W, Rosenfeld BD, Passik SD, McDonald NV, Thaler H, Portenoy RK. The undertreatment of pain in ambulatory AIDS patients. Pain 1996;65:243-9.

35. The SUPPORT Principal Investigators. A controlled trial to improve care for seriously ill hospitalized patients. JAMA 1995;274:1591-8.

36. Seale C, Cartwright A. The year before death. Hants, England: Avebury, 1994.

37. Von Roenn JH, Cleeland CS, Gonin R, Hatfield AK, Pandya KJ. Physician attitudes and practice in cancer pain management: a survey from the Eastern Cooperative Oncology Group. Ann Intern Med 1993;119:121-6.

38. Portenoy RK. Pain and quality of life: clinical issues and implications for research. Oncology 1990;4:172-8.

39. Breitbart W. Suicide risk and pain in cancer and AIDS patients. In: Chapman CR, Foley KM, eds. Current and emerging issues in cancer pain. New York: Raven Press, 1993.

40. Chochinov H, Wilson KG, Enns M, Lander S. Prevalence of depression in the terminally ill: effects of diagnostic criteria and symptom threshold judgments. Am J Psychiatry 1994;151:537-40.

41. Passik S, McDonald M. Rosenfeld B, Breitbart W. End of life issues in patients with AIDS: clinical and research considerations. J Pharm Care Pain Symptom Control 1995;3:91-111.

42. NT "success" in easing rural fear of euthanasia. The Age, August 31,1996:A7.

# POSTSCRIPT

## Should Doctors Ever Help Terminally Ill Patients to Commit Suicide?

As our population ages and the incidence of certain diseases, such as cancer and AIDS, continues to increase, it appears that the ranks of the dying and suffering will grow. In the past, there were limited means of prolonging life; however, due to advances in modern medicine and technology, the dying can be kept alive sometimes for lengthy time periods. Although some doctors are beginning to speak more often of euthanasia, the American Medical Association has unequivocally reaffirmed its opposition to the practice.

In the Netherlands officials have taken a different viewpoint: Although Dutch law still refers to euthanasia as a crime, the highest courts there have determined that doctors may practice it if they follow specific guidelines set up by the Royal Dutch Medical Association. See "Euthanasia in the Netherlands," *The New England Journal of Medicine,* (vol. 335, 1996).

Articles that support euthanasia include "Suicide: Should the Doctor Ever Help?" *Harvard Health Letter* (August 1991); "What Quinlan Can Tell Kevorkian About the Right to Die," *The Humanist* (March/April 1997); and "The Promise of a Good Death," *The Lancet* (May 16, 1998).

Opponents of euthanasia and physician-assisted suicide argue that all life has value and that doctors do not have the right to end it. These include Leon R. Kass, in "Neither for Love Nor Money: Why Doctors Must Not Kill," *The Public Interest* (December 1989); Richard Momeyer, in "Does Physician Assisted Suicide Violate the Integrity of Medicine?" *Journal of Medicine and Philosophy* (vol. 20, 1995); and Ezekiel Emanuel and Margaret Battin in "What Are the Potential Cost Savings from Legalizing Physician-Assisted Suicide?" *The New England Journal of Medicine* (July 16, 1998).

Other articles that discuss the issue include "Should Physicians Aid Their Patients in Dying?" *Journal of the American Medical Association* (May 20, 1992); "Assisted Suicide: Should Doctors Help Hopelessly Ill Patients Take Their Lives?" *CQ Researcher* (February 21, 1992); "Are Laws Against Assisted Suicide Unconstitutional?" *Hastings Center Report* (May/June 1993); "The Euthanasia Follies," *Commonweal* (June 3, 1994); "Attitudes Toward Assisted Suicide and Euthanasia Among Physicians in Washington State," *The New England Journal of Medicine* (July 14, 1994); "Assisted Suicide Controversy: Should Physicians Help the Dying to End Their Lives?" *CQ Researcher* (May 5, 1995); "Whose Right to Die?" *The Atlantic Monthly* (March 1997); "A National Survey of Physician-Assisted Suicide and Euthanasia in the United States," *The New England Journal of Medicine* (April 23, 1998); and "Clear Thinking About Morally Complex Questions," *The World & I* (July 1998).

# ISSUE 3

## Should Health Care for the Elderly Be Limited?

**YES: Daniel Callahan,** from "Setting Limits: A Response," *The Gerontologist* (June 1994)

**NO: Patricia Lanoie Blanchette,** from "Age-Based Rationing of Healthcare," *Generations* (Winter 1996–1997)

### ISSUE SUMMARY

**YES:** Hastings Center director Daniel Callahan contends that medical care for elderly people who have lived their natural life expectancy should consist only of pain relief rather than expensive health care services that serve only to forestall death.

**NO:** Patricia Lanoie Blanchette, a physician and a professor of medicine and public health, argues that health care should not be rationed by age and that age bias should be recognized and confronted.

In 1980, 11 percent of the U.S. population was over age 65, but they utilized about 29 percent ($219 billion) of the total American health care expenditures. By the end of the decade, the percentage of the population over 65 had risen to 12 percent, which consumed 31 percent of total health care expenditures, or $450 billion. The costs of Medicare, the government insurance for the elderly, are expected to increase to $114 billion by the year 2000. It has been projected that by the year 2040, people over 65 will represent 21 percent of the population and consume 45 percent of all health care expenditures.

Medical expenses at the end of life appear to be extremely high in relation to other health care costs. Studies have shown that nearly one-third of annual Medicare costs are for the 5–6 percent of beneficiaries who die that year. Expenses for dying patients increase significantly as death nears, and payments for health care during the last weeks of life make up 40 percent of the medical costs for the entire last year of life. Some studies have shown that up to 50 percent of the medical costs incurred during a person's entire life are spent during their last year!

Many surveys have indicated that most Americans do not want to be kept alive if their illness is incurable and irreversible, for both economic and humanitarian reasons. Many experts believe that if physicians stopped using high technology at the end of life to prevent death, then we would save billions of dollars, which could be used to insure the uninsured and provide basic health care to millions.

In England the emphasis of health care is on improving the quality of life through primary care medicine, well-subsidized home care, and institutional programs for the elderly and those with incurable illnesses, rather than through life-extending acute care medicine. The British seem to value basic medical care for all rather than expensive technology for the few who might benefit from it. As a result, the British spend a much smaller proportion of their gross national product (6.2 percent) on health services than do Americans (10.8 percent) for a nearly identical health status and life expectancy.

In the following selection, Daniel Callahan argues that using medical technologies to extend the lives of the terminally ill or individuals who have lived out their natural life spans is an expensive and inappropriate use of modern medicine. Technology, he feels, should be used to avoid premature death and to relieve suffering, not to prolong full and complete lives. Callahan also states that the attempt to indefinitely extend life can be an economic disaster. This goal also fails to put health in its proper place as only one among many human values, and it discourages the acceptance of aging and death as part of life.

In the second selection, Patricia Lanoie Blanchette maintains that health care must be appropriate, not rationed. She stresses that covert rationing of medical care based on age is a serious concern and must be addressed.

# YES

## Daniel Callahan

## SETTING LIMITS: A RESPONSE

Some six years ago, in the fall of 1987, I published *Setting Limits: Medical Goals in an Aging Society* (Callahan, 1987). I argued that we would have to rethink once again the place of aging in the life cycle and that, in the future, scarcity of resources could force an age limit on medical entitlements for the elderly. That was not a popular thesis. I expected controversy and I got it, ranging from scholarly debates conducted with academic decorum to nasty public and media exchanges. Some six books of commentary and criticism, and an issue of a law review, were directly or indirectly inspired by *Setting Limits* (St. Louis University Law Journal, 1989; Homer & Holstein, 1990; Binstock & Post, 1991; Jecker, 1991; Barry & Bradley, 1991; Winslow & Walters, 1993; Hackler, in press).

The birth of *Setting Limits* came about because, beginning in the mid-1980s, I became aware of the striking demographic trends being reported, often accompanied by worries about their economic and social impact in the decades ahead (Preston, 1984). I saw us moving—through no one's fault, and surely not the elderly—toward a potential tragic dilemma of the first order. Something would have to give somewhere. We could not possibly guarantee indefinitely to the growing number and proportion of the elderly all of the potentially limitless fruits of medical progress at public expense without seriously distorting sensible social priorities. Where and how could we set some sensible and fair limits?

### WHAT I TRIED TO SAY

*Setting Limits* was the result of my effort to think through that problem. I argued that we should begin now, *before* the crisis is fully upon us, to change our expectations about elderly care in the future. I stressed in the book the *trend* in the development of expensive technologies, not their present costs, and the likely need for *future* change in entitlement policies, not at present. As a way into these likely changes, I said that we need to rethink two deeply imbedded ideas, widely if not universally held. The first is the cherished notion that we should try endlessly through medical progress to modernize

From Daniel Callahan, "Setting Limits: A Response," *The Gerontologist*, vol. 34, no. 3 (June 1994), pp. 373–398. Copyright © 1994 by The Gerontological Society of America. Reprinted by permission.

old age, to turn it into a more or less permanent middle age. We should instead accept aging as a part of life, not just another medical obstacle to be overcome. The valuable and necessary campaign against ageism, highly individualistic in its premises, runs the risk of emptying age as a stage in life of meaningful content and, with the help of science, trying to turn it into a kind of repairable biological accident. The second idea I criticized was the view that there should be no limits to the claims of the elderly as a group to expensive life-extending medicine under *public* entitlement programs, that only their individual needs should count, and count in an age-blind way.

After criticizing those two ideas, I offered a different picture of what a future health care policy for the elderly might look like, one designed to balance the new limits with some enriched entitlements. I was seeking a public policy that: (1) would guarantee the elderly, along with everyone else, access to universal health care; (2) would help everyone to avoid an early, premature death; (3) would achieve a better balance of caring and curing to overcome the powerful bias toward the latter (whose effect is to undermine the former), and in particular to greatly strengthen long-term and home care support; and (4) would use age as a categorical standard to cut off life-extending technologies under the Medicare entitlement program—but using it as a standard *if and only if the* other reforms were put in place first.

I proposed the idea of a "natural life span" as a rough way of determining such a cut-off point. I would have been wise to have chosen a different word than "natural," since I meant by that concept a biographical not a biological standard,

that is, a notion of when it might be said that most people will have lived an adequately full, if not necessarily totally full, life. I drew that notion from my own experience, and the traditions of most cultures, which perceives an important moral and social distinction between the sadness but fittingness of death in old age and the tragedy or outrage of an avoidable early, particularly, childhood death. I did not specify an exact age but suggested that the "late 70s or early 80s" would be an appropriate age range in which to look for it.

The great need is to find a type of limit that would dampen the potent trend to apply ever more expensive technologies to saving and extending the life of the elderly. That trend has seen a steady rise in the age of various surgical and other medical procedures, and in particular a rise often marked by successful results (Hosking, Warner, Lobdell, Offord, & Melton, 1989; Latta & Keene, 1989; Breidenbaugh, Sarsitis, & Milam, 1990). But it is the success, I argued, that was creating the problem for us, not the failures, and I did not foresee us going backwards in care for the elderly, but radically slowing up and eventually plateauing the forward march of expensive medical progress.

I held, finally, that the needed changes should be effected, not by compulsion —the young imposing it by force on the unwilling old—but democratically, preceded by a decades-long period of changing our thinking, attitudes, and expectations about elderly health care. Those of us still reasonably young should be prepared in the future to impose an age limit on ourselves. As I noted in the Preface to my book, in a passage often overlooked, "what I am looking for is not any quick change but the beginning of a long-term discussion, one that will lead people to change their thinking and, most important, their expectations, about old age and death" (Callahan, 1987, p. 10).

## RESPONSES TO CRITICS

Let me take up, in turn, the major objections leveled at my argument. Since there were well over 100 papers written about the book, and I was given the back of someone's hand in at least that many more, I will consolidate here the criticisms.

**The Use of Age as a Standard for Limiting Health Care Would Be Ageist and Unjust.** There are two discordant ways of thinking about the place and relevance of age from an individual and from a policy perspective. From an individual perspective, it is said, age as such should have no place in resource allocation. It is not a good predictor of health, mental or physical. True. Yet the difficulty here is obvious from a policy perspective: Age *is* a relevant and conspicuous variable in health care costs, and the elderly are more costly as a group than people of younger ages. The fact that many elderly people remain healthy most of their final years—and that there is a heterogeneous pattern of health care usage—does not change the fact that the average per capita costs of the elderly are significantly higher than for younger people. Public policy must take account of, and work with, those averages. They are what count in devising programs, in projecting future costs, and in estimating different health care needs. Age matters.

If age matters, how does it matter? It matters when, as we can now see, meeting the health care costs of the elderly as a group begins to threaten the possibility of meeting the needs of other age groups. In the nature of the case, moreover, there are no fixed boundaries to the amount of money that can be spent combating the effects of biological aging and attempting to forestall death in old age. It is an unlimited frontier. One could say exactly the same thing about trying to save the life of low birthweight infants. We can go from the present 450–500 grams and 24–25 weeks gestation to 400 to 300 grams, and 20–21 weeks gestation, and so on. There are no end of possibilities there as well, and thus some very good reasons to set limits to those efforts, using either weight or gestational age as a categorical standard (Callahan, 1990). It is no more an anti-aging act than it is an anti-baby act to set limits (for instance, on neonatal care) in order to avoid pursuing unlimited, potentially ruinous possibilities.

Aging and death in old age are inevitable, and there should be no unlimited claim on public resources to combat them. But premature death, and bad schools, and blighted urban areas of great poverty, are not inevitable. The first health task of a society is that the young should have the chance to become old. That should always take priority over helping, at great cost, those who are already old from becoming still older. That is exactly what we can look forward to, as we throw more and more money into the fight to cure the chronic and degenerative diseases of aging, but not to care well for those who cannot be saved.

But if we set a limit on public entitlement for the elderly would this not be unfair and ageist? I believe we cannot achieve perfect equality in this world, much less in a health care system, without some harmful consequences. No country in the world, save the communist countries, has achieved any such goal, and the price they paid was rampant corruption and bribery; the wealthy and powerful still got better care. An age limit on entitlement benefits would of course perpetuate a two-tier system, with the rich able to buy health benefits not available to the poor, but that need not be the disaster many fear. The test should not be whether everyone receives exactly the same level of care. It should instead be whether the poorest and worst off receive decent health care. I believe the system I propose, guaranteeing universal care, a powerful effort to beat back premature death, a full range of health services through the late 70s or early 80s, a good range of social and caring services thereafter for one's entire life, and then (and only then) an age limit on expensive life-extending therapies, would be decent. If combined, moreover, with other kinds of limits in the health care systems for all groups, it would not be ageist even if it used age as a standard. It would use age as a standard simply because, as argued above, age does matter from a policy perspective.

**It Is Unduly Pessimistic to Take Seriously the Projections That Show a Steadily Increasing Burden of Elderly Health Care Costs.** "Callahan," one commentator said, "is overly alarmist about the relative burden of older persons..." (Lawlor, 1992, p. 132). I have never known quite what to make of that charge. I have used the standard research available on demographic trends and projected health care costs. I have never been able to find *any* optimistic projections based on historical and current demographic and economic projections. Even the critic who said I was "alarmist" concluded that paragraph by

criticizing the optimists for failing to note that "the arithmetic of compound growth is at work in the increase of health expenditures (prices, demographic change, and increasing intensity of care)" (Lawlor, 1992, p. 132). Since I wrote *Setting Limits,* moreover, the "pessimistic" data have continued to pour forth, even from those who are my critics on other grounds (Schneider & Guralnik, 1990).

Since I have been unable to locate *any* optimistic data and reassuring projections, nor have any been cited in rebuttal, I can only observe that those who find me pessimistic rely on hopeful, but essentially still imaginary, scenarios about the future. One scenario is that in the future there will be a "compression of morbidity" and thus a decrease in the costs of elderly morbidity. That is a most invigorating hope, but the present evidence has moved in exactly the opposite direction, to greater not lesser morbidity, even if there is at least one recent report suggesting a slight amelioration of that trend (Manton, Corder, & Stallard, 1993). The second scenario is that advances in medical research will find cures or inexpensive treatments for the degenerative diseases of aging (Schneider & Guralnik, 1990). I hope that is true, but there is no evidence so far to support that hope as a likely outcome. The third scenario is that the elderly in the future will retire later and work longer, thus contributing more and much later to their health care costs. That could surely happen, and may by force happen, but it will as such not do a great deal about the disproportion of resources that could go to the elderly, although it surely might help. It is not likely to be helpful with the large number of people who live beyond 85, a rapidly growing group.

**It Is Only Because Our Health Care System Is Wasteful, Capitalistic, and Paternalistic That We Are Even Thinking of Rationing and Limits on Care for the Elderly.** There is no doubt that ours is a wasteful, fragmented, and excessively costly system, and that we could spend more on the elderly if we reduced waste elsewhere (Estes, 1988). The amount of money we spend in comparison with other developed countries, which get as good and often better outcomes for considerably less money, establishes that point well enough (though it does not establish that the money saved should go to the elderly as distinguished, say, from improving the schools). There are two points to consider here. The first is that, after more than 20 years of trying, we have not discovered in this country how, short of the universal health care and global budgeting we have been slow to embrace, to significantly control our costs; they just keep rising.

The second point is that, even if we can achieve those needed reforms, the problem will still not go away. The experience of other developed countries is already showing how an aging population can continue to push costs and demand up even in efficient, cost-effective, non-market health care systems (Hollander & Becker, 1987; Loriaux, 1990; Jouvenel, 1989). Those countries, controlling the fees of health care workers, rationing technology, keeping a lid on drug and equipment costs, still have a growing age-related problem even so. Better health care systems can delay the problem, or ameliorate it; but they are not going to be a solution to it.

A popular proposal to reduce elderly costs is the promotion of "advance directives" to allow the elderly to voluntarily forgo expensive, useless, and undesired care at the end of life. Could that make a difference? The evidence is mixed on that point and still scanty. One study found that advance directives made no difference in the medical treatment or in the medical costs (Schneiderman, Kronick, Kaplan, Anderson, & Langer, 1992), while another found evidence of dramatic savings (Chambers, Diamond, Perkel, & Lasch, 1994). My own guess is that advance directives will in the long run make some economic difference in relatively clear-cut cases of terminal illness for some classes of patients. There are two problems, however, which will make the greatest difference over time. One of them is the number of people who will execute advance directives, now still a significant minority. The other is the extent of expensive medical treatments that successfully avert the need to invoke advance directives, putting them off to another day; that's where the real bill is likely to add up, even if money can be saved in the last illness. To save money in the last days of life is not identical with saving money in the last years of life.

**Even If It Becomes Necessary to Set Limits on Public Expenditures for Elderly Health Care, That Should Be Done on a Case-by-Case Basis Rather Than Categorically by Age.** Should rationing or limits be necessary, almost everyone's ideal would be a system that was simultaneously individualized, fair, and effective. Each patient would be considered on his or her medical merits, not on the basis of some categorical standard. Rejecting categorical standards, "the impersonal application of a rule to a faceless group," Dr. Norman G. Levinsky has written that "society must not insulate itself from the agony of each decision to forgo beneficial treatment as it is experienced by patients, families, and care givers" (Levinsky, 1990, p. 1815).

I can well understand the sentiment behind Dr. Levinsky's thinking, but I have simply never been able to understand how it would be possible to limit health care in general while individualizing it in particular. If the assumption is that people should receive care on the basis of its individual efficacy for them, then we will run afoul of what I would call the "efficacy fallacy," that is, the notion that those treatments that are individually efficacious are therefore socially affordable. But precisely the problem we are likely to face is this: It will be the efficacious, not wasteful, treatments that will cause us the most financial grief, simply because it will be all the harder to deny people such treatment. There is a related fallacy, what I will dub the "hidden hand fallacy," that is, the view that the aggregate impact of meeting individual needs will turn out to be identical with the available common resources. Why should that be the case?

My assumption, by contrast—using the available projections—is that we will be forced to limit some proven, efficacious treatments, of a kind that people will want and that would extend their lives. The choices we will have to make will then be genuinely tragic choices. The pain of such choices is that they allow us no happy way out. It is an easy exercise to measure age-limit proposals against the standard of unlimited resources and no hard choices; and, naturally, an age limit looks terrible by that standard. But if we understand that we may one day be faced only with nasty options, then our task will be to compare those options with each other, not compare them against a world where no unpleasant choices are needed.

**The Idea of Using a "Natural Life Span" as a Basis for Setting an Age Limit is Too Vague, and Too Controverted, to Be Useful.** With great frequency I felt my proposal ran up against the individualism of our culture, not only in the repeated assertion about the heterogeneity of the elderly, but also in the rejection of a use of the life cycle as a place to look for an age limit. Yet I find it hard to know where else we might fruitfully look. If our standard is simply individual benefit, regardless of age, then there is no possible way we could effectively limit elderly health care costs; they will inexorably rise as technology improves. My alternative approach is to ask: How can we design a health care and entitlement system that would allow each of us to live a long and full life, but would not entail unlimited public support for whatever technology turned up at whatever cost?

I turned to the idea of a "natural life span" in order to capitalize on a common culture sentiment, still alive in the United States. It is that, while all death is a cause for sadness, a death in old age after a long and full life is, given the inevitability of death, the most acceptable kind of death. Unlike the death of a child, or a young adult, death in old age is part of our biology and part of the life cycle. It is no accident, think, that there is less weeping at the death of a very old person than at the death of a child. Although the idea of a "natural life span" as a biographical notion was thoroughly assaulted by many of my critics, a recent survey indicates that the idea is still strong in our society, even if most people would at present probably resist using it for rationing purposes (Zweibel, Cassel, & Karvison, 1993). Increased financial pressure, certain in the years ahead, may perhaps change the public bias against an age-based rationing standard.

I come back to a fundamental question. Do the elderly have an unlimited medical claim on public resources? No, they have only a reasonable and thus limited claim. What is a "reasonable" claim? I take it to be a claim to live a long life with public support, but not indefinitely long, and not at the price of potential harm to others. If we can agree with that proposition, then a "natural life span" is one that is highly useful—though admittedly not precise —allowing us a way of talking about what should count as a premature death, and as the basis for a claim on the public purse. It will surely work better than, say, "individual need," which is subject to technological escalation and intractable subjective desires. If we agree, for instance, that the preservation of life is a basic medical need, then in the nature of the case with the aging person there are no necessary limits at all, scientific or economic, to what can be done to achieve that goal. To be sure, any specific age to invoke as a limit will be arbitrary, but not necessarily capricious. That was true of age 65 when Medicare was established. It could have been 66 or 64. The point is that it was within a generally acceptable range of choices, and that is sufficient for fair public policy.

## SOME TELLING POINTS

My response so far might indicate that I have been unwilling to give way to my critics or to admit any validity to what they say. Up to a point that is true. Nonetheless, on the old principle that much of life and policy lies in the details, some telling points have been made against me. They are worth further thought.

The most powerful criticism is political: Whatever the rational arguments in its favor, neither the public nor legislators would ever accept an open, explicit use of age as a criterion for cutting off life-extending medical care. One critic called this assumption on my part a "blunder," and (in some sympathy with my general argument about the need for limits) said that we might be forced to covertly have an age standard (Moody, 1991). I have no doubt that an age limit would, politically, be obnoxious to politicians, at least at present. Even those countries known for using age as a norm (such as England and Switzerland) have done so tacitly and quietly, out of the public eye. Yet, if it is true that an explicit age standard is now and will remain for some time politically unacceptable as public policy, then we will be left with another dilemma. We will either have to come up with some other standard, bound to be unwanted also if it has any bite, or resign ourselves to euphemism and evasion, using age privately but never admitting it publicly.

There is a telling scientific criticism also. One of my goals with an age limit is to discourage the kind of scientific "progress" that endlessly generates new, almost always expensive, ways of extending the lives of elderly people. If those modalities were not going to be reimbursed, that would be a powerful disincentive to developing them in the first place. The problem here, as many noted, is that most of the technologies now used with the elderly were first developed with younger people in mind; few life-extending technologies are created for the elderly as such.

I cannot deny the force of those contentions. But that leaves us with another dilemma: If scientific progress moves along in an unchecked fashion, generating still more expensive ways of saving life, our tragic dilemma will become all the more painful. The gap between what we know we can or could do to save life will all the more harshly and conspicuously clash with our economic limitations. My own preference would be for a sharp increase in research designed to decrease morbidity and disability, discouraging when possible explicit efforts to develop more life-extending technologies.

Still another criticism might, for lack of a better name, be called the repugnance argument. It takes a number of forms. One of them is that we would find it repugnant to deny reimbursement to someone for a form of care that would clearly save that person's life; we could not just stand by and let the person die for lack of money. Another form is that, however nice my theory of justice between age groups, it would *look* like we were devaluing the worth of the elderly if we used age as an exclusive standard for denying care; we would find that hard to stand.

I agree that most people would find these consequences of an age limit repugnant. But again we are left with a dilemma, indeed more than one. What will we do about the repugnance that could well result from seeing a larger and larger, and even more disproportionate, share of resources going to the elderly while the needs of younger groups are going unmet? Or placing heavier and heavier economic burdens on the young to sustain the old? If we leave all choices about resource allocation to doctors and families at the bedside, what will we do about the repugnance regarding the variations in treatment that method will

bring, with some getting too much treatment and others getting too little? If we find the open use of an age limit repugnant, will we feel any better about a covert use, one that could be forced by a shortage of money?

Another telling point, in some ways the most fundamental, leaves me with a deep and unresolved problem. In an unpublished paper Per Anderson suggests that the "high quality aging that Callahan wants medicine and society to support will serve to make the idea of the life cycle increasingly implausible ... one can wonder whether Callahan would have us adopt an ethic of limits because it is the human good or because it is the grim necessity to which we must be resigned" (Anderson, 1991, p. 3). On this point, a profound one for medicine in general and not just for care of the aged, I am deeply ambivalent.

My own reading of history is that those people and cultures who live with some sense of intrinsic limits, whether natural or culturally inspired, better adapt to the human situation, and to aging and mortality, than do those who want to carry out endless warfare against human finitude. Yet I cannot ignore the other side of that coin, which is that we have enormously benefited from many efforts to transcend what earlier generations took to be fixed limits. I might not now be alive but for those efforts. How do we find the right balance here, between acceptance and acquiescence and the desire to struggle against our human condition? It is open to my critics to make a good case for fighting the ravages of age and to seek to further postpone death. I will respond by asking: Why should we believe that will necessarily increase our human satisfaction and sense of well-being? We will, I am sure, go back and forth on that point—and no doubt so will future generations.

## WHAT ABOUT THE FUTURE?

There were three reasons why I was drawn to the use of an age limit as a likely way to eventually control health care allocation to the elderly. One reason was that it seems to me better in general for human beings to live with a strong sense of their mortality and to be willing to understand that their lives must come to an end. A second reason is that it seems to me merely the prejudice of an affluent, hyper-individualistic, technologically driven society to think that a denial of reimbursement for life-extending care beyond a certain point is tantamount to a denial of value and dignity to the elderly. The third reason for being drawn to age was that I simply could not imagine—and still cannot imagine—any other way of decisively and effectively and uniformly drawing a clear policy line than the use of age. It is precisely because it cuts through, and transcends, our individual differences that it is attractive for policy purposes.

That of course is precisely its greatest liability in the eyes of my critics, and I am more persuaded than I was initially that, for both symbolic and practical reasons, an age-based policy will appear, and well could be, obnoxious. Yet, having conceded that, I must then add: Show me an equally decisive alternative, one that will work to hold down costs, that does not depend upon variable bedside judgments, and that takes with full seriousness the need to find a solution —and a solution that does not depend on evading the problem altogether by invoking some yet-to-be-seen hopeful scientific or economic miracle.

If we agree on the eventual need for limits, does it follow that only an age limit would work? Not at all, and it may well be that the various repugnances I noted above will stand forever in the way of using an age limit. But in that case it will be necessary to come up with some plausible alternatives. Robert Veatch and Norman Daniels have suggested some interesting and alternative ways of using age, less stark than mine. They can be debated. Nancy S. Jecker and Robert A. Pearlman, after criticizing Harry R. Moody, Norman Daniels, and myself for our willingness to consider an age limit, conclude their article with a brief review of some possible alternatives—and find them full of problems as well! (See Jecker & Pearlman, 1989). No doubt anyway, as they say, we will have to explore those alternatives. I offer a simple test as we try to think about one alternative or another: If it seems to avoid the need for nasty choices altogether, or seems painless and congenial (like just cutting out unwanted treatment), we should have a hard time taking it seriously. In the best of all possible worlds, what the elderly want and need would fit perfectly with the available resources. Ours is not, nor is likely to be, such a world. Any solution that seems to imply such a world merits the same suspicion as offers of free trips to Europe or Florida just by placing a phone call.

Time and again I was accused of "blaming the elderly" for our present allocation problems. How nice it would be to find identifiable villains here, but I see no fault here *at all* with the elderly. Instead, we are only now beginning to see some of the costs and pitfalls of the great medical advances that have been made in recent decades, and some of the unforeseen and probably unforeseeable hazards of pursuing medical progress. It is the success of medicine, not its failures, that has created the problem of sustaining and paying for decent health care for the elderly. It is the success of the campaign against ageism, increasing the expectations of everyone for a medically and socially transformed old age, that have added to that problem. If there is any blame to be apportioned it should be directed at our dreams, some of which have come true. It is just that we did not know what that would mean. Now we are finding out.

## REFERENCES

Anderson, P. (1991). On the "ragged edge" of medical progress: Daniel Callahan and problems of limits. Unpublished paper.

Barry, R. L., & Bradley, G. V. (Eds.). (1991). Set no limits: A rebuttal to Daniel Callahan's proposal to limit health care for the elderly. Urbana: University of Illinois Press.

Binstock, R. H., & Post, S. G. (Eds.). (1991). Too old for health care: Controversies in medicine, law, economics, and ethics. Baltimore: The Johns Hopkins University Press.

Breidenbaugh, M. Z., Sarsitis, I. M., & Milam, R. A. (1990). Medicare end stage renal disease population, Health Care Financing Review, 12, 101–104.

Callahan, D. (1987). Setting limits: Medical goals in an aging society. New York: Simon and Schuster.

Callahan, D. (1990). What kind of life: The limits of medical progress. New York: Simon and Schuster.

Callahan, D. (1993). The troubled dream of life: Living with mortality. New York: Simon and Schuster.

Chambers, C. V., Diamond, J. J., Perkel, R. L., & Lasch, L. A. (1994). Relationship of advance directives to hospital charges in a Medicare population. Archives of Internal Medicine, 154, 541–547.

Estes, C. L. (1988). Cost containment and the elderly: Conflict or challenge? Journal of the American Medical Association, 36, 68–72.

Hackler, C. (Ed.). (In press). Health care for an aging population: Planning for the twenty-first century. Albany: State University of New York Press.

Holahan, J., & Palmer, J. L. (1988). Medicare's fiscal problems: An imperative for reform. Journal of Health, Politics, Policy and Law, 13, 53–81.

Hollander, C. F., & Becker, H. A., (Eds.). (1987). Growing old in the future. Dordrecht: Martinius Nijhoff Publishers.

Homer, P., & Holstein, M., (Eds.). (1990). A good old age: The paradox of setting limits. New York: Simon and Schuster.

Hosking, M. P., Warner, M. A., Lobdell, C. M., Offord, K. P., & Melton, J. L. (1989). Outcome of surgery in patients 90 years of age and older. Journal of the American Medical Association, 261, 1909–1915.

Jecker, N. S., (Ed.). (1991). Ethics and aging. Clifton, NJ: Humana Press.

Jecker, N. S. (1991). Age-based rationing and women. Journal of the American Medical Association, 266, 3012–3015.

Jecker, N. S., & Pearlman, R. A. (1989). Ethical constraints on rationing medical care by age. Journal of the American Geriatrics Society, 37, 1067–1075.

Jouvenel, H. de. (1989). Europe's ageing population: Trends and challenges to 2025. Special co-publication of Futures and Futuribles. Guildford, UK: Butterworth.

Latta, V. B., & Keene, R. E. (1989). Leading surgical procedures for aged Medicare beneficiaries. Health Care Financing Review, 11, 99–100.

Lawlor, E. F. (1992). What kind of medicine? The Gerontologist, 32, 131–133.

Levinsky, N. G. (1990). Age as a criterion for rationing health care. New England Journal of Medicine, 322, 1813–1815.

Loriaux, (1990). Il Sera une fois... la revolution gruse jeux at enjeux autour d'une profunde mutation societale (Someday it will happen... the revolution of aging and the profound social change at stake). Université Catholique de Louvain. Louvain-la-Neuve, Claco: Institut de Démographie.

Manton, K. G., Corder, L., & Stallard, S. (1993). Changes in the use of personal assistance and special equipment from 1982 to 1989: Results from the 1982 and 1989 NLTCS. The Gerontologist, 33, 168–176.

Moody, H. R. (1991). Allocation, yes; Age-based rationing, no. In R. H. Binstock & S. G. Post, (Eds.), Too Old for Health Care. Baltimore: The Johns Hopkins University Press, pp. 180–203.

Preston, S. (1984). Children and the elderly: Divergent paths for America's dependents. Demography, 21, 455–491.

St. Louis University. (1989). Health care for the elderly. Symposium in the St. Louis University Law Journal, 33, 557–710.

Schneider, E. L., Guralnik, J. M. (1990). The aging of America: Impact on health care costs. *Journal of the American Medical Association, 263,* 2335–2340.

Schneiderman, L., Kronick, R., Kaplan, R. M., Anderson, J. P., & Langer, R. D. (1992). Effects of offering advance directives on medical treatment and costs. *Annals of Internal Medicine, 117,* 599–606.

Winslow, G. R., & Walters, J. W. (Eds.). (1993). *Facing limits: Ethics and health care for the elderly.* Boulder, CO: Westview Press.

Zweibel, N. R., Cassel, C. K., & Karvison, T. (1993). Public attitudes about the use of chronological age as a criterion for allocating health care resources. *The Gerontologist, 36,* 74–80.

# NO

Patricia Lanoie Blanchette

# AGE-BASED RATIONING
# OF HEALTHCARE

Given the temporal relationship between the increasing numbers of older people and the nation's focus on the costs of healthcare, it might seem evident that aging is the major determinant of increasing costs. The image of demented oldsters avariciously consuming the legacy of our children springs to mind, and indeed, an incomplete and biased recitation of healthcare statistics would appear to support this conclusion, leading to serious proposals to ration healthcare for older people (Callahan, 1987). A careful examination of the facts begins with an acknowledgement of the potential for bias, the willingness to question what appears obvious, and a search beyond those data that are assembled to support a predetermined conclusion. Decisions about healthcare must be guided by objective information and by the ethical and moral principles that can enlighten decisions about limits on the public money allocated for people of all ages.

In considering the costs of healthcare, it is easy to be drawn into a debate that labels this an intergenerational contest, pitting the costs of providing increasingly sophisticated care to increasingly younger, potentially chronically impaired neonates, for example, against the costs of caring for the nation's elders. In such a debate, it might be argued that although the potential life expectancy of babies in general is much longer than that of elders, this is often not true when individual lives are compared. It is also possible to make the argument that elders may have contributed to the public good for many years and are now more deserving of care. However, basing decisions on whether an individual is deserving of care presupposes a wisdom that we have not yet attained and is to be strenuously avoided.

Another issue that might be raised in such a debate is that in a country concerned with overpopulation, we may question the use of public monies or health insurance for infertility treatment. However, our culture is one that cherishes children and families, and the social benefits of establishing families with children may return the output in full measure. We are most likely to

From Patricia Lanoie Blanchette, "Age-Based Rationing of Healthcare," *Generations,* vol. 20, no. 4 (Winter 1996–1997), pp. 60–63. Copyright © 1996 by The American Society on Aging, San Francisco, CA. Reprinted by permission.

accept the costs of raising a child and seldom stop to total up the costs of the years of dependency. We are less likely to appreciate the personal fulfillment, redefinition of productivity, and intergenerational significance in old age. The importance of completing psychological development and establishing roots for successive generations by the presence of elders as well as children is undervalued.

However, in considering the allocation of resources it is futile and intellectually inadequate to pursue the avenues of intergenerational conflict. People's lives are priceless at any age. A fully developed society must be guided by principles equally valid across an age spectrum. A consideration of the allocation of resources requires that we examine the quality of the data, guard against the old-age prejudice that exists in our culture, and be primarily guided by the ethical bases for limiting care at any age.

## POPULATION AGING AND COSTS

Is there a primary cause-and-effect relationship between the rapid aging of the population and healthcare costs? People over age 65 today constitute something over 12 percent of the U.S. population and account for one-third of the nation's annual federal healthcare expenditures, or $300 billion of an estimated $900 billion in 1993 (National Academy on Aging, 1994). By 2020, when baby boomers will be in their mid to late 70s, the population over 65 is estimated to be 20 percent of the total population, with the actual number of people over 65 doubling from today.

However, when examined closely, less than 10 percent of the increased costs of healthcare can be accounted for by population aging (National Academy on Aging, 1994; Newhouse, 1996). Further,

while it would appear that 12 percent of the population is using one-third of all public resources, state and local governments spend ten times the amount on education and children's programs than is spent on programs benefitting elders, including Medicaid (Gist, 1992).

## FUTILITY AND THE COSTS OF CARING FOR THE DYING

It has become a widespread belief that a majority of healthcare resources are spent on high-technology care for elderly people in their last year of life. However, the facts show that medical costs in the last year of life for people aged 80 and older are less than for younger people. In 1989, 2,150,466 persons died in the United States. Of these, 29 percent were younger than 65, 22 percent were aged 65–74, 28 percent were aged 75–84, and 21 percent were aged 85 and older. In one study of 500 persons who died, people over 80 had only half the hospital costs of those at younger ages, and costs for those age 65 to 79 were only slightly higher than for those under age 65 (Scitovsky, 1988). The beliefs about the costs of caring for the dying come from a series of papers showing that about 30 percent of Medicare costs are spent on about 6 percent of people who die (Lubitz and Prikoda, 1994; Lubitz and Riles, 1993). However, only 6 percent of those who died had costs of over $15,000, and in all age groups, a high proportion of costs are incurred for a small number of beneficiaries who are either sick enough to be at risk of dying or chronically ill. This is not an exclusive old-age phenomenon (Cohen, 1994).

There is also the argument that precious healthcare resources are squandered on demented elders who would be better off dead and that caring for older people is generally not only expensive, but futile.

Although the exact prevalence of dementia is still to be determined, it probably is present in 10 percent of people over age 65. It increases in prevalence with age, usually doubling in prevalence with each decade over 65, so that by age over 85, estimates of the proportion with dementia range between 30 and 50 percent. Conversely, then, from 50 to 70 percent of people over age 85 are not demented. Even in those who have dementia, with forgetfulness and disorientation as prominent features, the quality of life can be quite acceptable with proper assistance. Those whose lives are more burdensome than pleasurable would be best served by providing care according to their self-determined wishes and advanced directives than by an external application of rationing standards. Although advanced directives, such as living wills, have been developed to further autonomy and privacy, early studies of costs are beginning to show some savings, without the need to impose rationing (Goldstein, 1994).

If the cost of care is spread over an entire age spectrum, it still might seem obvious that there would be poorer outcomes of treatment in people of advanced age. But again, we see the value of hard data. In numerous studies of outcomes from surgical procedures and renal dialysis, counter to intuition, chronological age drops out as an independent predictor of results of treatment. Outcomes are more closely tied to the presence of several diseases or conditions and functional status (Cassel, 1991). Past studies on the results of cancer treatment showing poorer outcomes in older patients have now been shown to be flawed by a systematic undertreatment of elders. One

study of the impact of eliminating aggressive, life-prolonging treatments for patients beyond certain ages revealed that if the age limit for treatment were set at 80, the overall costs would be reduced 11 percent; if set at 90 years, the charges would be reduced only 0.4 percent. The study points out the wide range in fitness among individuals of the same age, with some at 80 years comparing favorably to others at 65, and some at 65 more like others at 95 (Goldstein, 1994). Although age may be a marker for co-morbidity and poorer functional status, the results of these studies underline the need to assess individuals one-by-one for appropriateness of treatment, and they caution against an across-the-board age exclusion.

## OVERT RATIONING

Despite the lack of data to support age-based rationing of care, it is common to hear or read comments about holding down healthcare costs by overtly withholding high-tech, high-cost services for older people. As noted above, there are no data to support chronological age as an independent criterion for the effectiveness of treatment. There is also the concern that a limitation of high-tech care will lead to a limitation on other types of care—the "slippery slope" phenomenon. In 1994, the British newspapers spotlighted the story of a 73-year-old man refused physiotherapy for arthritis. Subsequently, the Royal College of Physicians published its study of equity care for the elderly. They declared that "there is no biological rationale for separating older people from the rest of the human race: they should get the same quality of care as anyone else." In both the United States in the 1960s and in Great Britain until the 1980s there is a history of people over age 45 being excluded from renal dialysis (Moss, 1994). Subsequently, this age was gradually increased. In the early days of renal dialysis, in both places, with few resources to offer, an age bias was overt. It was assumed that older people would have a reduced life expectancy and derive less overall benefit from treatment. Subsequent information has shown that as a group, older people do have a shorter life expectancy in treatment, but, after careful study, the Institute of Medicine Committee for the Study of the Medicare ERSD (End-Stage Renal Disease) Program (Levinsky and Rettig, 1991) has specifically rejected age as a criterion for patient acceptance to dialysis, noting that comorbidities and functional status are the primary predictors of benefits from treatment, not age. Data influencing the decision include, as predicted, the finding that one-year and five-year survival of people on dialysis decreases with age. However, this decrease is to be expected because, of course, older people on or off dialysis have a shorter life expectancy than do younger people. In addition, the likelihood that other major medical events will occur is greater in the elderly, leading to a greater prevalence of older people voluntarily choosing to go off dialysis and dying from withdrawal of dialysis. However, whereas older people's life expectancy may be less, studies have shown that older people may value their continued lives on dialysis more than younger people do, with a higher well-being index, more positive feelings, and a greater life satisfaction in general, including being more satisfied with their marriages, family life, savings and investments, and standard of living (Office of Technology Assessment, 1987).

## COVERT RATIONING

As carefully as we must defend against unwarranted, overt age-based rationing, we must be evermore vigilant against covert rationing. Consider the following actual case:

A 75-year-old married man in overall good health except for mild emphysema chooses to be admitted to a long-term-care facility with his wife, who has severe, crippling arthritis and frail health. They have been married for over fifty years, and he would rather be admitted to a nursing home to be with her than remain at home alone. In addition, the nursing facility is run by a religious organization and offers the further opportunity to study and to live his faith and culture. While at the facility, he chances upon the occurrence of a friend receiving cardiopulmonary resuscitation. He is frightened by the event, and in counseling him staff take the opportunity to discuss advance directives. After careful consideration, with lots of questions asked and answered, he decides that his life is of high quality, and that he wishes to receive medical intensive care if he should ever need it, but without chest compressions. Some time later, he suffers a relatively uncomplicated inferior myocardial infarction and is transferred to the hospital. He is expected to recover fully, but, because of the emphysema and some respiratory fatigue, it is decided to "rest him" for a short while with elective pulmonary intubation (insertion of a breathing tube). He fully agrees to this plan with the stipulation that if weaning cannot be accomplished easily within a few days, he not be allowed to remain on the ventilator indefinitely. According to hospital policy, the intensive care unit medical director, who does not know the patient, becomes the attending physician of record. The next day, the patient is visited by his primary physician who finds him without the ventilator, cyanotic (bluish because of lack of oxygen), and near death, having been discharged from the intensive care unit.

The following explanation is offered to the primary physician by the unit resident trainee who was on duty the previous night. It was he who decided, without consultation, to extubate the patient. "Our society cannot afford to keep these elderly nursing home residents alive indefinitely. Besides, he's a 'no code' patient [meaning a notation of 'do not resuscitate' was on his chart]; what's he doing in an ICU?" The patient died shortly thereafter, leaving a grieving wife who fully expected to have him back with her within a few weeks and a stunned family and primary physician who were not consulted in the ICU decision.

While there are many aspects to criticize about this case, among them poor supervision of the unit trainee and the lack of consultation with the family and primary physician, the main factor at work was age discrimination. In-depth discussion with this misinformed and dangerously unsupervised trainee revealed a person who was both lacking in judgment and profoundly influenced by the comments he had heard and read about the cost and futility of healthcare for the elderly.

Covert actions to withdraw care are dangerous, must be anticipated, and must result in policies to prevent such situations as the above. Even more dangerous are the more concealed, less dramatic, case-by-case decisions in which healthcare providers choose to limit the treatment options they offer older people, strictly because of age, that erode options presented to older people. These providers may be well-intentioned, erroneously believing that the treatments will fail to have an acceptable outcome, or they may be responding to an excessive concern for costs. There is a growing concern that the pressure to tightly control costs in managed-care settings in particular will result in limits being placed on the marketing of these plans to older people or will stay the hand of care once these individuals are enrolled. We must guard against both systematized and individual discrimination.

## THE ANSWER: APPROPRIATE CARE

The concerns regarding costs and rationing are usually phrased in the context of the allocation of limited resources among individuals within a group. In cultures where personal autonomy and rights of the individual are priorities, the discussion of allocation of resources according to age is unsettling. In other cultures, utilitarianism, in which the interests of the individual are secondary to the interests of the group, predominates, and different ethical decisions are made. Despite the current substantial percentage of the national resources allocated to healthcare, some would question whether we are near the actual limits of the resources. They raise the "guns versus butter" argument, noting " ... the cost of stealth bombers," for example, as compared to health-related expenditures. But given that the amount of resources available for healthcare does have some reasonable limit, and assuming that we are at or near maximum, the argument about allocation rages. The issue at hand is how to control costs within an acceptable ethical and cultural framework.

There is every reason to believe that good care, self-determination, and autonomy can prevail at the same time that costs are reduced. This desirable combination can be achieved by focusing on providing the most appropriate care. Appropriate care requires the following: careful and comprehensive assessment; prevention as well as intervention; clinicians enlightened with evidence-based, unbiased data; and liberation from financial or other incentives to provide excessive care. A major concern at present is the lack of integration of geriatric principles and knowledge into the usual healthcare of many elders, and the limited geriatrics training received by many primary and specialist providers. Promoting quality care and self-determination and autonomy while containing costs also requires a systematic way to encourage patients to understand and to choose the extent of care they desire.

Healthcare should be appropriate, not rationed. Appropriate care requires that (1) decisions to accept or reject care be truly informed with good data, (2) the tendency to an age bias be recognized and confronted, and (3) advance directives and health proxies or surrogate decision-makers be explained and recommended for adults of all ages. While there does not appear to be any move to institute overt rationing by age in the United States, the possibility of covert rationing is of serious concern. Health policy must be enlightened so that the possibility of overt or covert rationing to people of all ages who may need appropriate high-cost care will be acknowledged and rejected.

*This work was supported in part by a Geriatric Education Center grant from the U.S. Public Health Service, Department of Health and Human Services, Health Resources and Services Administration, Bureau of Health Professions.*

## REFERENCES

Callahan, D. 1987. *Setting Limits: Medical Goals in an Aging Society.* New York: Simon and Schuster.

Cassel, C.K., et al. 1991. "Ethical Issues.' In R. A. Rettig and N. Levinsky, eds., *Kidney Failure and the Federal Government.* Washington, D.C.: National Academy Press.

Cohen, G.D. 1994. "Health Care at an Advanced Age: Myths and Misconceptions." *Annals of Internal Medicine* 121:146–47.

Gist, J. 1992. "Entitlements and the Federal Budget Deficit: Setting the Record Straight." Washington, D.C.: AARP Public Policy Institute.

Goldstein, M. K. 1994. *Reduction in Health Care Costs in the Last-Year-of-Life: Impact of Three Alternative Policies.* Master's thesis, Department of Health, Research and Policy, Stanford University.

Levinsky, N., and Rettig, R. A. 1991. "The Medicare End-Stage Renal Disease Program: A Report from the Institute of Medicine." *New England Journal of Medicine* 324:1143.

Lubitz, J., and Prikoda, R. 1994. "The Use and Costs of Medicare Services in the Last Two Years of Life." *Health Care Financing Review* 5:117–31.

Lubitz, J., and Riles, G. 1993. "Trends in Medicare Payments in the Last Year of Life." *New England Journal of Medicine* 328:1092–96.

Moss, A. H. 1994. "Dialysis Decisions and the Elderly." *Clinics in Geriatric Medicine* (August): 56–9.

Newhouse, J. P. 1996. "An Iconoclastic View of Healthcare Cost Containment." *Generations* 10(2):61–3.

National Academy on Aging. 1994. *Old Age in the 21st Century: A Report to the Assistant Secretary for Aging.* U.S. Department of Health and Human Services. Syracuse, N.Y.: The Maxwell School, Syracuse University.

Office of Technology Assessment. 1987. "Dialysis for Chronic Renal Failure." In *Life-Sustaining Technologies and the Elderly.* OTA-BA-306. Washington, D.C.: Government Printing Office.

Scitovsky, A. A. 1988. "Medical Care in the Last Twelve Months of Life: The Relation Between Age, Functional Status, and Medical Care Expenditures." *Milbank Memorial Fund Quarterly: Health and Society* 66: 40–60.

# POSTSCRIPT

## Should Health Care for the Elderly Be Limited?

In October 1986 Dr. Thomas Starzl of Pittsburgh, Pennsylvania, transplanted a liver into a 76-year-old woman at a cost of over $200,000. Soon after that, Congress ordered organ transplantation to be covered under Medicare, which ensured that more older persons would receive this benefit. At the same time these events were taking place, a government campaign to contain medical costs was under way, with health care for the elderly targeted.

Not everyone agrees with this means of cost cutting. In "Public Attitudes About the Use of Chronological Age as a Criterion for Allocating Health Care Resources," *The Gerontologist* (February 1993), the authors report that the majority of older people surveyed accept the withholding of life-prolonging medical care from the hopelessly ill but that few would deny treatment on the basis of age alone. Two publications that express opposition to age-based health care rationing are "Rationing by Any Other Name," *The New England Journal of Medicine* (June 5, 1997) and "Fighting for Health Care," *Newsweek* (March 30, 1998).

Currently, about 40 million Americans have no medical insurance and are at risk of being denied basic health care services. At the same time, the federal government pays most of the health care costs of the elderly. While it may not meet the needs of all older people, the amount of medical aid that goes to the elderly is greater than any other demographic group, and the elderly have the highest disposable income.

Most Americans have access to the best and most expensive medical care in the world. As these costs rise, some difficult decisions may have to be made regarding the allocation of these resources. As the population ages and more health care dollars are spent on care during the last years of life, medical services for the elderly or the dying may become a natural target for reduction in order to balance the health care budget. Additional readings on this subject include "Use of Medical Services by Older Patients Increases," *Geriatrics* (October, 1997); "Who Won't Pull the Plug?" *The Washington Post* (January 2, 1994); and "What Do We Owe the Elderly: Allocating Social and Health Care Resources," *Hastings Center Report* (March/April 1994). Articles dealing with age bias include "Recognizing Bedside Rationing: Clear Cases and Tough Calls," *Annals of Internal Medicine* (January 1, 1997); "Measuring the Burden of Disease: Healthy Life-Years," *American Journal of Public Health* (February 1998); "Rationing Health Care," *British Medical Journal* (February 28, 1998); and "Truth or Consequences," *The New England Journal of Medicine* (March 26, 1998).

# ISSUE 4

## Is Gun Control a Public Health Issue?

**YES: Josh Sugarmann,** from "Reverse Fire," *Mother Jones* (January/February 1994)

**NO: Don B. Kates, Henry E. Schaffer, and William C. Waters IV,** from "Public Health Pot Shots: How the CDC Succumbed to the Gun 'Epidemic,'" *Reason* (April 1997)

### ISSUE SUMMARY

**YES:** Josh Sugarmann, executive director of the Violence Policy Center, an education foundation that researches firearm violence and advocates gun control, argues that guns increase the costs of hospitalization, rehabilitation, and lost wages, making them a serious public health issue.

**NO:** Attorney Don B. Kates, professor of genetics Henry E. Schaffer, and William C. Waters IV, a physician, counter that most gun-related violence is caused by aberrants, not ordinary gun owners.

More and more people in the United States are buying guns to protect themselves and their families in response to increasing crime rates. There are currently over 216 million firearms—close to 900,000 assault weapons—in private hands in the United States, more than double the number in 1970. Also, each year more than 24,000 Americans are killed with handguns in homicides, suicides, and accidents (an average of 65 people each day). Firearms are used in 70 percent of all murders committed in the United States. These statistics raise important questions: Does gun ownership afford protection against crime or increase the risk of gun-related death? And are gun control and gun ownership public health concerns? Gun owners and opponents of gun control claim that weapons kept at home will prevent crime. Proponents of gun control claim that weapons kept at home are involved in too many fights that lead to injury or death, accidental shootings, and suicides.

To attempt to resolve these issues, Arthur Kellermann, an emergency room physician at the University of Tennessee, and his associates conducted a study, "Gun Ownership as a Risk Factor for Homicide in the Home," *The New England Journal of Medicine* (October 7, 1993). Kellermann's study concluded that people who keep guns in their homes are much more likely to kill or injure another family member than use the gun in self-defense against a criminal. Kellermann believes that a gun almost automatically makes any fight potentially more dangerous and that the risks of having a gun outweigh the benefits. Many supporters of gun control say that the study confirmed their warnings about the basic dangers of owning guns and keeping them in the home.

The contention that gun ownership is more dangerous than beneficial is not without its critics. The Kellermann et al. study, for instance, only measured risks associated with gun ownership. They did not study cases in which guns actually deterred crime. Kellermann et al. also did not discuss the possibility that the guns may not have caused the violence; the violence may have caused the use of guns. For instance, in areas of high crime, citizens are more likely to arm themselves for self-protection.

Although it is unclear whether guns deter crime or cause it, gun control in one form or another has been around since the early part of the twentieth century. The first major gun control act strengthening restrictions on handguns followed the assassinations of John F. Kennedy, Dr. Martin Luther King, Jr., and Robert Kennedy in the 1960s. Other laws banning the sale of handguns and the manufacture and sale of certain types of assault weapons followed. In 1993 President Bill Clinton signed the Brady Bill, which imposed a five-day waiting period for handgun purchases. (The bill was named for James Brady, aide to former president Ronald Reagan. Both Brady and Reagan were shot during an assassination attempt in the early 1980s). Unfortunately for gun control advocates, in June 1997 the Supreme Court ruled that the Brady gun control law violated "the very principle of separate state sovereignty" by requiring state officials to conduct background checks of prospective handgun buyers. In a 5-to-4 decision, the Court invalidated the background check of the 1993 law. This decision did not address, however, a separate portion of the Brady Bill that imposes a five-day waiting period before a gun sale can be completed.

Gun control is a controversial issue in the United States. Its opponents claim that it infringes on the constitutional rights of Americans to bear arms as granted by the Second Amendment. The gun lobby also pictures America under stricter gun controls as a country where honest citizens would be helpless against well-armed criminals. Many advocates of gun control, however, regard the deaths and injuries related to guns as a public health problem that can be treated only by getting rid of guns themselves.

In the following selections, Josh Sugarmann asserts that guns are definitely a public health issue and supports stricter gun control. He feels that guns offer no protective benefit even in homicide cases that follow forced entry. Don B. Kates, Henry E. Schaffer, and William C. Waters IV argue that violence is not a matter of honest citizens killing simply because a gun is nearby but of criminals committing violent acts. The authors also maintain that health organizations, such as the Centers for Disease Control, should focus on true public health issues and not veer off into social policy.

# YES                           Josh Sugarmann

# REVERSE FIRE

For seven years gun-control advocates have lobbied for the Brady Bill, which
mandates a national waiting period for buying handguns. But ironically,
the bill's passage may actually benefit the gun industry. Oversold by its
supporters, the Brady Bill has become synonymous in American minds with
gun control itself. If violence continues once a national waiting period goes
into effect (as it likely will), the gun lobby will offer the Brady Bill as proof
that gun control doesn't work.

## A LACK OF REGULATION

With its passage in 1993, gun-control advocates find themselves at a cross-
roads. We can continue to push legislation of dubious effectiveness. Or we
can acknowledge that gun violence is a public-health crisis fueled by an inherently dangerous consumer product. To end the crisis, we have to regulate
—or, in the case of handguns and assault weapons, completely ban—the
product.

The romantic myths attached to gun ownership stop many people from
thinking of them as a consumer product. As a result, the standard risk analysis
applied to other potentially dangerous products—pesticides, prescription
drugs, or toasters—has never been applied to firearms.

Yet guns are manufactured by corporations—with boards of directors, marketing plans, employees, and a bottom line—just like companies that manufacture toasters. What separates the gun industry from other manufacturers
is lack of regulation.

For example, when a glut in the market caused handgun production to
plummet from 2.6 million in 1982 to 1.4 million in 1986, the industry retooled
its product line. To stimulate sales, manufacturers added firepower, technology, and capacity to their new models. The result: assault weapons, a switch
from six-shot revolvers to high-capacity pistols, and increased use of plastics
and high-tech additions like integral laser sights.

The industry was free to make these changes (most of which made the
guns more dangerous) because guns that are 50 caliber or less and not fully

automatic can be manufactured with virtually no restrictions. The Bureau of Alcohol, Tobacco, and Firearms (ATF) lacks even the common regulatory powers—including safety-standard setting and recall—granted government agencies such as the Consumer Product Safety Commission, the Food and Drug Administration, and the Environmental Protection Agency.

## A DEADLY PRODUCT

Yet guns are the second most deadly consumer product (after cars) on the market. In Texas and Louisiana the firearms-related death rate already exceeds that for motor vehicles, and by the year 2000 firearms will likely supplant automobiles as the leading cause of product-related death throughout the United States.

But since Americans view firearm suicides, murders, and fatal accidents as separate problems, the enormity of America's gun crisis goes unrecognized. In 1990, American guns claimed an estimated 37,000 lives. Federal Bureau of Investigation data shows that gun murders that year reached an all-time high of 15,377; a record 12,489 involved handguns.

## THE HUMAN TOLL

In 1990 (the most recent year for which statistics are available), 18,885 Americans took their own lives with firearms, and an estimated 13,030 of those deaths involved handguns. Unlike pills, gas, or razor blades—which are of limited effectiveness—guns are rarely forgiving. For example, self-inflicted cutting wounds account for 15 percent of all suicide attempts but only 1 percent of all successful suicides. Poisons and drugs account

for 70 percent of suicide attempts but less than 12 percent of all suicides. Conversely, nonfatal, self-inflicted gunshot wounds are rare—yet three-fifths of all U.S. suicides involve firearms.

In addition to the human toll, the economic costs of not regulating guns are staggering. The Centers for Disease Control (CDC) estimated that the lifetime economic cost—hospitalization, rehabilitation, and lost wages—of firearms violence was $14.4 billion in 1985, making it the third most expensive injury category The average lifetime cost per person for each firearms fatality—$373,520 —was the highest of any injury.

Such human and economic costs are not tolerated for any other product. Many consumer products from lawn darts to the Dalkon Shield have been banned in the United States, even though they claimed only a fraction of the lives guns do in a day. The firearms industry is long overdue for the simple, regulatory oversight applied to other consumer products. For public safety, the ATF must be given authority to control the design, manufacture, distribution, and sale of firearms and ammunition.

Under such a plan, the ATF would subject each category of firearm and ammunition to an unreasonable-risk analysis to weed out products whose potential for harm outweighs any possible benefit. This would result in an immediate ban on the future production and sale of handguns and assault weapons because of their high risk and low utility.

Because they are easily concealed and accessed, handguns hold the dubious honor of being our number-one murder and suicide tool. Assault weapons—high-capacity, semiautomatic firearms designed primarily for the military and police—pose a public-safety risk as the result of their firepower. A 1989 study of ATF data conducted by Cox Newspapers found that assault firearms were twenty times more likely to turn up in crime traces than conventional firearms.

In addition, a regulatory approach to firearms would exert far greater control over the industry and its distribution network. It would not, however, affect the availability of standard sporting rifles and shotguns, which would continue to be sold because of their usefulness and relatively low risk.

## A PUBLIC-HEALTH ISSUE

Such an approach is the industry's worst nightmare—conjuring images of an all-powerful "gun czar." And in a sense, gun manufacturers would be right: the ATF would become a gun czar in the same way that the EPA is a pesticide czar, the FDA is a prescription-drug-and-medical-device czar, and the Consumer Product Safety Commission is a toaster czar. Yet it is just such a regulatory approach that has dramatically reduced motor-vehicle deaths and injuries over the past twenty years.

Gun-control advocates cannot afford to spend another seven years battling over piecemeal measures that have little more to offer than good intentions. We are far past the point where registration, licensing, safety training, background checks, or waiting periods will have much effect on firearms violence. Tired of being shot and threatened, Americans are showing a deeper understanding of gun violence as a public-health issue, and are becoming aware of the need to restrict specific categories of weapons.

As America's health-care debate continues, discussion of the role of guns—from the human price paid in mortality to the dollars-and-cents cost of uninsured gunshot victims—can only help clarify that gun violence is not a crime issue but a public-health issue. This shift in attitude is apparent in the firearms component of Bill Clinton's domestic violence prevention group, which is co-chaired not only by a representative from the Justice Department—as expected—but also by a CDC official.

Even if the only legacy of this current wave of revulsion is that gun violence will now be viewed as a public-health issue, America will still have taken a very large first step toward gun sanity.

# NO

## Don B. Kates, Henry E. Schaffer, and William C. Waters IV

# PUBLIC HEALTH POT SHOTS: HOW THE CDC SUCCUMBED TO THE GUN "EPIDEMIC"

Last year Congress tried to take away $2.6 million from the U.S. Centers for Disease Control and Prevention. In budgetary terms, it was a pittance: 0.1 percent of the CDC's $2.2 billion allocation. Symbolically, however, it was important: $2.6 million was the amount the CDC's National Center for Injury Prevention and Control had spent in 1995 on studies of firearm injuries. Congressional critics, who charged that the center's research program was driven by an anti-gun prejudice, had previously sought to eliminate the NCIPC completely. "This research is designed to, and is used to, promote a campaign to reduce lawful firearms ownership in America," wrote 10 senators, including then–Majority Leader Bob Dole and current Majority Leader Trent Lott. "Funding redundant research initiatives, particularly those which are driven by a social-policy agenda, simply does not make sense."

After the NCIPC survived the 1995 budget process, opponents narrowed their focus, seeking to pull the plug on the gun research specifically, or at least to punish the CDC for continuing to fund it. At a May 1996 hearing, Rep. Jay Dickey (R-Ark.), co-sponsor of the amendment cutting the CDC's budget, chastised NCIPC Director Mark Rosenberg for treating guns as a "public health menace," suggesting that he was "working toward changing society's attitudes so that it becomes socially unacceptable to own handguns." In June the House Appropriations Committee adopted Dickey's amendment, which included a prohibition on the use of CDC funds "to advocate or promote gun control," and in July the full House rejected an attempt to restore the money.

Although the CDC ultimately got the $2.6 million back as part of a budget deal with the White House, the persistent assault on the agency's gun research created quite a stir. *New England Journal of Medicine* Editor Jerome Kassirer, who has published several of the CDC-funded gun studies, called it "an attack that strikes at the very heart of scientific research." Writing in *The Washington Post*, CDC Director David Satcher said criticism of the firearm research did

From Don B. Kates, Henry E. Schaffer, and William C. Waters IV, "Public Health Pot Shots: How the CDC Succumbed to the Gun 'Epidemic,'" *Reason* (April 1997). Copyright © 1997 by The Reason Foundation, 3415 S. Sepulveda Boulevard, Suite 400, Los Angeles, CA 90034. www.reason.com. Reprinted by permission.

not bode well for the country's future: "If we question the honesty of scientists who give every evidence of long deliberation on the issues before them, what are our expectations of anyone else? What hope is there for us as a society?" Frederick P. Rivara, a pediatrician who has received CDC money to do gun research, told *The Chronicle of Higher Education* that critics of the program were trying "to block scientific discovery because they don't like the results. This is a frightening trend for academic researchers. It's the equivalent of book burning."

That view was echoed by columnists and editorial writers throughout the country. In a *New York Times* column entitled "More N.R.A. Mischief," Bob Herbert defended the CDC's "rigorous, unbiased, scientific studies," suggesting that critics could not refute the results of the research and therefore had decided "to pull the plug on the funding and stop the effort altogether." Editorials offering the same interpretation appeared in *The Washington Post* ("NRA: Afraid of Facts"), *USA Today* ("Gun Lobby Keeps Rolling"), the *Los Angeles Times* ("NRA Aims at the Messenger"), *The Atlanta Journal* ("GOP Tries to Shoot the Messenger"), the *Sacramento Bee* ("Shooting the Messenger"), and the *Pittsburgh Post-Gazette* ("The Gun Epidemic").

Contrary to this picture of dispassionate scientists under assault by the Neanderthal NRA and its know-nothing allies in Congress, serious scholars have been criticizing the CDC's "public health" approach to gun research for years. In a presentation at the American Society of Criminology's 1994 meeting, for example, University of Illinois sociologist David Bordua and epidemiologist David Cowan called the public health literature on guns "advocacy based on political beliefs rather than scientific fact." Bordua and Cowan noted that *The New England Journal of Medicine* and the *Journal of the American Medical Association*, the main outlets for CDC-funded studies of firearms, are consistent supporters of strict gun control. They found that "reports with findings not supporting the position of the journal are rarely cited," "little is cited from the criminological or sociological field," and the articles that are cited "are almost always by medical or public health researchers."

Further, Bordua and Cowan said, "assumptions are presented as fact: that there is a causal association between gun ownership and the risk of violence, that this association is consistent across all demographic categories, and that additional legislation will reduce the prevalence of firearms and consequently reduce the incidence of violence." They concluded that "[i]ncestuous and selective literature citations may be acceptable for political tracts, but they introduce an artificial bias into scientific publications. Stating as fact associations which may be demonstrably false is not just unscientific, it is unprincipled." In a 1994 presentation to the Western Economics Association, State University of New York at Buffalo criminologist Lawrence Southwick compared public health firearm studies to popular articles produced by the gun lobby: "Generally the level of analysis done on each side is of a low quality.... The papers published in the medical literature (which are uniformly anti-gun) are particularly poor science."

\* \* \*

As Bordua, Cowan, and Southwick observed, a prejudice against gun ownership pervades the public health field. Deborah Prothrow-Stith, dean of the Harvard School of Public Health, nicely summarizes the typical attitude of her colleagues in a recent book. "My own view on gun control is simple," she writes. "I hate guns and cannot imagine why anybody would want to own one. If I had my way, guns for sport would be registered, and all other guns would be banned." Opposition to gun ownership is also the official position of the U.S. Public Health Service, the CDC's parent agency. Since 1979, its goal has been "to reduce the number of handguns in private ownership," starting with a 25 percent reduction by the turn of the century.

Since 1985 the CDC has funded scores of firearm studies, all reaching conclusions that favor stricter gun control. But CDC officials insist they are not pursuing an anti-gun agenda. In a 1996 interview with the *Times-Picayune*, CDC spokeswoman Mary Fenley adamantly denied that the agency is "trying to eliminate guns." In a 1991 letter to CDC critic Dr. David Stolinsky, the NCIPC's Mark Rosenberg said "our scientific understanding of the role that firearms play in violent events is rudimentary." He added in a subsequent letter, "There is a strong need for further scientific investigations of the relationships among firearms ownership, firearms regulations and the risk of firearm-related injury. This is an area that has not been given adequate scrutiny. Hopefully, by addressing these important and appropriate scientific issues we will eventually arrive at conclusions which support effective, preventive actions."

Yet four years *earlier*, in a 1987 CDC report, Rosenberg thought the area adequately scrutinized, and his understanding sufficient, to urge confiscation of all firearms from "the general population," claiming "8,600 homicides and 5,370 suicides could be avoided" each year. In 1993 *Rolling Stone* reported that Rosenberg "envisions a long term campaign, similar to [those concerning] tobacco use and auto safety, to convince Americans that guns are, first and foremost, a public health menace." In 1994 he told *The Washington Post*, "We need to revolutionize the way we look at guns, like what we did with cigarettes. Now it [sic] is dirty, deadly, and banned."

As Bordua and Cowan noted, one hallmark of the public health literature on guns is a tendency to ignore contrary scholarship. Among criminologists, Gary Kleck's encyclopedic *Point Blank: Guns and Violence in America* (1991) is universally recognized as the starting point for further research. Kleck, a professor of criminology at Florida State University, was initially a strong believer that gun ownership increased the incidence of homicide, but his research made him a skeptic. His book assembles strong evidence against the notion that reducing gun ownership is a good way to reduce violence. That may be why *Point Blank* is never cited in the CDC's own firearm publications or in articles reporting the results of CDC-funded gun studies.

Three Kleck studies, the first published in 1987, have found that guns are used in self-defense up to three times as often as they are used to commit crimes. These studies are so convincing that the doyen of American criminologists, Marvin Wolfgang, conceded in the Fall 1995 issue of *The Journal of Criminal Law and Criminology* that they pose a serious challenge to his own anti-gun views. "I am as strong a gun-control advocate as can be found among the criminologists in this country... What troubles me is the article by Gary Kleck and Mark Gertz. The reason I am troubled is that they have provided an almost clear-cut case of methodologically sound research in support of something I have theoretically opposed for years, namely, the use of a gun against a criminal perpetrator."

Yet Rosenberg and his CDC colleague James Mercy, writing in *Health Affairs* in 1993, present the question "How frequently are guns used to successfully ward off potentially violent attacks?" as not just open but completely unresearched. They cite neither Kleck nor the various works on which he drew.

When CDC sources do cite adverse studies, they often get them wrong. In 1987 the National Institute of Justice hired two sociologists, James D. Wright and Peter H. Rossi, to assess the scholarly literature and produce an agenda for gun control. Wright and Rossi found the literature so biased and shoddy that it provided no basis for concluding anything positive about gun laws. Like Kleck, they were forced to give up their own prior faith in gun control as they researched the issue.

But that's not the story told by Dr. Arthur Kellermann, director of Emory University's Center for Injury Control and the CDC's favorite gun researcher. In a 1988 *New England Journal of Medicine* article, Kellermann and his co-authors cite Wright and Rossi's book *Under the Gun* to support the notion that "restricting access to handguns could substantially reduce our annual rate of homicide." What they actually said was: "There is no persuasive evidence that supports this view." In a 1992 *New England Journal of Medicine* article, Kellermann cites an *American Journal of Psychiatry* study to back up the claim "that limiting access to firearms could prevent many suicides." But the study actually found just the opposite—i.e., that

people who don't have guns find other ways to kill themselves.

At the same time that he misuses other people's work, Kellermann refuses to provide the full data for any of his studies so that scholars can evaluate his findings. His critics therefore can judge his results only from the partial data he chooses to publish. Consider a 1993 *New England Journal of Medicine* study that, according to press reports, "showed that keeping a gun in the home nearly triples the likelihood that someone in the household will be slain there." This claim cannot be verified because Kellerman will not release the data. Relying on independent sources to fill gaps in the published data, SUNY-Buffalo's Lawrence Southwick has speculated that Kellermann's full data set would actually vindicate defensive gun ownership. Such issues cannot be resolved without Kellermann's cooperation, but the CDC has refused to require its researchers to part with their data as a condition for taxpayer funding.

Even without access to secret data, it's clear that many of Kellermann's inferences are not justified. In a 1995 *JAMA* study that was funded by the CDC, he and his colleagues examined 198 incidents in which burglars entered occupied homes in Atlanta. They found that "only three individuals (1.5%) employed a firearm in self-defense"—from which they concluded that guns are rarely used for self-defense. On closer examination, however, Kellermann et al.'s data do not support that conclusion. In 42 percent of the incidents, there was no confrontation between victim and offender because "the offender(s) either left silently or fled when detected." When the burglar left silently, the victim was not even aware of the crime, so he did not have the opportunity to use a gun in self-defense (or to call the police, for that matter). The intruders who "fled when detected" show how defensive gun ownership can protect all victims, armed and unarmed alike, since the possibility of confronting an armed resident encourages burglars to flee.

These 83 no-confrontation incidents should be dropped from Kellermann et al.'s original list of 198 burglaries. Similarly, about 50 percent of U.S. homes do not contain guns, and in 70 percent of the homes that do, the guns are kept unloaded. After eliminating the burglaries where armed self-defense was simply not feasible, Kellermann's 198 incidents shrink to 17, and his 1.5 percent figure for defensive use rises to 17 percent. More important, this study covers only burglaries reported to the police. Since police catch only about 10 percent of home burglars, the only *good* reason to report a burglary is that police documentation is required to file an insurance claim. But if no property was lost because the burglar fled when the householder brandished a gun, why report the incident? And, aside from the inconvenience, there are strong reasons *not* to report: The gun may not be registered, or the householder may not be certain that guns can legally be used to repel unarmed burglars. Thus, for all Kellermann knows, successful gun use far exceeds the three incidents reported to police in his Atlanta study.

Similar sins of omission invalidate the conclusion of a 1986 *New England Journal of Medicine* study that Kellermann coauthored with University of Washington pathologist Donald T. Reay, another gun researcher who has enjoyed the CDC's support. (This particular study was funded by the Robert Wood Johnson Foundation.) Examining gunshot deaths in King County, Washington, from 1978 to 1983, Kellermann and Reay found that, of 398 people killed in a home where a gun was kept, only two were intruders shot while trying to get in. "We noted 43 suicides, criminal homicides, or accidental gunshot deaths involving a gun kept in the home for every case of homicide for self-protection," they wrote, concluding that "the advisability of keeping firearms in the home for protection must be questioned."

* * *

But since Kellermann and Reay considered only cases resulting in death, which Gary Kleck's research indicates are a tiny percentage of defensive gun uses, this conclusion does not follow. As the researchers themselves conceded, "Mortality studies such as ours do not include cases in which burglars or intruders are wounded or frightened away by the use or display of a firearm. Cases in which would-be intruders may have purposely avoided a house known to be armed are also not identified." By leaving out such cases, Kellermann and Reay excluded almost all of the lives saved, injuries avoided, and property protected by keeping a gun in the home. Yet advocates of gun control continue to use this study as the basis for claims such as, "A gun in the home is 43 times as likely to kill a family member as to be used in self-defense."

Another popular factoid—"having a gun in the home increases the risk of suicide by almost five times"—is also based on a Kellermann study, this one funded by the CDC and published by *The New England Journal of Medicine* in 1992. Kellermann and his colleagues matched each of 438 suicides to a "control" of the same race, sex, approximate age, and neighborhood. After controlling for arrests, drug abuse, living alone, and use of psychotropic medication (all of which were more common among the suicides), they found that a household with one or more guns was 4.8 times as likely to be the site of a suicide.

Although press reports about gun research commonly treat correlation and causation as one and the same, this association does not prove that having a gun in the house raises the risk of suicide. We can imagine alternative explanations: Perhaps gun ownership in this sample was associated with personality traits that were, in turn, related to suicide, or perhaps people who had contemplated suicide bought a gun for that reason. To put the association in perspective, it's worth noting that living alone and using illicit drugs were both better predictors of suicide than gun ownership was. That does not necessarily mean that living alone or using illegal drugs leads to suicide.

Furthermore, Kellermann and his colleagues selected their sample with an eye toward increasing the apparent role of gun ownership in suicide. They started by looking at all suicides that occurred during a 32-month period in King County, Washington, and Shelby County, Tennessee, but they excluded cases that occurred outside the home—nearly a third of the original sample. "Our study was restricted to suicides occurring in the victim's home," they explained with admirable frankness, "because a previous study has indicated that most suicides committed with guns occur there."

* * *

Kellermann also participated in CDC-funded research that simplistically compared homicide rates in Seattle and Vancouver, attributing the difference to Canada's stricter gun laws. This study, published in *The New England Journal of Medicine* in 1988, ignored important demographic differences between the two cities that help explain the much higher incidence of violence in Seattle. Furthermore, the researchers were aware of nationwide research that came to strikingly different conclusions about Canadian gun control, but they failed to inform their readers about that evidence.

Two years later in the same journal, the same research team compared suicide rates in Seattle and Vancouver. Unfazed by the fact that Seattle had a *lower* suicide rate, they emphasized that the rate was higher for one subgroup, adolescents and young men—a difference they attributed to lax American gun laws. Gary Mauser, a criminologist at Simon Fraser University, called the Seattle/Vancouver comparisons "a particularly egregious example" of "an abuse of scholarship, inventing, selecting, or misinterpreting data in order to validate *a priori* conclusions."

These and other studies funded by the CDC focus on the presence or absence of guns, rather than the characteristics of the people who use them. Indeed, the CDC's Rosenberg claims in the journal *Educational Horizons* that murderers are "ourselves—ordinary citizens, professionals, even health care workers": people who kill only because a gun happens to be available. Yet if there is one fact that has been incontestably established by homicide studies, it's that murderers are not ordinary gun owners but extreme aberrants whose life histories include drug abuse, serious accidents, felonies, and irrational violence. Unlike "ourselves," roughly 90 percent of adult murderers have significant criminal records, averaging an adult criminal career of six or more years with four major felonies.

Access to juvenile records would almost certainly show that the criminal careers of murderers stretch back into their adolescence. In *Murder in America* (1994), the criminologists Ronald W. Holmes and Stephen T. Holmes report that murderers generally "have histories of committing personal violence in childhood, against other children, siblings, and small animals." Murderers who don't have criminal records usually have histories of psychiatric treatment or domestic violence that did not lead to arrest.

Contrary to the impression fostered by Rosenberg and other opponents of gun ownership, the term "acquaintance homicide" does not mean killings that stem from ordinary family or neighborhood arguments. Typical acquaintance homicides include: an abusive man eventually killing a woman he has repeatedly assaulted; a drug user killing a dealer (or vice versa) in a robbery attempt; and gang members, drug dealers, and other criminals killing each other for reasons of economic rivalry or personal pique. According to a 1993 article in the *Journal of Trauma*, 80 percent of murders in Washington, D.C., are related to the drug trade, while "84% of [Philadelphia murder] victims in 1990 had antemortem drug use or criminal history." A 1994 article in *The New England Journal of Medicine* reported that 71 percent of Los Angeles children and adolescents injured in drive-by shootings "were documented members of violent street gangs." And University of North Carolina-Charlotte criminal justice scholars Richard Lumb and Paul C. Friday report that 71 percent of adult gunshot wound victims in Charlotte have criminal records.

As the English gun control analyst Colin Greenwood has noted, in any society there are always enough guns available, legally or illegally, to arm the violent. The true determinant of violence is the number of violent people, not the availability of a particular weapon. Guns contribute to murder in the trivial sense that they help violent people kill. But owning guns does not turn responsible, law-abiding people into killers. If the general availability of guns were as important a factor in violence as the CDC implies, the vast increase in firearm ownership during the past two decades should have led to a vast increase in homicide. The CDC suggested just that in a 1989 report to Congress, where it asserted that "[s]ince the early 1970s the year-to-year fluctuations in firearm availability has [sic] paralleled the numbers of homicides."

But this correlation was a fabrication: While the number of handguns rose 69 percent from 1974 to 1988, handgun murders actually dropped by 27 percent. Moreover, as U.S. handgun ownership more than doubled from the early 1970s through the 1990s, homicides held constant or declined for every major population group except young urban black men. The CDC can blame the homicide surge in this group on guns only by ignoring a crucial point: Gun ownership is far less common among urban blacks than among whites or rural blacks.

The CDC's reports and studies never give long-term trend data linking gun sales to murder rates, citing only carefully selected partial or short-term correlations. If murder went down in the first and second years, then back up in the third and fourth years, only the rise is mentioned. CDC publications focus on fluctuations and other unrepresentative phenomena to exaggerate the incidence of gun deaths and to conceal declines. Thus, in its *Advance Data from Vital and Health Statistics* (1994), the CDC melodramatically announces that gun deaths now "rival" driving fatalities, as if gun murders were increasing. But this trend simply reflects the fact that driving fatalities are declining more rapidly than murders.

While the CDC shows a selective interest in homicide trends, it tends to ignore trends in accidental gun deaths— with good reason. In the 25 years from 1968 to 1992, American gun ownership increased almost 135 percent (from 97 million to 222 million), with handgun ownership rising more than 300 percent. These huge increases coincided with a two-thirds *decline* in accidental gun fatalities. The CDC and the researchers it funds do not like to talk about this dramatic development, since it flies in the face of the assumption that more guns mean more deaths. They are especially reluctant to acknowledge the drop in accidental gun deaths because of the two most plausible explanations for it: the replacement of rifles and shotguns with the much safer handgun as the main weapon kept loaded for self-defense, and the NRA's impressive efforts in gun safety training.

\* \* \*

The question is, why hasn't it been studied? The answer illustrates how the CDC's political agenda undermines its professed concern for saving lives. In the absence of an anti-gun animus, a two-thirds decrease in accidental gun deaths would surely have been a magnet for studies, especially since it coincided with a big increase in handgun ownership. But the CDC wants to reduce gun deaths only by banning guns, not by promoting solutions that are consistent with more guns. So the absence of studies is an excuse to dismiss gun safety training rather than an incentive for research.

Taken by itself, any one of these flaws —omission of relevant evidence, misrepresentation of studies, questionable methodology, overreaching conclusions —could be addressed by a determination to do better in the future. But the consistent tendency to twist research in favor of an anti-gun agenda suggests that there is something inherently wrong with the CDC's approach in this area. Implicit in the decision to treat gun deaths as a "public health" problem is the notion that violence is a communicable disease that can be controlled by attacking the relevant pathogen.

Dr. Katherine Christoffel, head of the Handgun Epidemic Lowering Plan, a group that has received CDC support, stated this assumption plainly in a 1994 interview with *American Medical News:* "Guns are a virus that must be eradicated.... They are causing an epidemic of death by gunshot, which should be treated like any epidemic—you get rid of the virus.... Get rid of the guns, get rid of the bullets, and you get rid of the deaths."

In the same article, the CDC's Rosenberg said approvingly, "Kathy Christoffel is saying about firearms injuries what has been said for years about AIDS: that we can no longer be silent. That silence equals death and she's not willing to be silent anymore. She's asking for help." Similarly, in a 1993 *Atlanta Medicine* article on the public health approach to violence, Arthur Kellermann subtitled part of his discussion "The Bullet as Pathogen."

It is hardly surprising that research based on this paradigm would tend to indict gun ownership as a cause of death. The inadequacy of the disease metaphor, which some public health specialists seem to take quite literally, is readily apparent when we consider Koch's postulates, the criteria by which suspected pathogens are supposed to be judged: 1) The microorganism must be observed in all cases of the disease; 2) the microorganism must be isolated and grown in a pure culture medium; 3) microorganisms from the pure culture must reproduce the disease when inoculated in a test animal; and 4) the same kind of microorganism must be recovered from the experimentally diseased animal. A strict application of these criteria is clearly impossible in this case. But applying the postulates as an analogy, we can ask about the consistency of the relationship between guns and violence. Gun ownership usually does not result in violence, and violence frequently occurs in the absence of guns. Given these basic facts, depicting violence as a disease caused by the gun virus can only cloud our thinking.

It may also discredit the legitimate functions of public health. "The CDC has got to be careful that we don't get into social issues," Dr. C.J. Peters, head of the CDC's Special Pathogens Branch, told the *Pittsburgh Post-Gazette* last year, in the midst of the controversy over taxpayer-funded gun research. "If we're going to do that, we ought to start a center for social change. We should stay with medical issues."

If treating gun violence as a public health issue invites confusion and controversy, why is this approach so popular? The main function of the disease metaphor is to lend a patina of scientific credibility to the belief that guns cause violence—a belief that is hard to justify on empirical grounds. "We're trying to depoliticize the subject," Rosenberg told *USA Today* in 1995. "We're trying to transform it from politics to science." What they are actually trying to do is disguise politics as science.

# POSTSCRIPT

## Is Gun Control a Public Health Issue?

Between 1960 and 1970 both the murder rate in the United States and the rate of handgun ownership doubled. Was it coincidence that violence and gun ownership grew at nearly the same pace? Can it be assumed from this fact that more guns cause more violence? The conventional wisdom is that guns and violence are related in the same sense that owning a gun increases the risk that the *gun owner*, rather than the criminal, will be hurt.

In several major studies, Dr. Arthur Kellermann attempted to prove just that. In 1986 he published "Protection or Peril? An Analysis of Firearm-Related Deaths in the Home," *The New England Journal of Medicine* (vol. 314). His other publications on guns as a public health issue include "Validating Survey Responses to Questions About Gun Ownership Among Owners of Registered Handguns," *American Journal of Epidemiology* (vol. 131, 1990); "Men, Women, and Murder: Gender-Specific Differences in Rates of Fatal Violence and Victimization," *Journal of Trauma* (vol. 33, 1992); "Suicide in the Home in Relation to Gun Ownership," *The New England Journal of Medicine* (vol. 327, 1992); and "Gun Ownership as a Risk Factor for Homicide in the Home," *The New England Journal of Medicine* (vol. 329, 1993). Kellermann, quoted in "Should You Own a Gun?" *U.S. News and World Report* (August 15, 1994), says, "Most gun homicides occur in altercations among family members, friends or acquaintances. In a heated dispute, few carefully weigh the legal consequences of their actions. They are too busy reaching for a weapon. If it's a gun, death is more likely to result." Kellermann and his colleagues are not the only physicians who consider homicide and gun ownership public health issues. In *Mother Jones* (May/June 1993), Mark Rosenberg, an epidemiologist at the Centers for Disease Control, maintains that violence is a public health issue and that violence prevention should be pushed to the top of the public health agenda.

Is violence really a *health* issue? Each year, more than 500,000 Americans, including children, are brought to hospital emergency rooms for treatment of a violent injury. These injuries, including shootings and assaults, add over $5 billion dollars in direct medical costs to current health care expenditures. Lifetime costs of violent injuries, which include medical care and loss of productivity, is over $45 billion. And since many gunshot victims are uninsured, the public at large pays the bill. Gunshot wounds can also strain the health care system by diverting resources away from other illnesses and injuries.

Articles on the relationship between guns and public health include "Loaded Guns in the Home," *Journal of the American Medical Association* (June 10, 1992); "Handgun Control, M.D.," *Weekly Standard* (April 15, 1996); "Gun

Violence Remains a Public Health Risk That's Still Hard to Track," *Nation's Health* (November 1996); "Gun Availability and Violent Death," *American Journal of Public Health* (June 1997); and "Private Arsenals and Public Peril," *The New England Journal of Medicine* (May 7, 1998).

Doctors who treat gunshot victims may feel that controlling gun ownership will reduce the number of shootings, but there is opposition to controlling the sale or possession of guns in the United States. Despite this opposition, a majority of gun owners and the general public favor stricter gun controls, including safety classes for gun owners. Only 39 percent of the American public backs a total ban on handguns, according to an article in *USA Today* (December 17, 1993). And although gun control may save some lives, the availability of guns can never be truly stemmed. In "The False Promise of Gun Control," *The Atlantic Monthly* (March 1994), law professor Daniel Polsby argues that gun control also diverts attention away from the roots of the crime problem in America: lack of job opportunities, inadequate education, and the breakdown of families. Polsby compares gun control with Prohibition. Jacob Sullum, senior editor of *Reason*, presents evidence that crime rates increase in countries that do not recognize a right to carry a weapon in "Gun Shy," *Reason* (April 1998). However, an article in *Health Letter on the CDC* (May 4, 1998) reports on the results of the Centers for Disease Control's study on firearm death rates among 36 nations. This study shows that the highest rate of gun-related death occurs in the United States.

Overviews of the gun control issue include "Gun Control: Will It Help Reduce Violent Crime in the US?" *CQ Researcher* (June 10, 1994); *The Mounting Threat of Home Intruders: Weighing the Moral Option of Armed Self-Defense* (Charles C. Thomas Publishers, 1993); "Guns and Poses," *The New Republic* (October 11, 1993); "Struggling Against Common Sense: The Pluses and Minuses of Gun Control," *The World & I* (February 1997); and "Still Under the Gun," *Time* (July 6, 1998).

# ISSUE 5

## Should Human Cloning Ever Be Permitted?

**YES: John A. Robertson,** from "Human Cloning and the Challenge of Regulation," *The New England Journal of Medicine* (July 9, 1998)

**NO: George J. Annas,** from "Why We Should Ban Human Cloning," *The New England Journal of Medicine* (July 9, 1998)

### ISSUE SUMMARY

**YES:** Attorney John A. Robertson contends there are many benefits to cloning and that a ban on privately funded cloning research is unjustified.

**NO:** Attorney and medical ethicist George J. Annas argues that cloning devalues people by depriving them of their uniqueness.

The idea that humans may someday be cloned (created from a cell without sexual reproduction) is now closer to reality. In 1996 a Scottish veterinarian named Ian Wilmut was able to produce a sheep by transferring the nucleus of an adult sheep mammary cell into a sheep egg from which the nucleus had been removed. The sheep was named "Dolly," and it possessed the genetic material of only one parent. This experiment increased the prospect of the creation of a new individual genetically identical to an existing or previously living person. Interest in cloning following the birth of Dolly escalated when Richard Seed, a physicist, announced that he would clone humans for a fee. Fear that unregulated cloning of humans would begin before anyone had the chance to evaluate the implications of this new technology sent Congress into action. Legislation to ban cloning was introduced to both houses of Congress. The Bond-Frist bill in the Senate and the Ehlers bill in the House were designed to prohibit or delay cloning indefinitely. This was the first time Congress introduced legislation to stop a single type of medical or scientific research, despite the fact that many medical groups and scientists were opposed to the ban. These bills are currently being reviewed. In addition, some states are now contemplating legislative action of their own. In 1997 Florida considered a law that would have barred the cloning of human DNA, a routine procedure in biomedical research. As of early 1998, 19 European nations have signed a treaty banning cloning.

While most people are comfortable with a moritorium on cloning to allow the implications to be studied, the congressional bills would go beyond restricting the cloning of humans. These bills would end research into what is known as somatic-cell nuclear-transfer technology. This technology involves transferring a human nucleus into a human egg that has had its nucleus removed. Research in this area is believed by some to be instrumental in disease and organ transplantation management. A compromise bill was introduced by Senators Edward Kennedy (D-Massachusetts) and Dianne Feinstein (D-California). This bill would ban the implantation of an embryo developed by the technology into a human uterus in order to create a child but would protect research to clone molecules, cells, and tissues.

Cloning-related research has already been accomplished using laboratory animals. Scientists have simulated models of human disease in cells from mouse embryos and placed these cells into recipient embryos. Some argue that the resulting offspring are valuable tools for studying the roles that genes play in disease. Similar reseach may yield other benefits, including information about the causes of cancer or the mechanics of aging. It is asserted that cloning could also be a source of material for the transplantation of human tissue. The treatment of diseases, such as diabetes or leukemia, and of genetic disorders may significantly improve with the availability of healthy, cloned cells. These cells would less likely be rejected by the body as foreign. Cloning may also help couples who carry genes for serious disorders to have healthy children. Although these benefits are theoretically possible, much research is still needed. A ban on research would not allow us to understand the full benefits of cloning.

Currently, some critics argue that it is immoral to experiment on human embryonic cells. The arguments against this technology are similar to those against abortion. Cloned organs would probably have to develop within human fetuses, which would be aborted when the organs are ready to be harvested. However, many people feel that a fetus is a viable life with rights that need to be protected. It has also been contended that cloning could create serious potential abuses, such as the destruction of embryos and the creation of master races.

In the following selections, John A. Robertson argues that there are many potential benefits of cloning and that the research should only be regulated, not banned. George J. Annas counters that cloning humans would devalue them and deprive them of their uniqueness.

# YES
## John A. Robertson

# HUMAN CLONING AND THE CHALLENGE OF REGULATION

The birth of Dolly, the sheep cloned from a mammary cell of an adult ewe, has initiated a public debate about human cloning. Although cloning of humans may never be clinically feasible, discussion of the ethical, legal, and social issues raised is important. Cloning is just one of several techniques potentially available to select, control, or alter the genome of offspring.[1-3] The development of such technology poses an important social challenge: how to ensure that the technology is used to enhance, rather than limit, individual freedom and welfare.

A key ethical question is whether a responsible couple, interested in rearing healthy offspring biologically related to them, might ethically choose to use cloning (or other genetic-selection techniques) for that purpose. The answer should take into account the benefits sought through the use of the techniques and any potential harm to offspring or to other interests.

The most likely uses of cloning would be far removed from the bizarre or horrific scenarios that initially dominated media coverage.[4] Theoretically, cloning would enable rich or powerful persons to clone themselves several times over, and commercial entrepreneurs might hire women to bear clones of sports or entertainment celebrities to be sold to others to rear. But current reproductive techniques can also be abused, and existing laws against selling children would apply to those created by cloning.

There is no reason to think that the ability to clone humans will cause many people to turn to cloning when other methods of reproduction would enable them to have healthy children. Cloning a human being by somatic-cell nuclear transfer, for example, would require a consenting person as a source of DNA, eggs to be enucleated and then fused with the DNA, a woman who would carry and deliver the child, and a person or couple to raise the child. Given this reality, cloning is most likely to be sought by couples who, because of infertility, a high risk of severe genetic disease, or other factors, cannot or do not wish to conceive a child.

Several plausible scenarios can be imagined. Rather than use sperm, egg, or embryo from anonymous donors, couples who are infertile as a result

From John A. Robertson, "Human Cloning and the Challenge of Regulation," *The New England Journal of Medicine*, vol. 339, no. 2 (July 9, 1998), pp. 119–122. Copyright © 1998 by The Massachusetts Medical Society. Reprinted by permission.

of gametic insufficiency might choose to clone one of the partners. If the husband were the source of the DNA and the wife provided the egg that received the nuclear transfer and then gestated the fetus, they would have a child biologically related to each of them and would not need to rely on anonymous gamete or embryo donation. Of course, many infertile couples might still prefer gamete or embryo donation or adoption. But there is nothing inherently wrong in wishing to be biologically related to one's children, even when this goal cannot be achieved through sexual reproduction.

A second plausible application would be for a couple at high risk of having offspring with a genetic disease.[5] Couples in this situation must now choose whether to risk the birth of an affected child, to undergo prenatal preimplantation diagnosis and abortion or the discarding of embryos, to accept gamete donation, to seek adoption, or to remain childless. If cloning were available, however, some couples, in line with prevailing concepts of kinship, family, and parenting, might strongly prefer to clone one of themselves or another family member. Alternatively, if they already had a healthy child, they might choose to use cloning to create a later-born twin of that child. In the more distant future, it is even possible that the child whose DNA was replicated would not have been born healthy but would have been made healthy by gene therapy after birth.

A third application relates to obtaining tissue or organs for transplantation. A child who needed an organ or tissue transplant might lack a medically suitable donor. Couples in this situation have sometimes conceived a child coitally in the hope that he or she would have the correct tissue type to serve, for example, as a bone marrow donor for an older sibling.[6,7] If the child's disease was not genetic, a couple might prefer to clone the affected child to be sure that the tissue would match.

It might eventually be possible to procure suitable tissue or organs by cloning the source DNA only to the point at which stem cells or other material might be obtained for transplantation, thus avoiding the need to bring a child into the world for the sake of obtaining tissue.[8] Cloning a person's cells up to the embryo stage might provide a source of stem cells or tissue for the person cloned. Cloning might also be used to enable a couple to clone a dead or dying child so as to have that child live on in some closely related form, to obtain sufficient numbers of embryos for transfer and pregnancy, or to eliminate mitochondrial disease.[5]

Most, if not all, of the potential uses of cloning are controversial, usually because of the explicit copying of the genome. As the National Bioethics Advisory Commission noted, in addition to concern about physical safety and eugenics, somatic-cell cloning raises issues of the individuality, autonomy, objectification, and kinship of the resulting children.[5] In other instances, such as the production of embryos to serve as tissue banks, the ethical issue is the sacrifice of embryos created solely for that purpose.

Given the wide leeway now granted couples to use assisted reproduction and prenatal genetic selection in forming families, cloning should not be rejected in all circumstances as unethical or illegitimate. The manipulation of embryos and the use of gamete donors and surrogates are increasingly common. Most fetuses conceived in the United States and Western Europe are now screened for genetic or chromosomal anomalies. Before conception, screening to identify carriers of genetic diseases is widespread.[9] Such practices also deviate from conventional notions of reproduction, kinship, and medical treatment of infertility, yet they are widely accepted.

Despite the similarity of cloning to current practices, however, the dissimilarities should not be overlooked. The aim of most other forms of assisted reproduction is the birth of a child who is a descendant of at least one member of the couple, not an identical twin. Most genetic selection acts negatively to identify and screen out unwanted traits such as genetic disease, not positively to choose or replicate the genome as in somatic-cell cloning.[3] It is not clear, however, why a child's relation to his or her rearing parents must always be that of sexually reproduced descendant when such a relationship is not possible because of infertility or other factors. Indeed, in gamete donation and adoption, although sexual reproduction is involved, a full descendant relation between the child and both rearing parents is lacking. Nor should the difference between negative and positive means of selecting children determine the ethical or social acceptability of cloning or other techniques. In both situations, a deliberate choice is made so that a child is born with one genome rather than another or is not born at all.

Is cloning sufficiently similar to current assisted-reproduction and genetic-selection practices to be treated similarly as a presumptively protected exercise of family or reproductive liberty?[10] Couples who request cloning in the situations I have described are seeking to rear healthy children with whom they will have a genetic or biologic tie, just as couples who conceive their children sexually do. Whether described as "replication" or as "reproduction," the resort to cloning is similar enough in purpose and effects to other reproduction and genetic-selection practices that it should be treated similarly. Therefore, a couple should be free to choose cloning unless there are compelling reasons for thinking that this would create harm that the other procedures would not cause.[10]

The concern of the National Bioethics Advisory Commission about the welfare of the clone reflects two types of fear. The first is that a child with the same nuclear DNA as another person, who is thus that person's later-born identical twin, will be so severely harmed by the identity of nuclear DNA between them that it is morally preferable, if not obligatory, that the child not be born at all.[5] In this case the fear is that the later-born twin will lack individuality or the freedom to create his or her own identity because of confusion or expectations caused by having the same DNA as another person.[5,11]

This claim does not withstand the close scrutiny that should precede interference with a couple's freedom to bear and rear biologically related children.[10] Having the same genome as another person is not in itself harmful, as widespread experience with monozygotic twins shows. Being a twin does not deny either twin his or her individuality or freedom, and twins often have a special intimacy or closeness that few non-twin siblings can experience.[12] There is no reason to think that being a later-born identical twin resulting from cloning would change the overall assessment of being a twin.

Differences in mitochondria and the uterine and childhood environment will undercut problems of similarity and minimize the risk of overidentification with the first twin. A clone of Smith may look like Smith, but he or she will not be Smith and will lack many of Smith's phenotypic characteristics. The effects of having similar DNA will also depend on the length of time before the second twin is born, on whether the twins are raised together, on whether they are informed that they are genetic twins, on whether other people are so informed, on the beliefs that the rearing parents have about genetic influence on behavior, and on other factors. Having a previously born twin might in some circumstances also prove to be a source of support or intimacy for the later-born child.

The risk that parents or the child will overly identify the child with the DNA source also seems surmountable. Would the child invariably be expected to match the phenotypic characteristics of the DNA source, thus denying the second twin an "open future" and the freedom to develop his or her own identity?[5,11,13] In response to this question, one must ask whether couples who choose to clone offspring are more likely to want a child who is a mere replica of the DNA source or a child who is unique and valued for more than his or her genes. Couples may use cloning in order to ensure that the biologic child they rear is healthy, to maintain a family connection in the face of gametic infertility, or to obtain matched tissue for transplantation and yet still be responsibly committed to the welfare of their child, including his or her separate identity and interests and right to develop as he or she chooses.

The second type of fear is that parents who choose their child's genome through somatic-cell cloning will view the child as a commodity or an object to serve their own ends.[5] We do not view children born through coital or assisted reproduction as "mere means" just because people reproduce in order to have company in old age, to fulfill what they see as God's will, to prove their virility, to have heirs, to save a relationship, or to serve other selfish purposes.[14] What counts is how a child is treated after birth. Self-interested motives for having children do not prevent parents from loving children for themselves once they are born.

The use of cloning to form families in the situations I have described, though closely related to current assisted-reproduction and genetic-selection practices, does offer unique variations. The novelty of the relation—cloning in lieu of sperm donation, for example, produces a later-born identical twin raised by the older twin and his spouse—will create special psychological and social challenges. Can these challenges be successfully met, so that cloning produces net good for families and society? Given the largely positive experience with assisted-reproduction techniques that initially appeared frightening, cautious optimism is justified. We should be able to develop procedures and guidelines for cloning that will allow us to obtain its benefits while minimizing its problems and dangers.

In the light of these considerations, I would argue that a ban on privately funded cloning research is unjustified and likely to hamper important types of research.[8] A permanent ban on the cloning of human beings, as advocated by the Council of Europe and proposed in Congress, is also unjustified.[15,16] A more limited ban—whether for 5 years, as proposed by the National Bioethics Advisory Commission and enacted in California, or for 10 years, as in the bill of Senator Dianne Feinstein (D-Calif.) and Senator Edward M. Kennedy (D-Mass.) that is now before Congress—is also open to question.[5,17,18] Given the early state of cloning science and the widely shared view that the transfer of cloned embryos to the uterus before the safety and efficacy of the procedure has been established is unethical, few responsible physicians are likely to offer human cloning in the near future.[5] Nor are profit-motivated entrepreneurs, such as Richard Seed, likely to have many customers for their cloning services until the safety of the procedure is demonstrated.[19] A ban on human cloning for a limited period would thus serve largely symbolic purposes. Symbolic legislation, however, often has substantial costs.[20,21] A government-imposed prohibition on privately funded cloning, even for a limited period, should not be enacted unless there is a compelling need. Such a need has not been demonstrated.

Rather than seek to prohibit all uses of human cloning, we should focus our attention on ensuring that cloning is done well. No physician or couple should embark on cloning without careful thought about the novel relational issues and child-rearing responsibilities that will ensue. We need regulations or guidelines to ensure safety and efficacy, fully informed consent and counseling for the couple, the consent of any person who may provide DNA, guarantees of parental rights and duties, and a limit on the number of clones from any single source.[10] It may also be important to restrict cloning to situations where there is a strong likelihood that the couple or individual initiating the procedure will also rear the resulting child. This principle will encourage a stable parenting situation and minimize the chance that cloning entrepreneurs will create clones to be sold to others.[22] As our experience grows, some restrictions on who may serve as a source of DNA

for cloning (for example, a ban on cloning one's parents) may also be defensible.[10]

Cloning is important because it is the first of several positive means of genetic selection that may be sought by families seeking to have and rear healthy, biologically related offspring. In the future, mitochondrial transplantation, germ-line gene therapy, genetic enhancement, and other forms of prenatal genetic alteration may be possible.[3,23,24] With each new technique, as with cloning, the key question will be whether it serves important health, reproductive, or family needs and whether its benefits outweigh any likely harm. Cloning illustrates the principle that when legitimate uses of a technique are likely, regulatory policy should avoid prohibition and focus on ensuring that the technique is used responsibly for the good of those directly involved. As genetic knowledge continues to grow, the challenge of regulation will occupy us for some time to come.

## REFERENCES

1. Silver LM. Remaking Eden: cloning and beyond in a brave new world. New York: Avon Books, 1997.
2. Walters L, Palmer JG. The ethics of human gene therapy. New York: Oxford University Press, 1997.
3. Robertson JA. Genetic selection of offspring characteristics. Boston Univ Law Rev 1996; 76:421–82.
4. Begley S. Can we clone humans? Newsweek. March 10, 1997:53–60.
5. Cloning human beings: report and recommendations of the National Bioethics Advisory Commission. Rockville, Md.: National Bioethics Advisory Commission, June 1997.
6. Robertson JA. Children of choice: freedom and the new reproductive technologies. Princeton, N.J.: Princeton University Press. 1994.
7. Kearney W, Caplan AL. Parity for the donation of bone marrow: ethical and policy considerations. In: Blank RH, Bonnicksen Al, eds. Emerging issues in biomedical policy: an annual review.

Vol. 1. New York: Columbia University Press, 1992:262–85.

8. Kassirer JP, Rosenthal NA. Should human cloning research be off limits? N Engl J Med 1998; 338:905–6.

9. Holtzman NA. Proceed with caution: predicting genetic risks in the recombinant DNA era. Baltimore: Johns Hopkins University Press, 1989.

10. Robertson JA. Liberty, identity, and human cloning. Texas Law Rev 1998;77:1371–456.

11. Davis DS. What's wrong with cloning? Jurimetrics 1997;38:83–9.

12. Segal NL. Behavioral aspects of intergenerational human cloning: what twins tell us. Jurimetrics 1997;38:57–68.

13. Jonas H. Philosophical essays: from ancient creed to technological man. Englewood Cliffs, N.J.: Prentice-Hall, 1974:161.

14. Heyd D. Genethics: moral issues in the creation of people. Berkeley: University of California Press, 1992.

15. Council of Europe. Draft additional protocol to the Convention on Human Rights and Biomedicine on the prohibition of cloning human beings with explanatory report and Parliamentary Assembly opinion (adopted September 22, 1997). XXXVI International Legal Materials 1415 (1997).

16. Human Cloning Prohibition Act, H.R. 923, S.1601 (March 5, 1997).

17. Act of Oct. 4, 1997, ch. 688, 1997 Cal. Legis. Serv. 3790 (West, WESTLAW through 1997 Sess.).

18. Prohibition on Cloning of Human Beings Act, S.1602, 105th Cong. (1998).

19. Stolberg SG. A small spark ignites debate on laws on cloning humans. New York Times, January 19, 1998:A1.

20. Gusfield J. Symbolic crusade: status politics and the American temperance movement. Urbana: University of Illinois Press, 1963.

21. Wolf SM. Ban cloning? Why NBAC is wrong. Hastings Cent Rep 1997;27(5):12.

22. Wilson JG. The paradox of cloning. The Weekly Standard. May 26, 1997:23–7.

23. Zhang J, Grifo J, Blaszczyk A, et al. In vitro maturation of human preovulatory oocytes recontrructed by germinal visicle transfer. Fertil Steril 1997;68:Suppl:S1. abstract.

24. Bonnicksen AL. Transplanting nuclei between human eggs: implications for germ-line genetics. Politics and the Life Sciences. March 1998:3–10.

# NO
George J. Annas

## WHY WE SHOULD BAN
## HUMAN CLONING

In February the U.S. Senate voted 54 to 42 against bringing an anticloning bill directly to the floor for a vote.[1] During the debate, more than 16 scientific and medical organizations, including the American Society of Reproductive Medicine and the Federation of American Societies for Experimental Biology, and 27 Nobel prize-winning scientists, agreed that there should be a moratorium on the creation of a human being by somatic nuclear transplants. What the groups objected to was legislation that went beyond this prohibition to include cloning human cells, genes, and tissues. An alternative proposal was introduced by Senator Edward M. Kennedy (D-Mass.) and Senator Dianne Feinstein (D-Calif.) and modeled on a 1997 proposal by President Bill Clinton and his National Bioethics Advisory Commission. It would, in line with the views of all of these scientific groups, outlaw attempts to produce a child but permit all other forms of cloning research.[2,3] Because the issue is intimately involved with research with embryos and abortion politics, in many ways the congressional debates over human cloning are a replay of past debates on fetal-tissue transplants[4] and research using human embryos.[5] Nonetheless, the virtually unanimous scientific consensus on the advisability of a legislative ban or voluntary moratorium on the attempt to create a human child by cloning justifies deeper discussion of the issue than it has received so far.

It has been more than a year since embryologist Ian Wilmut and his colleagues announced to the world that they had cloned a sheep.[6] No one has yet duplicated their work, raising serious questions about whether Dolly the sheep was cloned from a stem cell or a fetal cell, rather than a fully differentiated cell.[7] For my purposes, the success or failure of Wilmut's experiment is not the issue. Public attention to somatic-cell nuclear cloning presents an opportunity to consider the broader issues of public regulation of human research and the meaning of human reproduction.

### CLONING AND IMAGINATION

In the 1970s, human cloning was a centerpiece issue in bioethical debates in the United States.[8,9] In 1978, a House committee held a hearing on human cloning in response to the publication of David Rorvik's *In His Image: The Cloning of a Man*.[10] All the scientists who testified assured the committee that the supposed account of the cloning of a human being was fictional and that the techniques described in the book could not work. The chief point the scientists wanted to make, however, was that they did not want any laws enacted that might affect their research. In the words of one, "There is no need for any form of regulation, and it could only in the long run have a harmful effect."[11] The book was an elaborate fable, but it presented a valuable opportunity to discuss the ethical implications of cloning. The failure to see it as a fable was a failure of imagination. We normally do not look to novels for scientific knowledge, but they provide more: insights into life itself.[12]

This failure of imagination has been witnessed repeatedly, most recently in 1997, when President Clinton asked the National Bioethics Advisory Commission to make recommendations about human cloning. Although acknowledging in their report that human cloning has always seemed the stuff of science fiction rather than science, the group did not commission any background papers on how fiction informs the debate. Even a cursory reading of books like Aldous Huxley's *Brave New World*, Ira Levin's *The Boys from Brazil*, and Fay Weldon's *The Cloning of Joanna May*, for example, would have saved much time and needless debate. Literary treatments of cloning inform us that cloning is an evolutionary dead end that can only replicate what already exists but cannot improve it; that exact replication of a human is not possible; that cloning is not inherently about infertile couples or twins, but about a

technique that can produce an indefinite number of genetic duplicates; that clones must be accorded the same human rights as persons that we grant any other human; and that personal identity, human dignity, and parental responsibility are at the core of the debate about human cloning.

We might also have gained a better appreciation of our responsibilities to our children had we examined fiction more closely. The reporter who described Wilmut as "Dolly's laboratory father,"[13] for example, probably could not have done a better job of conjuring up images of Mary Shelley's *Frankenstein* if he had tried. Frankenstein was also his creature's father and god; the creature told him, "I ought to be thy Adam." As in the case of Dolly, the "spark of life" was infused into the creature by an electric current. Shelley's great novel explores virtually all the noncommercial elements of today's debate.

The naming of the world's first cloned mammal also has great significance. The sole survivor of 277 cloned embryos (or "fused couplets"), the clone could have been named after its sequence in this group (for example, C-137), but this would only have emphasized its character as a laboratory product. In stark contrast, the name Dolly (provided for the public and not used in the scientific report in *Nature*, in which she is identified as 6LL3) suggests a unique individual. Victor Frankenstein, of course, never named his creature, thereby repudiating any parental responsibility. The creature himself evolved into a monster when he was rejected not only by Frankenstein, but by society as well. Naming the world's first mammal clone Dolly was meant to distance her from the Frankenstein myth both by making her something she is not (a doll) and by accepting "parental" responsibility for her.

Unlike Shelley's world, the future envisioned in Huxley's *Brave New World*, in which all humans are created by cloning through embryo splitting and conditioned to join a specified worker group, was always unlikely. There are much more efficient ways of creating killers or terrorists (or even soldiers and workers) than through cloning. Physical and psychological conditioning can turn teenagers into terrorists in a matter of months, so there is no need to wait 18 to 20 years for the clones to grow up and be trained themselves. Cloning has no real military or paramilitary uses. Even clones of Adolf Hitler would have been very different people because they would have grown up in a radically altered world environment.

## CLONING AND REPRODUCTION

Even though virtually all scientists oppose it, a minority of free-marketers and bioethicists have suggested that there might nonetheless be some good reasons to clone a human. But virtually all these suggestions themselves expose the central problem of cloning: the devaluing of persons by depriving them of their uniqueness. One common example suggested is cloning a dying or recently deceased child if this is what the grieving parents want. A fictional cover story in the March 1998 issue of *Wired*, for example, tells the story of the world's first clone.[14] She is cloned from the DNA of a dead two-week-old infant, who died from a mitochondrial defect that is later "cured" by cloning with an enucleated donor egg. The closer one gets to the embryo stage, the more cloning a child looks like the much less problematic method of

cloning by "twinning" or embryo splitting. And proponents of cloning tend to want to "naturalize" and "normalize" asexual replication by arguing that it is just like having "natural" twins.

Embryo splitting might be justified if only a few embryos could be produced by an infertile couple and all were implanted at the same time (since this does not involve replicating an existing and known genome). But scenarios of cloning by nuclear transfer have involved older children, and the only reason to clone an existing human is to create a genetic replica. Using the bodies of children to replicate them encourages all of us to devalue children and treat them as interchangeable commodities. For example, thanks to cloning, the death of a child need no longer be a singular human tragedy but, rather, can be an opportunity to try to replicate the no longer priceless (or irreplaceable) dead child. No one should have such dominion over a child (even a dead or dying child) as to use his or her genes to create the child's child.

Cloning would also radically alter what it means to be human by replicating a living or dead human being asexually to produce a person with a single genetic parent. The danger is that through human cloning we will lose something vital to our humanity, the uniqueness (and therefore the value and dignity) of every human. Cloning represents the height of genetic reductionism and genetic determinism.

Population geneticist R. C. Lewontin has challenged my position that the first human clone would also be the first human with a single genetic parent by arguing that, instead, "a child by cloning has a full set of chromosomes like anyone else, half of which were derived from a mother and half from a father. It happens that these chromosomes were passed through another individual, the cloning donor, on the way to the child. That donor is certainly not the child's 'parent' in any biological sense, but simply an earlier offspring of the original parents."[15] Lewontin takes genetic reductionism to perhaps its logical extreme. People become no more than containers of their parents' genes, and their parents have the right to treat them not as individual human beings, but rather as human embryos—entities that can be split and replicated at their whim without any consideration of the child's choice or welfare. Children (even adult children), according to Lewontin's view, have no say in whether they are replicated or not, because it is their parents, not they, who are reproducing. This radical redefinition of reproduction and parenthood, and the denial of the choice to procreate or not, turns out to be an even stronger argument against cloning children than its biologic novelty. Of course, we could require the consent of adults to be cloned—but why should we, if they are not becoming parents?

Related human rights and human dignity would also prohibit using cloned children as organ sources for their father or mother original. Nor is there any constitutional right to be cloned in the United States that is triggered by marriage to someone with whom an adult cannot reproduce sexually, because there is no tradition of asexual replication and because permitting asexual replication is not necessary to safeguard any existing conception of ordered liberty (rights fundamental to ordered liberty are the rights the Supreme Court sees as essential to individual liberty in our society).

Although it is possible to imagine some scenarios in which cloning could be used for the treatment of infertility, the use of cloning simply provides parents another choice for choice's sake, not out of necessity. Moreover, in a fundamental sense, cloning cannot be a treatment for infertility. This replication technique changes the very concept of infertility itself, since all humans have somatic cells that could be used for asexual replication and therefore no one would be unable to replicate himself or herself asexually. In vitro fertilization, on the other hand, simply provides a technological way for otherwise infertile humans to reproduce sexually.

John Robertson argues that adults have a right to procreate in any way they can, and that the interests of the children cannot be taken into account because the resulting children cannot be harmed (since without cloning the children would not exist at all).[16] But this argument amounts to a tautology. It applies equally to everyone alive; none of us would exist had it not been for the precise and unpredictable time when the father's sperm and the mother's egg met. This biologic fact, however, does not justify a conclusion that our parents had no obligations to us as their future children. If it did, it would be equally acceptable, from the child's perspective, to be gestated in a great ape, or even a cow, or to be composed of a mixture of ape genes and human genes.

The primary reason for banning the cloning of living or dead humans was articulated by the philosopher Hans Jonas in the early 1970s. He correctly noted that it does not matter that creating an exact duplicate of an existing person is impossible. What matters is that the person is chosen to be cloned because of some characteristic or characteristics he or she possesses (which, it is hoped, would also be possessed by the genetic copy or clone). Jonas argued that cloning is always a crime against the clone, the crime of depriving the clone of his or her "existential right to certain subjective terms of being"—particularly, the "right to ignorance" of facts about his or her origin that are likely to be "paralyzing for the spontaneity of becoming himself" or herself.[17] This advance knowledge of what another has or has not accomplished with the clone's genome destroys the clone's "condition for authentic growth" in seeking to answer the fundamental question of all beings, "Who am I?" Jonas continues: "The ethical command here entering the enlarged stage of our powers is: never to violate the right to that ignorance which is a condition of authentic action; or: to respect the right of each human life to find its own way and be a surprise to itself."[17]

Jonas is correct. His rationale, of course, applies only to a "delayed genetic twin" or "serial twin" created from an existing human, not to genetically identical twins born at the same time, including those created by cloning with use of embryo splitting. Even if one does not agree with him, however, it is hypocritical to argue that a cloning technique that limits the liberty and choices of the resulting child or children can be justified on the grounds that cloning expands the liberty and choices of would-be cloners.[18]

## MORATORIUMS AND BANS ON HUMAN CLONING

Members of the National Bioethics Advisory Commission could not agree on much, but they did conclude that any current attempt to clone a human being should be prohibited by basic ethical principles that ban putting human subjects at substantial risk without their informed consent. But danger itself will not prevent scientists and physicians from performing first-of-their-kind experiments—from implanting a baboon's heart in a human baby to using a permanent artificial heart in an adult—and cloning techniques may be both safer and more efficient in the future. We must identify a mechanism that can both prevent premature experimentation and permit reasonable experimentation when the facts change.

The mechanism I favor is a broad-based regulatory agency to oversee human experimentation in the areas of genetic engineering, research with human embryos, xenografts, artificial organs, and other potentially dangerous boundary-crossing experiments.[19] Any such national regulatory agency must be composed almost exclusively of nonresearchers and nonphysicians so it can reflect public values, not parochial concerns. Currently, the operative American ethic seems to be that if any possible case can be imagined in which a new technology might be useful, it should not be prohibited, no matter what harm might result. One of the most important procedural steps Congress should take in setting up a federal agency to regulate human experimentation would be to put the burden of proof on those who propose to undertake novel experiments (including cloning) that risk harm and call deeply held social values into question.

This shift in the burden of proof is critical if society is to have an influence over science.[20] Without it, social control is not possible. This model applies the precautionary principle of international environmental law to cloning and other potentially harmful biomedical experiments involving humans. The principle requires governments to protect the public health and the environment from realistic threats of irreversible harm or catastrophic consequences even in the absence of clear evidence of harm.[21] Under this principle, proponents of human cloning would have the burden of proving that there was some compelling contravailing need to benefit either current or future generations before such an experiment was permitted (for example, if the entire species were to become sterile). Thus, regulators would not have the burden of proving that there was some compelling reason not to approve it. This regulatory scheme would depend on at least a de facto, if not a de jure, ban or moratorium on such experiments and a mechanism such as my proposed regulatory agency that could lift the ban. The suggestion that the Food and Drug Administration (FDA) can substitute for such an agency is fanciful. The FDA has no jurisdiction over either the practice of medicine or human replication and is far too narrowly constituted to represent the public in this area. Some see human cloning as inevitable and uncontrollable.[22,23] Control will be difficult, and it will ultimately require close international cooperation. But this is no reason not to try—any more than a recognition that controlling terrorism or biologic weapons is difficult and uncertain justifies making no attempt at control.

On the recommendation of the National Bioethics Advisory Commission, the White House sent proposed anticloning legislation to Congress in June 1997. The Clinton proposal receded into obscurity until early 1998, when a Chicago physicist, Richard Seed, made national news by announcing that he intended to raise funds to clone a human. Because Seed acted like a prototypical "mad scientist," his proposal was greeted with almost universal condemnation.[24] Like the 1978 Rorvik hoax, however, it provided another opportunity for public discussion of cloning and prompted a more refined version of the Clinton proposal: the Feinstein–Kennedy bill. We can (and should) take advantage of this opportunity to distinguish the cloning of cells and tissues from the cloning of human beings by somatic nuclear transplantation[25] and to permit the former while prohibiting the latter. We should also take the opportunity to fill in the regulatory lacuna that permits any individual scientist to act first and consider the human consequences later, and we should use the controversy over cloning as an opportunity to begin an international dialogue on human experimentation.

## REFERENCES

1. U.S. Senate. 144 Cong. Rec. S561–S580, S607–S608 (1998).
2. S.1611 (Feinstein–Kennedy Prohibition on Cloning of Human Beings Act of 1998).
3. Cloning human beings: report and recommendations of the National Bioethics Advisory Commission. Rockville, Md.: National Bioethics Advisory Commission, June, 1997.
4. Annas GJ, Elias S. The politics of transplantation of human fetal tissue. N Engl J Med 1989; 320:1079–82.
5. Annas GJ, Caplan A, Elias S. The politics of human embryo research—avoiding ethical gridlock. N Engl J Med 1996;334:1329–32.
6. Wilmut I, Schnieke AE, McWhir J, Kind AJ, Campbell KH. Viable offspring derived from fetal and adult mammalian cells. Nature 1997; 385:810–3.
7. Butler D. Dolly researcher plans further experiments after challenges. Nature 1998;391:825–6.
8. Lederberg J. Experimental genetics and human evolution. Am Naturalist 1996;100:519–31.
9. Watson JD. Moving toward the clonal man. Atlantic Monthly. May 1971:50–3.

10. Rorvik DM. In his image: the cloning of a man. Philadelphia: J.B. Lippincott, 1978.

11. Development in cell biology and genetics, cloning. Hearings before the Subcommittee on Health and the Environment of the Committee on Interstate and Foreign Commerce of the U.S. House of Representatives, 95th Congress, 2d Session, May 31, 1978.

12. Chomsky N. Language and problems of knowledge: the Managua lectures. Cambridge, Mass.: MIT Press, 1988.

13. Montalbano W. Cloned sheep is star, but not sole project, at institute. Los Angeles Times. February 25, 1997:A7.

14. Kadrey R. Carbon copy: meet the first human clone. Wired. March 1998:146–50.

15. Lewontin RC. Confusion over cloning. New York Review of Books. October 23, 1997:20–3.

16. Robertson JA. Children of choice: Freedom and the new reproductive technologies. Princeton, N.J.: Princeton University Press, 1994:169.

17. Jonas H. Philosophical essays: From ancient creed to technological man. Englewood Cliffs, N.J.: Prentice-Hall, 1974:162–3.

18. Annas GJ. Some choice: law, medicine and the market. New York: Oxford University Press, 1998:14–5.

19. Annas GJ. Regulatory models for human embryo cloning: the free market, professional guidelines, and government restrictions. Kennedy Inst Ethics J 1994;4:235–49.

20. Hearings before the U.S. Senate Subcommittee on Public Health and Safety, 105th Congress, 1st Session, March 12, 1997. (Or see: http://www-busph.bu.edu/depts/lw/clonetest.htm.)

21. Cross FD. Paradoxical perils of the precautionary principle. Washington Lee Law Rev 1996; 53:851–925.

22. Kolata GB. Clone: the road to Dolly, and the path ahead. New York: W. Morrow, 1998.

23. Silver LM. Remaking Eden: cloning and beyond in a brave new world. New York: Avon Books, 1997.

24. Knox RA. A Chicagoan plans to offer cloning of humans. Boston Globe. January 7, 1998:A3.

25. Kassirer JP, Rosenthal NA. Should human cloning research be off limits? N Engl J Med 1998; 338:905–6.

# POSTSCRIPT

## Should Human Cloning Ever Be Permitted?

Early in 1998 Senator Christopher Bond (R-Missouri) debated the issue of human cloning. He stated that "science has given us partial-birth abortions and Dr. Kevorkian's assisted suicide. We should say no to these scientific advances and no to the cloning of human embryos." Senator Bond, as well as other politicians and activists, are treating the issue of cloning as similar to the abortion issue. Some argue that cloning could result in the production of made-to-order humans and organ farming for money. The Bond-Frist bill and the Ehlers bill, recently submitted to Congress, call for a total ban on cloning and on research involving somatic-cell nuclear transfer. The monitoring required to enforce the ban could necessitate intruding into scientific labs and policing the intent of researchers. There are also concerns that the ban is to be imposed by Congress, not a scientific regulatory body. This brings cloning into a political rather than a scientific arena.

Are there ways to prevent potential abuses of cloning without banning all research involving somatic-cell nuclear transfer? Discussions about restricting research were held in the 1970s, when recombinant DNA technology was first introduced. Rather than ban this technology, scientists and representatives of the government and the public developed stringent voluntary standards and guidelines to regulate it. Since that time, the technology has yielded significant benefits in medicine and health. Although many scientists have announced a self-imposed five-year moritorium on the cloning of human beings, they have argued that research involving the use of somatic-cell nuclear transfer should continue. They state that this research could result in cures for cancer and other diseases and offer infertile couples another option to have a child. Articles that contain arguments in favor of continuing this research include "Fetal Positions," *Mother Jones* (May/June 1998); "Animal Cloning Technology Applied to Disease," *World Disease Weekly Plus* (May 11, 1998); "Should Human Cloning Research Be Off Limits?" *The New England Journal of Medicine* (March 26, 1998); and "The Case for Cloning," *Time* (February 9, 1998). In "Cooling Down Over Cloning," *Lancet* (January 17, 1998), the importance of carefully considered and informed decisions about cloning is discussed. In "Ban Cloning? Why the National Bioethics Advisory Commission Is Wrong," *Hastings Center Report* (September/October 1997), Susan Wolf states that the ban on cloning is unjustified, but she advocates strongly for regulation. E. V. Kontorovich, in "Asexual Revolution," *National Review* (March 9, 1998), asserts that even if cloning could actually improve human health, it should be rejected.

# *On the Internet . . .*

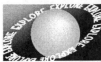

http://www.dushkin.com

## The StressFree Net Home Page
This is the StressFree Net home page and virtual offices for the StressFree Network. StressFree is a system of health care professionals providing solutions to stress. *http://www.stressfree.com*

## Kaplan Stress Management Links
This site offers dozens of links related to stress management under the headings Stress Management, Test Stress and Job Stress, Breathing Exercises, Yoga and Meditation, Other Stress-Busting Techniques, Fitness and Exercise, Diet and Nutrition Info., Stress Relief and Stress Test Games, and Anxiety and Panic. *http://www.kaplan.com/library/chill.html*

# PART 2

## Mind/Body Relationship

*Humans have long sought to extend life, eliminate disease, and prevent sickness. In modern times, people depend on technology to develop creative and innovative ways to improve health. However, as cures for diseases such as AIDS, cancer, and heart disease continue to elude scientists and doctors, many people question whether or not modern medicine has reached a plateau in improving health. As a result, over the last decade, an emphasis has been placed on prevention as a way to improve health. Managing stress is one way many individuals attempt to prevent and control illness, since many studies have linked stress with disease. The role of mind and body relationships is the key question regarding the issues debated in this section.*

■ Is Stress Responsible for Disease?

■ Can Spirituality Overcome Disease?

# ISSUE 6

## Is Stress Responsible for Disease?

**YES: Editors of *Harvard Health Letter*,** from "Can Stress Make You Sick?" *Harvard Health Letter* (April 1998)

**NO: Christopher Caldwell,** from "The Use and Abuse of Stress," *The Weekly Standard* (June 2, 1997)

### ISSUE SUMMARY

**YES:** The editors of the *Harvard Health Letter* maintain that there is evidence that individuals who are chronically stressed possess an increased risk of cancer and heart disease.

**NO:** Writer Christopher Caldwell argues that no one, including doctors, can come to an agreement on what stress is, so stress can not be blamed as the cause of disease.

In the 1930s Dr. Hans Selye, a stress researcher, asserted that the physical symptoms activated by stress can protect the body but can also cause disease and damage. Selye wrote that "it is immaterial whether the agent or situation we face is pleasant or unpleasant; all that counts is the intensity of the demand for adjustment and adaption." Stressful experiences include major life events such as divorce, trauma, or the birth of a child, and day-to-day events such as traffic jams, deadlines, or lost keys. The effects of chronic stress may be increased by drugs, a poor diet, and lack of exercise. Selye also described the response to stressors as a three-stage general adaptation syndrome. The three stages are alarm, resistance, and exhaustion. During the alarm stage the body's systems release the hormones cortisol and epinephrine, which enable the body to meet challenges caused by stress. In the resistance stage the body adapts to the challenge of stress by increasing strength and endurance. During the final stage, exhaustion, the body's psychological and physical energy is depleted and rest is necessary. If the body does not rest and the stress continues, illness may follow.

Several researchers have attempted to identify causes of stress, or specific factors that increase the liklihood of stress-related illness. In the early 1960s physicians Thomas Holmes and Richard Rahe developed a scale that identified certain stressful life events, both positive and negative. Individuals who scored high on the scale, the researchers determined, were more likely to become ill. In 1974 two California doctors, Meyer Friedman and Ray Rosenman, correlated people with hurried, hostile personalities to higher instances of stress-related heart disease. They maintained that people who have more easygoing and relaxed personalities are less likely to develop stress-related heart problems. A third stress theory, "psychological hardiness," was developed in the late 1970s. According to researcher Suzanne Kobasa, people who react positively to stress are less likely to develop illnesses since they possess psychological hardiness that helps them withstand the rigors of stress exposure. Kobasa defined hardiness as having a sense of challege when confronted with new events, a commitment to one's work, and a sense of control over one's environment, particularly the workplace.

Some argue that although an understanding of the causes of stress is important, understanding the physical and emotional harm that can result from exposure to stress is equally important. Assertions have been made that many physical symptoms such as high blood pressure, headaches, and irritable bowel syndrome have been linked to stress. Pregnant women exposed to severe stress may deliver a low-birth-weight or premature baby. Specific illnesses have also been linked to stress exposure. These include heart disease, certain cancers, and the common cold. Reported among the behavioral and emotional reactions to stress are anxiety, burnout, substance abuse, and nervousness.

People have always been exposed to stress. Early men and women faced physical stress daily in an effort to avoid dangerous animals, ensure enough food, and cope with harmful weather patterns. Modern humans experience different kinds of stressful events, such as job burnout, financial problems, and difficult interpersonal situations. It is argued that because modern life can be so hectic, it is easy to blame many illnesses and negative behaviors on stressful events.

To control stress, support groups, classes, and worksite health programs have been developed. These programs help individuals manage stress through a variety of methods, including relaxation techniques, meditation, and biofeedback. A technique called "stress inoculation training" consists of three phases: conceptualization, skill acquisition, and application and follow-through. Other programs teach time management to minimize the effects of stressful and debilitating deadlines. Some programs encourage exercise and nutritious eating to maintain a healthy body, which can better withstand stress. While many people have positive feelings about these programs and feel less stressed, the evidence linking stress management programs and disease reduction is not always clear. Is exposure to stress a legitimate concern that needs to be managed, or is it an inevitable part of life?

In the following articles, the editors of the *Harvard Health Letter* contend that emotions are tied to health. They also maintain that researchers who study stress and health conclude that many illnesses are related to problems with the body's reaction to stress. Writer Christopher Caldwell argues that stress is a part of life and that too many individuals claim that exposure to stress has made them sick.

# YES    Editors of *Harvard Health Letter*

## CAN STRESS MAKE YOU SICK?

Many people may recall reading newspaper accounts last year of a study which found that people with a wide variety of social ties were much less likely to catch colds than those who had limited contacts with friends, relatives, neighbors, and business associates.

The investigation, which was published in June 1997 in the Journal of the American Medical Association, revealed that a lack of diverse social contacts was a stronger risk factor for colds than smoking, low vitamin C intake, or elevated stress hormones.

The Carnegie Mellon University researchers who conducted the study say that interacting with a broad array of individuals likely tempers a person's physical response to stressful situations. Although it remains unproven, the investigators suspect that social support may somehow boost immune function.

### Age-Old Thinking

The idea that emotions are tied to health is not a new one. Before Hippocrates (500 B.C.) and until contemporary times, doctors believed that "the passions" played a role in causing disease. Modern scientists have had little reason to revisit this antiquated notion—until recently. As they have gained a greater understanding of the way the body functions at the cellular level, they have made the surprising discovery that certain molecules transmit signals between the nervous and immune systems.

Meanwhile, animal studies have demonstrated that impairing communication between the two systems—either by genetic engineering or with drugs —is associated with a susceptibility to inflammatory diseases, thyroid problems, and arthritis. Such research may one day explain why there are so many variations in people's vulnerability to infections, autoimmune disorders, and even cancer.

Most human research on stress and health has looked at the link between emotions, hypertension, and heart disease. A growing and convincing body of data suggest that chronic anger, anxiety, loneliness, or depression can be lethal to people with coronary artery disease. There is also some evidence that physically healthy people who experience frequent blow-ups, who are chronically depressed, or who are constantly anxious may be setting the stage for future heart disease.

Researchers point to the fact that some heart attacks are triggered by the sudden clumping together of blood platelets —one of the body's reactions to the evolutionary "fight or flight" response —which is evoked by fear or anger. When these emotions run high, platelets become stickier as the body prepares itself to stanch a potential wound.

Investigators who study the effects of stress on health believe that heart disease is only one of many ills that may ultimately be linked to disturbances of the flight or flight reaction.

## An Ongoing Struggle

Everyone experiences stress in one form or another. There is the acute stress of a traumatic event, such as the death or illness of a loved one or the loss of a job, or the day-to-day wear and tear from sitting in traffic jams, feeling angry or isolated, or constantly worrying about work, finances, or relationships.

When the brain perceives stress— either from an internal or external trigger —the flight or flight response kicks in. Initially, this reaction stimulates the release of two stress hormones: adrenalin, which is produced by the adrenal glands near the kidneys, and corticotrophin-releasing hormone (CRH), from nerve cells in the hypothalamus, at the base of the brain. CRH then travels to the pituitary gland, where it causes the release of adrenocorticotrophic hormone (ACTH); this triggers the production of cortisol by the adrenal gland.

In response, blood platelets aggregate, immune cells activate, blood sugar rushes to muscles to give them energy, the heart and breathing rate quickens, and blood pressure rises. Cortisol, a steroid hormone which at first sustains the stress response, later slows it down so the body can return to normal functioning.

Sometimes, however, this feedback loop goes awry. If stress hormones fail to turn off once the challenge has passed or if a person is subjected to chronic stress, cortisol and other hormones can get out of whack. Instead of providing protection, they may suppress the immune system by interfering with the regular repair and maintenance functions of the body, leaving people open to infections and disease.

## A Heavy Burden

In a report published in the January 15, 1998, issue of the New England Journal of Medicine, Bruce S. McEwen, a neuroscientist at Rockefeller University, uses the term allostatic load to refer to the long-term physical effects of the body's response to stress. Allostasis is derived from the Greek word that means "to achieve stability through change." However, the price our bodies pay for accommodating to stressful changes may be high; some people develop a hyperactivity or hypoactivity of the normal stress response.

Too little production of stress hormones can be just as harmful as too much, because it may trigger the secretion of other substances that compensate for the loss. For example, if cortisol does not increase in response to stress, inflammatory cytokines (signals), which are regulated by cortisol, will rise.

On the other hand, too much cortisol can predispose a person to infection, bone loss, muscle weakening, and increased insulin production. Women with a history of depression tend to have higher cortisol levels and lower bone mineral density than those who are not depressed. And studies on aging animals and humans suggest that chronic exposure to stress hormones may accelerate changes in the brain that lead to memory loss.

No one knows why stress hormones don't turn off in some people when the stressful event has passed. It is also unclear why some individuals lose the ability to produce stress hormones when they need them.

The Rockefeller researchers believe that regular, moderate exercise is probably the best way to counteract the deleterious effects of stress. Physical activity can reduce insulin levels raised by excessive cortisol secretion and also lowers blood pressure and the heart's resting rate. People who exercise regularly may find that they can more easily give up overeating or excessive alcohol consumption, which they had previously used to quell stress.

**The Cancer Connection**
There is some, but less conclusive, evidence that stress may somehow be linked to cancer. Over the past decade, studies have suggested that emotional support not only enhances the lives of cancer patients but also prolongs life. In a 1989 investigation, Stanford University researchers found that women with metastatic breast cancer who participated in support groups survived an average of 18 months longer than those who did not.

In January 1998, a published report by Ohio State University researchers indicated that breast cancer patients with high levels of anxiety about their disease experienced a 20%–30% reduction in the effectiveness of their natural killer (NK) cells compared to those with low levels of stress. NK cells fight infection and cancer.

Previous research has found that cancer patients who say they feel emotionally supported have highly active NK cells; experts speculate that emotional support boosts the activity of these white blood cells by decreasing stress.

However, only a few studies have ever looked at whether reducing stress can actually improve immune function and thus slow the progression of cancer. Now, several such investigations are under way. One, by the same Ohio State University reseachers, is measuring baseline levels of NK activity and other cellular reactions in 235 women with metastatic breast cancer who will undergo surgery. After their operations, one group will attend support groups for a year and learn ongoing coping skills; the other will not attend such sessions. Stress levels, immune and endocrine response, and cancer recurrence will be compared to the women's baseline measurements after five years.

The study will shed new light on the 1989 Stanford investigation, which was designed only to examine the impact of particular kinds of emotional support on quality of life; the investigators had not intended to look at survival rates and did not measure immune responses or tumor growth.

However, the same Stanford researchers are now in the process of replicating their previous study, but this time they are monitoring cortisol levels, NK cell activity, cancer recurrence, and survival rates. The final results are expected to be published in about two years.

**The Jury Is Out**
It's important to keep in mind that no one has yet proven that reducing stress alters immune function in a way that

influences cancer. In fact, the hypothesis itself is controversial: scientists don't fully understand the ways in which immune responses affect the progression of cancer.

And although the Ohio State and Stanford groups will track several indicators that predict a person's prognosis, such as whether cancer has spread to lymph nodes, they can't account for all factors that may alter the outcome. For example, researchers will not know if some of the participants' previous chemotherapy treatments suppressed immune function. Finally, it's possible that support groups have no effect on immune response; they may bolster health simply because they encourage participants to comply with drug or dietary regimens. Nevertheless, research suggests that people with or without the stress of illness enjoy better health and a better quality of life when they get emotional support through a network of friends, relatives, and associates or through structured groups.

When experts recommend that people reduce stress in their lives, it doesn't necessarily mean that you need to leave the city for the country, quit your job, or make other dramatic changes to avoid an early grave. It may simply mean exercising more, expanding your social circle, reaching out to others, joining a support group, or putting traffic jams in perspective.

Researchers who study stress and health suspect that many ills are linked to problems with the body's "fight or flight" reaction.

# NO

**Christopher Caldwell**

# THE USE AND ABUSE OF STRESS

Springfield, Massachusetts, home of the Merriam-Webster's Dictionary, has long been proud of its annual spelling bee. But in the first week of May, Springfield superintendent of schools Peter Negroni canceled the event forever, on the grounds that "the bee provided too much stress and too few rewards." He announced that henceforth the school system would replace it with Scrabble.

The local newspaper applauded, as well it might. For the problem Negroni cited—stress—is now viewed as a society-wide scourge, and efforts to battle it are expensive and intense. According to the journal of the Society for the Advancement of Management, stress is the cause of as many as 90 percent of all job-related doctors' visits, is responsible for over half the sick days American workers take, and is the culprit in up to 80 percent of on-the-job accidents. The total cost to American companies: up to $300 billion a year.

Companies now call for outside "stress audits," courts throughout the world are increasingly indulgent of stress-based awards, and "stress management" has become a multi-billion-dollar industry. A survey by stress expert Kenneth R. Pelletier found that stress-management plans are by far the leading priority for corporate health programs, cited four times as often as the next closest concern (cardiac care). What should alarm us, and lead us to distrust all of the statistics cited above, is that no one—not the doctors who study it, not the plaintiffs who claim it, not even the "stress-management consultants" who have become the ethicists of the stress trade—can come to any agreement on what stress *is*.

It's not that the medical study of stress is bogus and newfangled; quite the contrary. Hippocrates spoke of something like stress (*pónos*). Our current understanding of the problem has its beginnings with doctors Walter Bradford Cannon and Hans Selye, who, working separately between the wars, uncovered the syndrome Selye would name "stress." Cannon investigated the "fight-or-flight" response—the way in which the human body produces adrenaline and other hormones in response to outside stimuli. When activated, these hormones sharpen the attention, speed up the heart, and prepare the body for action. But the response also depletes the immune system and temporarily halts the normal function of certain of the body's regulatory networks. Cannon and Selye speculated that, in the 20th century, the fight-or-flight response was not being evoked at rare moments of extreme need, as it presumably was when prehistoric man had to outrun a lion, but that it had become a chronic condition. The irony was that 20th-century man, awash in conveniences and more divorced from nature than ever before, lived in a state of constant, or at least over-frequent, bodily vigilance that was causing his body to squander its whole bank account of self-protective resources.

Cannon and Selye were medical researchers, but their followers turned their research into an amalgam of social theory and psychiatric dogma. Now, it seems, practically *everything* causes stress. According to the Society for the Advancement of Management,

> causes of workplace stress include: schedules and deadlines, fear of failure, inadequate support, problems with the boss, job ambiguity, role conflict, change, new technology, work overload or underload, repetitive work, excess rules and regulations, lack of participation in decisions, poor interpersonal relationships, career development factors (obsolescence, under/over promotion, organizational structure, organizational leadership, culture), and poor working conditions that include the climate, overcrowding, politics, and communication problems.

(Sorry—did someone say "the climate"?) As if that weren't enough to worry about, *success* on the job— or the "success syndrome," as stress-management consultants put it—affects one in five managers, and can cause "apathy, irritability, uninvolvement in projects, decline in productivity, marital problems, and excessive drinking or smoking." Stress-management candidates include people dying of AIDS, hot-tempered adolescents, people scared of surgery, binge drinkers, undergraduates with exam anxiety, athletes who choke, vaguely defined "Type A personalities," and on and on.

The comprehensive nature of the stress theory is the first indication that we're in the presence of a racket. Stress-related lawsuits and claims are booming in courts across the country. Under the 1970 Occupational Safety and Health Act, companies are responsible for "all diseases arising out of and in the course of employment," and that is now taken to include stress. The National Institute for Occupational Safety and Health considers stress one of the 10 leading occupational diseases. Recent rulings on the Americans with Disabilities Act make it likely that that act, too, will be used to buttress stress-related claims. The U.S. Court of Appeals for the 6th Circuit recently ruled that a factory employee in Michigan could collect for a heart attack suffered on the factory floor and caused, he said, by the stress-inducing incompetence of one of his fellow workers and the unpleasant noise at work.

For all its American roots, stress is a global issue, at least in any country where people have grown impatient with modern life. Sweden's incredibly generous 1991 Work Environment Act makes it the responsibility of employers to make sure "that the employee is not exposed to physical *or mental* loads which may lead to ill health or accidents." One British citizen got a settlement for the stress of being stuck in an elevator. British papers have been in a panic about stress since 1994, when the social worker John Walker received £175,000 for being "severely mentally wounded" by the stress at work. More recently, the Scottish social worker Janet Ballantyne received a settlement of £66,000 for the stress caused by her "outspoken and abrasive" boss. (It's interesting that both these British stress collectors hail from UNISON, the same left-wing union of underpaid social workers. As one London businessman told the London *Times*, "I've yet to see a damages claim brought by a City stockbroker.")

Clearly, if we're looking for a synonym for stress it would be something like "modern life," and the current anti-stress activism is an ethical and political critique of it. University of Chicago anthropologist Richard Shweder thinks that stress is merely a synonym for unhappiness, much as people a century ago talked of angst and ennui. Others see it as similar to the 19th-century fad ailment of hysteria. But it is more than that, for unlike its forebears, stress is linked to treatments and to states and corporations that mandate them. As University of Montreal psychologist Ethel Roskies puts it, "The most distinctive characteristic of stress management as a treatment is its universality; there is no one for whom treatment is apparently unneeded or inappropriate." According to Roskies, "Essentially, the diagnosis of a clinical stress problem has less to do with the etiology or severity of the problem itself than with the prediction of its responsiveness to the teaching of coping skills."

That means that stress can degenerate into a hunt for problems to fit preexisting (and lucrative) solutions. Some commonsense techniques for stress reduction appear to work. Meditation, biofeedback, hypnosis, "visulization therapy," and relaxation coaching show results. But other techniques appear so commonsensical as

to be laughable: Stress consultant Ray Shelton has said his Awareness-Attitude-Action model relies in part on "avoiding excess coffee and junk food." And treatments can veer into charlatanism: "acupressure," "meridian energy flow," and something called "trampoline therapy." The *Washington Post's* Liza Mundy attended a Fred Pryor motivational seminar designed to fight stress and learned little more than that she ought to keep a "smile file" of happy thoughts and "take time out to just be." European American Bank, meanwhile, reportedly invited Jesse "Two Owls" Teasley of the Oglala Sioux tribe to talk about *tai chi*—not, to the best of anyone's knowledge, an American Indian cultural product.

The very idea of stress management, its opponents suggest, instills "learned helplessness"—the assumption that people don't have enough internal resources to quiet the storm within their own minds. Stress thus becomes the close relative of the "Twinkie Defense." If self-help methods don't work, then obviously society has the obligation to protect us from our own adrenaline.

The great pop-psych expression of this attitude is the Social Readjustment Rating Scale, devised by two psychologists in 1967. It ranks stressful events using a point system. Death of a spouse is 100, pregnancy is 40, problems with the law is 29, etc. If your tally rises above 150 points, you have a 50 percent possibility of suffering stress.

The effect of such a scale is to muddy all *moral* claims—the notion that maybe you ought to feel bad if you do something wrong. By assuming that a tragedy, like the death of a spouse, can be ranked on the same scale as a pregnancy makes the very idea of stress itself arbitrary. Is it worse than initiating a divorce or changing your diet? Where does "having an incompetent co-worker" (the problem that allegedly caused a heart attack) fit in?

The current conception of "stress" is a way of micromanaging fairness. It's just unfair that someone's stress rating should rise above 150 points, and there's no reason it should! If a guy gets up to 300 points and flies off the handle, who can blame him? The goal of the Social Readjustment Rating System is to quantify moral, physical, and spiritual well-being so that they can be redistributed, as money and goods are in a socialist society.

Stress is now the preserve of those unacknowledged legislators of the world: social workers and other members of the caring professions. It is they, not the wider public, who decide the stress agenda. While 74 percent of corporate managers in one survey felt that the responsibility for stress management "should lie with the individual rather than the organization," institutional stress professionals continue to extend their reach and their agenda. That agenda is, not to put too fine a point on it, pro-feminist, anti-competitive, and inclined to see a racist under every bed.

The classic idea of stress has been easily adapted to a feminized America. Much of the initial research on stress had to do with men; the fact that they were undeniably more susceptible to stress-related heart attacks made it likely they suffered more stress. But recent research, all of it sociological and psychological rather than medical, has sought to put women at center-stage. The prevailing theory is that "juggling work and home" *must* make women's lives more stressful than men's, whether or not there's any evidence to back it up. Too little attention has been paid, say the stress enthusiasts,

to women's stress, brought about by the fact that women have been "socialized to care for others."

From heart attacks to the woes of caring for others—yet again we see, even inside the world of stress management, a great leveling taking place. These days, women are increasingly considered the true victims of stress. Take NBC's "Stressed Out in America," a series of spots that ran on the network's weekend *Today* show throughout the month of April. "It's estimated that—get this— 75 percent of all doctor visits are due to stress-related disorders," said host Jodi Applegate. "Now there's evidence to suggest that women may be more prone to stress than men." Participants consistently favored stereotypical female coping mechanisms to stereotypical male ones. Take Xavier Amador of Columbia University: "Really what we mean is it's important to talk about how you feel, and —and the worst thing you can do if you're stressed out is to keep it inside and carry it with you." Then Amador talked about the importance of using "I" statements: "It's very important that you talk about how you feel, not what the other person is doing. So, if you're stressed out, you come home, the dishes aren't done, don't say, 'You don't do the dishes, why didn't you do the dishes?' Say, 'I would really appreciate it.'"

The who-does-the-dishes example hardly came out of thin air. Indeed, one commonplace assertion in the world of stress management is that stress in men is caused by their being too aggressive, while stress in women is caused by women's being too passive. Says Dr. Redford Williams, director of the Behavioral Medicine Research Center at Duke, "You should just cool out. Let it go." But what if the situation is amenable to change?

"That means you should really swing into action . . . and for women that often means being assertive."

The agenda of the stress industry also includes race. The most notorious recent example was a study by Harvard epidemiologists Nancy Krieger and Stephen Sidney on "Racial Discrimination and Blood Pressure," which appeared in last October's *American Journal of Public Health.* Blacks die on average seven years earlier than whites, from cancer, heart attacks, and a variety of diseases to which they have a higher propensity. The two researchers asked for responses about exposure to racial discrimination and plotted the results against high-blood-pressure statistics. There was no statistically significant relationship; in fact, those blacks who had faced zero episodes of discrimination had higher blood pressure than those who had faced one or more. But Krieger and Sidney assumed a relationship anyway, on the grounds that those with the highest blood pressure were probably *underreporting* the number of racist incidents they'd been exposed to, and that they were thus merely victims of "internalized oppression."

High stress, in the categories of race and gender, is seen as merely a stand-in for virtue. That's not the case with stress in the category of achievement— and the contrast is instructive. We all know about how dangerous it is to be a "Type A," shorthand for "Type A behavior syndrome," which researchers define as "characterized by competitive drive, impatience, hostility, and rapid speech and motor movements." For years, doctors and stress researchers have found a correlation between those behavioral qualities and a high incidence of coronary heart disease.

If, for physicians, the Type A is merely a cardiac-ward candidate who deserves attention, for stress professionals he's the vice president in the penthouse with the five secretaries and the attitude. An unmistakable note of righteous discipline, even divine wrath, can be heard in their discussions of Type A personalities. In their view, for Type As, excessive work is an "obsessive-compulsive disorder." NBC's "Stressed Out in America" suggested that Type As who are always nervously looking for the shortest line in a supermarket should instead seek out the *longest* one.

Here as elsewhere, "stress" is frequently an explicit indictment of competitiveness, and this means an implicit indictment of the economic status quo. Karen Nussbaum, the director of the working women's department at the AFL-CIO, told a *Newsday* reporter that "companies that really want to relieve stress should be more concerned with redistributing work, paying a decent wage, and creating a family-friendly environment." Stress thus serves as the ultimate pretext for gripes about the need for economic reorganization.

As a medical matter, the study of stress is an effort to examine the problem that the human animal lives under conditions of modernity to which his system has not adapted. It is a serious issue that deserves serious study. But that is not why America has become so addicted to talk about stress. "Stress" is a smoke screen —a cover for what is, at root, a political and moral movement aimed at fixing "inappropriate" ways of responding to modernity. Its agenda is large enough and its rationale vague enough that it ought to be drawing more skeptical interest, and meeting more resistance.

# POSTSCRIPT

## Is Stress Responsible for Disease?

Some physicians maintain that stress can make people sick. Some estimate that close to two-thirds of all physician visits are related to negative stress. In the early 1990s Sheldon Cohen, a professor at Carnegie Mellon University, conducted a study that showed the relationship between stress and the common cold. He measured the stress levels of nearly 400 men and women and then exposed them to cold viruses. Almost half of the subjects under the most stress became ill compared to 27 percent of the least stressed. The kind of stress that was most likely to increase the probability of developing a cold was related to extended conflict in personal relationships. Stress does not cause colds, but researchers hypothesize that it makes us more susceptible to cold viruses by negatively affecting the immune system. Similar studies have indicated that stress may play a major role in headaches, gastrointestinal distress, asthma, and skin disorders. Stress may even play a role in the aging process. A recent study found that cortisol, the major human stress hormone, can increase mental deterioration in healthy people. These findings appear in "Cortisol Levels During Human Aging Predict Hippocampal Atrophy and Memory Deficits," *Nature Neuroscience* (May 1998).

Many theories exist concerning the dual nature of stress. It is argued that exposure to stress is linked to illnesses, including heart disease, cancer, tuberculosis, and the common cold. However, when carefully managed and utilized, stress can serve as a positive force by increasing productivity. Stress is said to elevate the risk of illness, but it also increases the secretion of hormones that can help people become more effective and increase their energy. Many experts in the field of stress management claim that learning to relax, prioritize tasks, and maintain a sense of humor can help make stress work for everyone. See "Evidence for Mind-Body Connection Increases," *Lancet* (April 18, 1998).

However, we are all exposed to stressful situations. According to Christopher Caldwell, stress is blamed for too much that goes wrong in our lives. The definition of stress is too comprehensive, making "stress management" a multi-billion-dollar industry. Caldwell asserts that a more skeptical examination of the definition of stress is necessary. Further readings on the stress-illness relationship include "Stress and Atherosclerosis," *Harvard Health Letter* (February 1998); "Fight or Flight—Or Sit Tight?" *Consumer Reports on Health* (February 1998); "Protective and Damaging Effects of Stress Mediators," *The New England Journal of Medicine* (January 15, 1998); "How Stress Can Make You Sick," *Current Health* (November 1997); and "Stressed Out and Sick from It," *Redbook* (March 1997).

# ISSUE 7

## Can Spirituality Overcome Disease?

**YES: Herbert Benson and Marg Stark,** from *Timeless Healing: The Power and Biology of Belief* (Scribner, 1996)

**NO: William B. Lindley,** from "Prayer and Healing," *Truth Seeker* (vol. 122, no. 2, 1995)

### ISSUE SUMMARY

**YES:** Herbert Benson, an associate professor of medicine at Harvard Medical School, and journalist Marg Stark contend that faith and spirituality will enhance and prolong life.

**NO:** William B. Lindley, associate editor of *Truth Seeker*, counters that there is no scientific way to determine that spirituality can heal.

Practitioners of holistic medicine believe that people must take responsibility for their own health by practicing healthy behaviors and maintaining positive attitudes instead of relying on health providers. They also believe that physical disease has behavioral, psychological, and spiritual components. These spiritual components can be explained by the relationship between beliefs, mental attitude, and the immune system. Until recently, few studies existed to prove a relationship between spirituality—a feeling of connectedness to the greater self—and health.

Much of modern medicine has spent the past century ridding itself of mysticism and relying on science. Twenty years ago, no legitimate physician would have dared to study the effects of spirituality on disease. Recently, however, at the California Pacific Medical Center in San Francisco, California, Elisabeth Targ, clinical director of psychosocial oncology research, has recruited 20 faith healers to determine if prayer can affect the outcome of disease. Targ claims that her preliminary results are encouraging. In addition to Targ's study, other research has shown that religion and spirituality can help determine health and well-being. According to a 1995 investigation at Dartmouth College, one of the strongest predictors of success after open-heart surgery was the level of comfort patients derived from religion and spirituality. Other recent studies have linked health with church attendance, religious commitment, and spirituality. There are, however, other studies that have not been as successful; a recent one involving the effects of prayer on alcoholics found no relationship.

Can spirituality or prayer in relation to health and healing be explained scientifically? Prayer or a sense of spirituality may function in a similar manner as stress management or relaxation. Spirituality or prayer may cause the release of hormones that help lower blood pressure or produce other benefits. Though science may never be able to exactly determine the benefits of spirituality, it does appear to help some people.

In the following selections, Herbert Benson and Marg Stark state that spirituality can have a significant influence over the body. William B. Lindley argues that people do not become ill because their mental states, psyches, or attitudes negatively affect their biological systems.

# YES Herbert Benson and Marg Stark

# TIMELESS HEALING: THE POWER AND BIOLOGY OF BELIEF

At one time or another, I'm sure nearly everyone experiences extraordinary and magical events, the converging of time and circumstance so logic-defiant that one cannot help but feel these events were divinely directed. It could be a chance reunion with a long-lost friend, a life change that comes at precisely the time you need it, or an image you see in a cloud formation. It could be a clergyperson's sermon that seems eerily relevant to the problems you've been facing, something as dramatic as hearing a voice speak to you inspirationally or as quiet as a bliss that envelops you suddenly. Whatever the form, the more the incident means to us, the more we attach sacred status to it in our lives. We shake our heads, asking, "What are the chances?" all the while feeling a profound reverberation within that perhaps life is not random, that perhaps these are tangible signs that a mystical force contours our life.

But it's possible that the reverberation you feel within when an experience you deem magical or spiritual occurs may not be just emotional but physical as well. Not only did my research—and that of my colleagues—reveal that 25% of people feel more spiritual as the result of the elicitation of the relaxation response, but it showed that those same people have fewer medical symptoms than do those who reported no increase in spirituality from the elicitation.

I decided to call the combined force of these internal influences the *faith factor*—remembered wellness and the elicitation of the relaxation response. But it became clear that a person's religious convictions or life philosophy enhanced the average effects of the relaxation response in three ways: (1) People who chose an appropriate focus, that which drew upon their deepest philosophic or religious convictions, were more apt to adhere to the elicitation routine, looking forward to it and enjoying it; (2) affirmative beliefs of any kind brought forth remembered wellness, reviving top-down, nerve-cell firing patterns in the brain that were associated with wellness; (3) when present, faith in an eternal or life-transcending force seemed to make the fullest use of remembered wellness because it is a supremely soothing belief, disconnecting unhealthy logic and worries.

I already knew that eliciting the relaxation response could "disconnect" everyday thoughts and worries, calming people's bodies and minds more quickly and to a degree otherwise unachievable. It appeared that beliefs added to the response transported the mind/body even more dramatically, quieting worries and fears significantly better than the relaxation response alone. And I speculated that religious faith was more influential than other affirmative beliefs.

I want to emphasize that the benefits of the faith factor are not the exclusive domain of the devout. People don't have to have a professed belief in God to reap the psychological and physical rewards of the faith factor. With lead investigator Dr. Jared D. Kass, a professor at Lesley College Graduate School of Arts and Sciences in Cambridge, MA, my colleagues and I developed a questionnaire to quantify and describe the spiritual feelings that accompanied the relaxation response, to document their frequency and potential health effects.

Based on the survey responses, we calculated "spirituality scores." But because virtually all of our survey respondents reported a "belief in God," this statement could not be used to differentiate people. It was the more amorphous feeling of spirituality that could be linked to better psychological and physical well-being. However, there is one group that does seem more likely to have spiritual encounters. Indeed, women had higher spirituality scores than men, for reasons we don't yet understand.

As subjective as remembered wellness is, there are some definitive things I can say about incorporating healing beliefs and faith into your life. These are some of the principles and practical lessons I've drawn from my long medical quest for lasting truths. I hope they prove helpful to you:

**Let Faith, the Ultimate Belief, Heal You.** According to medical research, faith in God is good for us, and this benefit is not exclusive to one denomination or theology. You can believe in God in a quiet, introspective way or declare your convictions out loud to the world—either way, you'll still reap the physiologic rewards.

For many reasons, religious activity and churchgoing are also healthy. Religious groups encourage all kinds of health-affirming activities—fellowship and socializing perhaps first among them, but also prayer, volunteerism, familiar rituals and music. Prayer, in particular, appears to be therapeutic, the specifics of which science will continue to explore.

**Trust Your Instincts More Often.** People describe the process of finding out what is important to them, of tapping into their beliefs, in very different ways, sometimes calling it "soul-searching," "mulling it over," "listening to one's heart," "going inside of one's self," "praying," or "sleeping on it." Some people act on instincts or common sense; others find a truth or intuition emerges slowly. But most people know when something "feels right." Most people have a kind of internal radar that occasionally calls out to them.

The next time you're faced with a major decision, medical or otherwise, ask yourself, "What would I do if the choice were entirely up to me?" I'm not suggesting that you make decisions based on this factor alone, but at least let belief be a player. Honor your convictions and perceptions enough to make them a part of a hearty intellectual argument.

Let your instincts guide you. Follow them up with research. Put your health in good, trustworthy hands. Let your health have time to correct itself. Invest remembered wellness and a reasonable application of self-care, medications and surgery for maximum health returns.

**Practice and Apply Self-Care Regularly.** Work with your doctor, and with unconventional practitioners if you so choose, to learn self-care habits. I consider self-care anything an individual can do, independent of doctors or healers, to enhance his or her health. This includes mind/body reactions such as remembered wellness, the relaxation response and the faith factor. It also embraces good nutrition, exercise and other means of stress management.

I use the term "self-care" because it puts the onus on you, it shifts the emphasis from your role as passive patient to active participant—a shift that medicine has not always encouraged. However, I caution against becoming self-absorbed in self-care. Don't become fixated on your health or on the avoidance of aging, illness or death. Make your daily elicitation of the relaxation response, your jog or your salad at lunch a no-brainer, which you do not analyze or overthink. Simply delight in the event itself.

It's almost always valuable to seek the assistance of your physician to determine the difference between a condition that will benefit from self-care exclusively and one that requires drugs or procedures to treat. Learning about your body is an evolutionary process. You'll work toward a more independent attitude. Become acquainted with the warning signs of heart attacks, strokes, cancer and other life-threatening diseases. Over time, you'll develop a sense of what symptoms are important—those that are extreme or don't go away.

How influential can a coordinated contingent of self-care habits be? We honestly don't know, but *Prevention* advisor Dean Ornish, MD, president of the Preventive Medicine Research Institute in Sausalito, CA, found that heart disease could not only be relieved but reversed when patients made significant changes in diet, exercise and stress management. Our two programs will soon be compared in a groundbreaking research project sponsored by the Commonwealth of Massachusetts Group Insurance Commission and the John Hancock Insurance Company. In this comparison, patients with heart disease will be divided between our two clinics in hopes that we can gauge the adherence to and results of various self-care components and other treatments.

**Beware of People with All the Answers.** Be careful of any physician, nontraditional healer, spiritual guide, mind/body guru, or any adviser who claims to have all the answers or wants others to think so. Besides love and sex, writers and lecturers today take up few topics with as much evangelistic zeal as health and spirituality. It is no small task shielding these very personal matters from unhealthy speculation and overanalysis, but start with tuning out overly confident or all-knowing mentors and guides. Value your emotions and intuitions the same way your brain does; don't let someone manipulate your wiring for his or her gain.

Mind/body medicine should remind us of the precious nature of our minds, and of the importance of critiquing the messages we allow to become actualized in our brains/bodies.

Whether or not you believe in God, I believe that we are all wired to crave meaning in life, to assign profound power and sacredness to human experiences, and sometimes even to lend "god" status or "godliness" to humans and human endeavors. Be wary of this tendency, because it may rob spiritual life of its grandeur and of the wonderful transcendent qualities that cannot be accessed entirely by human intellect, and because it makes us very susceptible to human manipulation. Not only is your body a temple, but your mind is an architect, busy transforming the ideas you feed it. Protect it from those who exploit the power of remembered wellness for personal gain.

**Remember that the 'Nocebo' is Equally Powerful.** Unfortunately, remembered wellness has a flip side. It can have negative side effects, called the *nocebo* (as opposed to placebo). Our agitated minds may inappropriately trigger the fight-or-flight response in the body. Similarly, automatic negative thoughts, bad moods and compulsive worrying eventually take up physical residence in our bodies. Extreme examples of the nocebo effect include voodoo death, belief-engendered death, mass psychogenic illness, false memories and "memories" of alien abductions. People who dwell on worst-case scenarios, who exaggerate risks, or who project doubt and undue worry keep the nocebo effect busy in their physiologies. They signal their brains to send help when no physical sickness is present, persuading the body to get sick when there is no biologic reason sickness should occur.

**Remember that Immortality is Impossible.** While it's healthy to listen to your heart, it's also harmful to deny or duck the truth. No one lives forever. No matter how well-versed you become in mind/body medicine, no matter how far medical progress may be able to set back the clock, death is, like illness and pain, an unfortunate but natural fact of life.

I must sound as if I'm talking in circles, first telling you not to let a diagnosis define you, then warning you not to fall prey to denial. Nonetheless, some lecturers and New Age entrepreneurs imply that all disease is curable and that we can avoid death and aging if we only believe. These salespeople do great harm to people by fostering guilt, and they damage the field of mind/body medicine, which is legitimately trying to establish its findings and change the way Western medicine is practiced. No evidence exists that death can be denied its eventual toll.

Indeed, fear of death can bring out the worst in people, but the realization that death is an inevitable, natural occurrence can also propel healthy, impassioned living.

Living well, exercising and eating appropriately, seeing doctors when you need to but not overrelying on the medical system—these are all proven buffers against disease and illness.

**Believe in Something Good.** Even though we do not necessarily need all the pills and procedures that conventional medicine and unconventional medicine give us, these medicinal symbols retain an aura of effectiveness and often appease our desire for action. While we must learn to use medicine more appropriately for the conditions it can help, and to wean ourselves from excessive spending on unnecessary therapies, we'll often need some catalysts for belief, even if belief is really the healer.

So remember the vigor from the time you felt healthiest in your life. Remember the blessing your mother said to you before you left for school, the smell of incense at church, or the tranquility you felt picking up stones from the beach on Cape Cod. Remember the time the penicillin vanquished your ear infection, or the time the surgeon removed the splinter from deep in your foot and your pain immediately ceased. Remember how full-throated you sang in the choir or how long you stayed on the dance floor of a nightclub. Remember the doctor who really cared about you or the chaplain who prayed with you in the hospital. Remember the way you felt when you made love to your husband or wife, and the way you felt when your daughter or son was born.

Then let go, and believe. You've read all about your physiology, you've surrounded yourself with good caregivers who help you take a moderate, balanced approach to your health and health care. Now it's time to enjoy your endowment, this wiring for faith that makes the power of remembered wellness so enduring.

Believe in something good if you can. Or even better, believe in something better than anything you can fathom. Because for us mortals, this is very profound medicine.

# NO

William B. Lindley

# PRAYER AND HEALING

I was raised in Christian Science. That gives me somewhat of an inside perspective on prayer and healing. However, the Christian Science experience is far from typical. The "Scientific Statement of Being" begins: "There is no life, truth, intelligence nor substance in matter." Most Christians who offer prayers of petition for the healing of an illness believe that their bodies are real and the illness is real, but they want supernatural intervention, the sort of thing Jesus is reported to have done in the gospels. Christian Science, interpreting Jesus' work quite differently insists that reality lies elsewhere. The analogue to prayer is "knowing the truth." Christian Science insists that miracles are not "supernatural, but divinely natural."

As I grew up and matter made more sense to me, I drifted away from Christian Science. Then I began hearing about natural, nonmiraculous analogues to what I had been taught: psychosomatic diseases and cures, the placebo effect, and, more recently, the neurochemical connections between mood and the immune system. These, along with "spontaneous remission" of cancers, were attempts to explain "miracles" without invoking the supernatural or the paranormal. (Note that "spontaneous" (natural), and "God did it" (supernatural), are "explanations" that explain nothing. There's no "how.") Believers in miracles—evangelicals, Christian Scientists, miscellaneous New Agers, and so forth—continue as before.

## PRAYER AND HEALING

*Healing Words* by Larry Dossey, M.D., is a book devoted to prayer and healing, and its author believes firmly that prayer (communication with "the Absolute") brings about beneficial effects that are real and substantial and supernatural or paranormal in character. However, when he raises the question, "What is prayer?", the answer is so far-ranging that all sorts of things that would not ordinarily be considered prayer are included. He rejects the Christian concept of prayer! Of course he doesn't use such strong language as "reject," preferring slippery words like "redefine," tentative" and "reevaluate." He has a chart contrasting the "traditional Western model" with the "modern" model of prayer. Probably over 95% of the prayers for healing that are made in the United States would be of the "old" model, which Dossey considers obsolete. Interestingly enough, Christian Science prayer would fall under the 5% that he would approve of.

Even though Dossey seems to think little of traditional prayer, his citations of many experiments that allegedly demonstrate the efficacy of prayer do not indicate whether the style of prayer was traditional or otherwise. (He clearly expresses his opinion that all kinds work, some better than others.) The experiments are broken down into various categories of what was prayed over—barley seeds(!), mice, people, etc.—but not into categories of what kind of prayer was made.

Sometimes Dossey seems to be unaware of the implications of what he says. For example, he quotes psychologist Lawrence LeShan to the effect that healing through prayer is effective in perhaps 15 to 20% of cases and that nobody can tell in advance which cases will have happy outcomes. Somewhat disheartened by this, Dossey goes on to claim that prayer works anyway. Then he mentions the "bizarre," "perverted" use of prayer by high school football teams in Texas, where, of course, they offer up highly unsportsmanlike prayers for victory. Such prayers obviously "work" 50% of the time. (We might cut this to 48% or so for tie games.) Thus one can conclude that prayer for victory in football is three times as efficacious as prayer for healing!

## THE PROBLEMS OF PRAYER

Dossey wisely reminds us that if all prayers for healing led to success, population growth would be even more catastrophic than it is; 100% success rates for other kinds of prayer could have other horrible long-term effects. (Billy Graham put it a little differently: "God answers all prayers; sometimes the answer is 'no.'") However, once this is admitted—and note that it flatly contradicts Jesus' promise in Matthew 7:7,8: "Ask, and it will be given you; search, and you will find; knock, and the door will be opened for you. For everyone who asks receives, and everyone who searches finds, and for everyone who knocks, the door will be opened"—the result is indistinguishable from that of no prayer at all.

Another problem is the intent of the person praying. Others who have faced the incoherent attempts to define prayer have said that the essence of prayer, whether there be a Supreme Being or not, is that the person praying must intend, or want, or be praying for, a particular happy ending to the current crisis. However, Dossey rejects the concept of intent. He states: "For reasons I shall discuss later, never once did I pray for specific outcomes—for cancers to go away, for heart attacks to be healed, for diabetes to vanish." He reports on an interesting group, Spindrift, that provides many "proofs" that prayer works. This group had a number of Christian Scientists in it. (One was a Christian Science practitioner whose "license" was revoked after The First Church of Christ, Scientist found out what he was up to.) Spindrift took up the question of directed vs. undirected prayer, and found that the undirected prayer worked somewhat better. Most of the other experiments by other groups, for example, with barley seeds, were directed—the intent to have the seeds flourish was in the minds of the people who prayed over them.

## PRAYER EXPERIMENTS

Let's take a closer look at those experiments. There is a long list of them. The compiler is Daniel J. Benor, M.D. He published his survey in the journal *Complementary Medical Research* in 1990. The activity is called "spiritual healing," and this is defined as "the intentional influence of one or more people upon another living system without utilizing known physical means of intervention." (Note how this differs from the Spindrift effort cited above and from Dossey's preference for nondirected prayer.) Of 131 trials, five involved water, with three showing "significant results," but what was being prayed for in the water cases is not mentioned. There were ten trials of "enzymes," including trypsin, dopamine, and noradrenaline. (Are these enzymes? I think not.) There were seven trials on fungi and yeasts, with some prayers being for, some against, the prosperous growth of the culture. Similarly for the ten trials on bacteria, mainly E. coli and salmonella. Cells in vitro (tube or glass dish) were prayed over, including four trials on snail pacemaker cells. There were 19 trials on plants and seeds, including five on the above-mentioned barley seeds. Three of these involved different kinds of person praying: one with neurotic depression, one with psychotic depression, and one with a green thumb. As you might guess, the last showed the strongest beneficial effect. Other plants and seeds prayed over include: rye grass, wheat seeds, radish seeds, mung beans, potatoes and corn. The prayer trials on animals include 14 on anesthetized mice, with a variety of experimental conditions and effects sought. Humans were also prayed over for a total of 38 of the 131 trials. Some of the conditions prayed over are obviously psychosomatic, some less so. Clearly there is an enthusiastic "spiritual healing research" community doing many things we wouldn't ordinarily think of.

Something I was unable to find in all this is any breakdown by religion of the person praying. Christians would consider it vital to ask whether the words "In Jesus' name we pray, amen" were spoken. If they weren't, the Christians would be extremely skeptical of the efficacy of the prayers. If they were confronted by overwhelming evidence that a non-Christian prayer was highly effective, they would suspect Satanism and look for evidence of it. Similarly perhaps for Muslims. Catholics might accept evidence of efficacy of prayers invoking the Trinity while being skeptical of those with Protestant prayer tags. Regrettably, the 131 trials provide us with no information along these lines.

Another missing factor that I regret is a detailed skeptical review of the experimental methodology of some of the more impressive trials. The Committee for the Scientific Investigation of Claims of the Paranormal seems to be silent in this area. While they have offered some criticism of Therapeutic Touch, they seem to be silent on the question of religious prayer healing, except in "revivals," where some noteworthy frauds have been exposed. This is part of a pattern. Most of the subjects discussed in the *Skeptical Inquirer* are New Age phenomena, such as crop circles, UFOs, pyramid power, astrology, and so on. CSICOP seems to be leaving Christianity alone, at least for the time being. Dossey's book cries for skeptical attention. As in the other cases, such attention would have to be very painstaking, time-consuming, and expensive.

Meanwhile, prayers for healing continue, some effectively utilizing known psychosomatic processes, others producing remarkable placebo effects (the same thing, except that we don't know what's happening), and many more where supernatural claims are made, as well as those disappointing cases where God seems to have said "no."

# POSTSCRIPT

## Can Spirituality Overcome Disease?

Can we influence the course of our own illnesses? Can emotions, stress management, and prayer prevent or cure disease? In a telephone poll of 1,004 Americans conducted by TIME/CNN in June 1996, 82 percent indicated that they believed in the healing power of personal prayer. Three-fourths felt that praying for someone else could help cure their illness. Interestingly, fewer than two-thirds of doctors say they believe in God. Benson, who developed the "relaxation response," thinks there is a strong link between religious commitment and good health. He believes that people do not have to have a professed belief in God to reap the psychological and physical rewards of the "faith factor." Benson defined the faith factor as the combined force of the relaxation response and the placebo effect.

Dr. Bernard Siegel, writing in his bestseller *Love, Medicine and Miracles* (Harper & Row, 1986), argues that there are no "incurable diseases, only incurable people" and that illness is a personality flaw. In "Welcome to the Mind/Body Revolution," *Psychology Today* (July/August 1993), author Marc Barash further discusses how the mind and immune system influence each other. The *American Journal of Public Health* (1997) published a literature review entitled "The Spiritual Dimension of Health: A Review," which discussed many aspects of spirituality and health.

In *You Don't Have to Die: Unraveling the AIDS Myth* (Burton Goldberg Group, 1994), a chapter entitled "Mind-Body Medicine" discusses the body's innate healing capabilities and the role of self-responsibility in the healing process. A long-term AIDS survivor who traveled the country interviewing other long-term survivors found that the one thing they all shared was the belief that AIDS was survivable. They all also accepted the reality of their diagnosis but refused to see their condition as a death sentence.

Readings that address these issues include "Can Prayer Heal?" *Health* (March 1998); "Debate on Spirituality," *Ardell Wellness Report* (Winter 1998); "The Greatest Story Never Told," *Utne Reader* (March/April 1997); "Commentary: Into the Heart of Healing," *Making the Rounds in Health, Faith and Ethics* (May 20, 1996); "Faith and Healing," *Time* (June 24, 1996); "Healing Power of Prayer," *Family Circle* (January 9, 1996); "The New Millennium," *Fate* (May 1995); and "Mysterious Remission," *Vogue* (March 1995), which discusses cancer remission.

# On the Internet . . .

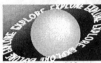

### INFACT: Campaigning for Corporate Accountability

Founded in 1977, INFACT is a national grassroots corporate watchdog organization. This page links to the organization's recently organized tobacco industry campaign and boycott. *http://www.boutell.com/infact/*

### The Alcohol Research Group

This is the home page of the Alcohol Research Group (ARG). Located in Berkeley, California, ARG has been engaged in alcohol studies and related research since 1959. Studies conducted at ARG are funded by grants from a variety of sources, including the National Institute on Alcohol Abuse and Alcoholism, the National Institute on Drug Abuse, and the Robert Wood Johnson Foundation. Current research focuses on alcohol and substance use and intervention in the general population and in specific populations, such as individuals in treatment, welfare recipients, and the homeless. *http://www.arg.org*

### Institute of Alcohol Studies

This is the home page of the U.K.–based Institute of Alcohol Studies (IAS). IAS is an educational body with the basic aims of increasing knowledge of alcohol and the social and health consequences of its misuse and encouraging and supporting the adoption of effective measures for the management and prevention of alcohol-related problems. This site provides fact sheets, publications, press releases, and links to related sites. *http://www.ias.org.uk*

# PART 3

## Substance Use and Abuse

*While millions of Americans use and abuse drugs ranging from marijuana to alcohol and tobacco, experts continue to seek solutions for the related problems and to find causes of addiction. According to some reports, marijuana helps AIDS and cancer patients' symptoms, and some people feel that this use of the drug should be legalized. Although excessive drinking is clearly associated with health problems, there are researchers who claim that moderate alcohol consumption may actually benefit health! Tobacco advertising is being debated as to its influence on teenage smoking. The issues in this section deal with the complex concerns about drugs in our society.*

■ Does Tobacco Advertising Influence Teens to Smoke?

■ Should Moderate Use of Alcohol Be Recommended?

■ Is Marijuana Dangerous and Addictive?

# ISSUE 8

## Does Tobacco Advertising Influence Teens to Smoke?

**YES: Richard W. Pollay,** from "Hacks, Flacks, and Counter-Attacks: Cigarette Advertising, Sponsored Research, and Controversies," *Journal of Social Issues* (vol. 53, no. 1, 1997)

**NO: Jacob Sullum,** from "Cowboys, Camels, and Kids," *Reason* (April 1998)

### ISSUE SUMMARY

**YES:** Professor of business Richard W. Pollay states that teens are influenced to smoke by advertising that appeals to them. He argues that the advertisements portray smokers as independent and successful in the quest for social approval.

**NO:** Editor and journalist Jacob Sullum argues that there is no evidence that advertising encourages people, particularly teens, to smoke.

Smoking has become an established part of our culture. When cigarette manufacturing became a major industry at the turn of the twentieth century, the typical smoker was a middle-class working man. Beginning in the 1920s, however, cigarettes began to be portrayed as sophisticated and even fashionable. Women in increasing numbers began to smoke. Then, as advertising successfully penetrated the youth market, the number of teenage smokers increased. By 1964, 40 percent of the adult population in the United States smoked. Despite the current health warnings, approximately one-fourth of Americans continue to smoke.

In 1964 the first major blow to smoking occurred. The surgeon general of the United States at that time, Luther L. Terry, released a report that positively linked smoking to lung cancer, heart disease, and other ailments. Other reports and stronger warnings on cigarette packs have contributed to a steady decline of smoking in the United States. The Public Health Cigarette Smoking Act, passed in 1970, prohibited cigarette advertisements on television and radio. Since the 1970 ban, cigarettes have been advertised only on billboards and in the print media.

Despite the warnings, smoking continues to be appealing to many teenagers. Teen smoking has risen from 27.5 percent of high school students in 1991 to 36.4 percent in 1997 according to figures from the Centers for Disease Control and Prevention. A recent bill drafted by Arizona senator John McCain may change those numbers. The bill is designed to significantly reduce teen smoking by prohibiting advertising, banning cigarette vending machines, and increasing cigarette taxes. This bill has been referred to the Committee on Commerce, Science, and Transportation for further study and review. According to a recent study entitled "Tobacco Industry Promotion of Cigarettes and Adolescent Smoking," *Journal of the American Medical Association* (February 18, 1998), there is a strong connection between marketing and teen smoking. Teenagers who owned or wanted a promotional item offered by a tobacco company, such as a cap or T-shirt, or who had a favorite tobacco ad were three times more likely to progress toward smoking. The McCain bill would force tobacco companies to abandon logos and icons such as the Marlboro Man and Joe Camel. The bill would also prohibit companies from placing a product logo or name on promotional items.

Why is curbing teen smoking via an advertising ban considered by some to be so important? It is maintained that the vast majority of adult smokers started smoking when they were teenagers, so if everyone could be shielded from cigarettes until the age of 18, virtually no one would smoke. This assumes that when people are old enough to make rational decisions about the health risks of smoking, they typically choose not to start. Tobacco use is also linked with the use of other drugs. It has been asserted that teenagers who smoke are more likely to experiment with alcohol, marijuana, and cocaine.

The tobacco industry disagrees with the contention that teenagers are influenced by tobacco advertisements. Spokesmen in the industry argue that there is no definitive evidence linking advertising with smoking initiation. Tobacco executives maintain that advertising is used to heighten brand loyalty or to entice existing smokers to switch to their brand. The companies also argue that they do not target their advertising specifically to young people. They state that banning cigarette ads violates free speech. See "Tobacco and Liberty," *Insight* (March 16, 1998).

In the following selections, Richard W. Pollay maintains that there should be greater regulation of the tobacco industry, particularly in advertising. He contends that cigarette ads influence the smoking behavior of young adults. Jacob Sullum argues that there is no evidence that advertising has a major impact on teen smoking.

# YES

Richard W. Pollay

## HACKS, FLACKS, AND COUNTER-ATTACKS: CIGARETTE ADVERTISING, SPONSORED RESEARCH, AND CONTROVERSIES

The tobacco industry is acknowledged as outstanding for its ability to promote "friendly" research, to denigrate research inimical to its interests as prohibitionist propaganda (Jones, 1996), and "to produce and manage uncertainty" (Proctor, 1995, p. 105). At their extreme, critics are denigrated as a conspiracy of overzealous crusaders exhibiting totalitarianism (Boddewyn, 1986b). The industry's strategy doesn't require winning or resolution of the debates its principals manage to create or inflame. It is enough to foster and perpetuate the illusion of controversy in order to "muddy the waters" around potentially damaging studies and streams of research. This serves at least two important ends: offering reassurance and a basis for rationalization to the otherwise concerned, thereby calming public opinion; and encouraging friendly, ignorant, or naive legislators away from relying on scientific findings threatening to the industry. These tactics are now being used on many fronts of the tobacco battlefield.

The tobacco industry's first major success with this strategy was in combating the so-called "health scare" from the early lung cancer studies of the 1950s. Industry leaders gathered seeds of doubt from around the world, and reproduced and disseminated these through a massive public relations machinery (Pollay, 1990b). Encouraged by that success, they have continued to muddy the waters around the scientific findings relevant to almost every aspect of tobacco and its control, including: heart disease; passive or second-hand smoke; addiction; the medical and larger social costs consequential to smoking; the economic consequences of regulation, etc. Where necessary, as in the case of indoor air quality, they have even turned small local businessmen into apparent international authorities (Mintz, 1996). Of course, they prefer to employ those who seem to be independent from the industry, because trade organizations like the Tobacco Institute are admittedly biased. "We don't pretend to be objective, unbiased or fair.... We represent a commercially vested interest" (Cosco, 1988, p. 8). It should be no surprise, then, that these tactics are also used to combat the issue of cigarette advertising and its effects, particularly its role in recruiting new smokers.

For example, when Fischer et al. (1991) measured product logo recognition of three-to-six-year-olds, they found over 90 percent of the six-year-olds could correctly match the cartoon Camel with cigarettes. So threatening was this result that industry-hired academic consultants attacked the study with or without the benefit of added research (Boddewyn, 1993; Martin, 1993; Mizerski, 1995). Their primary line of attack was to allege that this work was methodologically "inferior," in part because it had been authored, reviewed and published by and for medical experts, rather than marketing or advertising experts. The finding of high awareness among the very young has since been replicated by marketing academics (Henke, 1994), and even by the R. J. Reynolds–sponsored researcher (Mizerski, 1995), although this report is notable for downplaying this embarrassing fact and, instead, emphasizing allegations of methodological weaknesses of the original. More recently, Pollay's (1996) report that teens were three times as responsive to cigarette advertising as adults drew instant and inaccurate attacks from the Tobacco Institute as "a great deal of sound and fury signifying nothing" and "flatly contradicted" by a study sponsored by R. J. Reynolds (Stolberg, 1996).

The standard response of the industry to concerns about children and cigarette advertising has been to insist that "kids just don't pay attention to cigarette ads. . . . (Our advertising) purpose is to get smokers of competitive products to switch . . . virtually the only way a cigarette brand can meaningfully increase its business" (R. J. Reynolds, 1984), a thesis uncritically echoed by some others (e.g., Boddewyn. 1986b). The belief and assertion is that cigarette advertising is of little consequence, at least with respect to the young (e.g., Boddewyn, 1989; Reid, 1989; Ward, 1989). This assertion, so counter to common sense, is argued on theoretical grounds. Because cigarettes seem to be a so-called "mature" industry, i.e., one which has completed its dynamic growth and reached a stasis, it is claimed that its advertising and promotional activity can and does affect only brand-switching behavior among established adult smokers. By neither intent nor effect, tobacco industry magnates would have us believe, does cigarette advertising influence young people, reassure and retain existing smokers who might otherwise quit, or induce current smokers to smoke more—several of the ways in which advertising might conceivably influence primary demand. . . .

## No Known Industry Documents Employ the "Mature Market" Concept

To date, no corporate documents have been produced in litigation or research reports to verify that the "mature market" classification is relied upon by the industry in its internal strategic analyses, nor has any evidence of any kind been offered in support of the "mature market" opinions expressed by industry-advanced experts like Ward (1989). Reid (1989), when testifying for the industry, ignored the literature equivocal about the concept's validity, the literature specific to the cigarette industry, and the contradictory profit and advertising expenditure data. He ignored all the many corporate documents produced in the same litigation documenting the consumer research and advertising strategies focused on young starters (Pollay & Lavack, 1993). He even ignored his own observation, surely fitting cigarettes, that given "the existence of an undesirable image, advertising can play a major role" (Reid & Rotfeld, 1976, p. 26). Testimony like this that offers theoretical conjectures, while ignoring the relevant literature and the available case facts, is not merely speculative, but quite literally ignorant and prejudicial. . . .

## Enormous Promotional Budgets Cannot Be Justified by "Adult Brand Switching" Alone

The cigarette market may seem, to the naive, to be stable and, therefore, to be a so-called "mature market" because total sales seem nearly constant. This appearance, however, hides the dynamics of substantial rates of quitting attempts, quitting successes, and dying—and the countervailing rates of recruitment of hundreds of thousands of new smokers. Maintaining constancy of market size involves recruiting over a million new smokers a year, and almost all smokers are recruited as minors, not as consenting adults.

Brand-switching alone cannot easily justify the enormous advertising and promotional expenditures, over $6 billion a year in 1993, larger than Hollywood's gross income from the United States and Canada combined (Kilday & Thompson, 1995). Brand switchers are an unattractive market segment, as they are typically older, health-concerned, or symptomatic smokers, thus relatively frail in constitution, in addition to being fickle by definition. They are also few in number. Siegel et al. (1996), after noting that less than 10 percent of smokers will switch in any

given year, estimate that the total profit from all "company switching" was $362 million, small compared to the costs of the battle of these brands. Accounting for sales in future years, the net present value of a new smoker to the cigarette companies has been estimated as US $1,085 (Tye, Warner, & Glantz, 1987).

If cigarette advertising had no effect on smoking recruitment, as the industry contends, a ban on advertising expenditures of this magnitude should and would be welcomed by savvy oligopolists like the tobacco industry. Indeed, a ban would benefit the larger firms the most, by saving them the enormous promotional expense and helping to freeze their large market shares. Thus, if advertising had no effect on primary demand, profit-maximizing firms and industries would curtail advertising competition, just as they would refrain from cut-throat price competition, and the largest firms would be expected to act as leaders in this self-restraint. Failing a tacit collusion to this end, the industry would eagerly seize the opportunity provided by regulatory proposals to ban advertising, with the larger firms the most motivated to do so. The fact that cigarette companies, led by the largest, are lobbying so hard against advertising bans or controls of any kind is illogical —unless the advertising and promotion has the effect of enticing new smokers. As Davis (1996, p. 3) stated: "The reason for the industry's failure to support a federal ban on tobacco advertising must be that . . . the companies must indeed perceive an industry-wide benefit to advertising and promotion." Failing that, they could save themselves all the spending on advertising that only attacked or defended market shares.

## No Isolation or Immunity Protects Youth from Cigarette Ads

There is no way to isolate teens and pre-teens from popular culture and media, including cigarette advertising's inducements. The absence of a "magic curtain" around children obviates any "convincing defense of a view that would make young nonsmokers immune" (Cohen, 1990, p. 240–241). Those empowered with self-regulatory responsibilities in the National Association of Broadcasters (NAB) saw this vividly for the medium of television: "The difficulty in cigarette advertising is that commercials which have an impact upon an adult cannot be assumed to leave unaffected a young viewer, smoker or otherwise" (Bell, 1966, p. 30–31). Even a Marlboro ad man admitted after retiring, "I don't know any way of doing this that doesn't tempt young people to smoke" (Daniels, 1974, p. 245). Consistent with these views, newer research indicates that the likelihood of adolescent smoking is related to ad exposure rates (Botvin et al., 1993).

## Advertising Gives the Cigarette "Friendly Familiarity"

Cigarette advertising is so pervasive and ubiquitous that cigarettes are a cultural commonplace, taken for granted by the public, and treated as less risky than appropriate. We are all aware of the reverse of this, when we feel suspicion of the unfamiliar. This positive effect is called "friendly familiarity" by advertising professionals (Burnett, 1961, p. 217).

"The ubiquitous display of messages promoting tobacco use clearly fosters an environment in which experimentation by youth is expected, if not explicitly encouraged" (Bonnie & Lynch, 1994, p. 34). "The kind of advertising that is al-most everywhere makes cigarets (*sic*) respectable and is therefore reassuring," according to Social Research Inc. (*Cigarets: who buys,* 1952, p. 23). Repetition, oft referred to as the soul of persuasion, likely biases both risk and social perceptions, such as assessments of smoking prevalence, and/or the social acceptance experienced by smokers, according to both consumer behavior and psychology experts (e.g., Cohen, 1990; Fishbein, 1977). This phenomenon is well known to psychologists as the "familiarity effect" (Zajonc, 1980).

## The Perceptions and Judgments of Youth Are Known to Be Biased

The young do, in fact, overestimate the prevalence of cigarette smoking among both peers and adults, and the degree of this overestimation is among the strongest predictors of smoking initiation (e.g., Chassin et al., 1984). They also underestimate the negative attitudes of peers and the risks to which they personally are exposed should they smoke. Youths are also inclined to manifest an "invulnerability syndrome" (Greening & Dollinger, 1991). Youths tend to both "exaggerate the social benefit (by overestimating the prevalence and popularity of smoking among peers and adults) and to underestimate the risks (by underestimating the prevalence of negative attitudes toward smoking held by their peers)" (Bonnie & Lynch, 1994, p. 34). Another literature review concludes that "cigarette advertising appears to influence young people's perceptions of the pervasiveness, image, and function of smoking. Since misperceptions in these areas constitute psychosocial risk factors for the initiation of smoking, cigarette advertising appears to increase young people's risk of smoking" (USDHHS,

1994, p. 195). These facts seriously undermine the notion that the uptake of smoking is an informed choice or decision (Leventhal, Glynn, & Fleming, 1987). Irrespective of this naiveté, it is a misbehavior of minors, not consenting adults.

## Cigarette Imagery Appeals to Adolescents

Cigarette ads often feature veritable pictures of health, depicting bold and lively behavior typically in pure and pristine outdoor environments (Pollay, 1991, 1993a; USDHHS 1994). The images of cigarette ads portray themes known to appeal to young people, such as independence, adventure seeking, social approval, and sophistication. The theme of independence, in particular, so well captured by the Marlboro Man, strikes a responsive chord with the dominant psychological need of adolescents for autonomy and freedom from authority. Adolescent girls feel the same needs for autonomy as do boys, accounting for the otherwise surprising popularity of the Marlboro brand among girls. Motivation research confirms the insights of previous advertisers and public relations professionals in seeing smoking as an expression of freedom and worldliness for women (Martineau, 1957). It seems no coincidence that marketers of female brands "try to tap the emerging independence and self-fulfillment of women, to make smoking a badge to express that" (Waldman, 1989, p. 81).

In addition, some of the models in cigarette advertisements appear particularly youthful (Mazis et al., 1992). This isn't all that common, however, as cigarette firms know that teens desire symbols of adulthood, not symbols of youth (e.g., hard rock vs. "bubble gum" music). Imagery-based ads are potentially insidious, in contrast to verbal assertions which require cognitive processing. Imagery is taken in at a glance, experienced more than thought about, tending to "bypass logical analysis." Because of this, imagery advertising is deemed "transformational" rather than informational (Cohen, 1990). The old adage says "seeing is believing," and cigarette ads use carefully tuned images to create positive experiences, while being careful to avoid precipitating cognitive counter-argumentation.

## The Tobacco Industry Has Long Displayed a Strategic Interest in Youth

The industry has demonstrated an interest in the youth market in its planning documents, market research activities, and media plans for many decades (USDHHS, 1994, Pollay, 1995). Ads have been placed on billboards near schools and malls, and in after-school radio spots with effective reach into youth markets. The TV advertising schedules bought in the 1960s reflected a preference for those times with the higher proportions of delivered teenagers, not adults (Pollay, 1994a, 1994b). R. J. Reynolds' 1973 "Research Planning Document on Some Thoughts about New Brands for the Youth Market" described programs for appealing to "learning smokers" (Schwartz, 1995). Philip Morris found that almost half of the non-smoking girls "share many of the same values as the smokers and are highly exposed to the total smoking environment. We call them the 'Vulnerables' for, on the surface, they appear to be ready candidates for the next wave of new smokers" (Udow, 1976, H7664).

Copy concepts for many brands focus on independence, with the adolescent need for autonomy and self-reliance known by the industry to be a dominant one (USDHHS, 1994). The success of starter brands, according to trial evidence, is the result of carefully planned and executed strategies, guided throughout by extensive research (Pollay & Lavack, 1993). Corporate research documents discuss the behavior, knowledge, and attitudes of eleven-, twelve-, and thirteen-year-olds and media plans specify targets beginning at age fifteen, with willingness to pay as much for ad exposures to fifteen-year-old nonsmokers as to smokers. R. J. Reynolds' Canadian affiliate, for example, commissioned customization of "Youth Target Study '87" and got extensive data on subjects as young as fifteen.

The need to have a strategic interest in youth has long been recognized by the industry, and used to be freely admitted to. For example, just before the Surgeon General's Report of 1964, an advertising trade magazine, *Sponsor* ("What will happen," 1963), noted pro-health education with concern and asked: "If, however, impressionable youngsters are now approached mostly by the anti-smoking fraternity, how will cigarette sales fare 10 years hence?" Note, too, that this also demonstrates the long time spans appropriate in understanding cigarette advertising's effects, which are generational rather than instantaneous, inculcative rather than impulse-generating.

## Adolescence Is a Time of Identity Formation and Advertising Attentiveness

"Cigarette advertising's cultural function is much more than the selling of cigarettes. Its collective images represent a corpus of deeply rooted cultural mythologies that are not simply pieces of advertising creativity, but icons that pose solutions to real, experienced problems of identity" (Chapman & Fitzgerald, 1982, p. 494). The National Association of Broadcasters knew this when trying to help the industry self-regulate TV ads. "The adult world depicted in cigarette advertising very often is a world to which the adolescent aspires.... To the young, smoking indeed may seem to be an important step towards, and a help in growth from adolescence to maturity" (Bell, 1966, p. 30–31).

Youths are alert to popular culture for cues and clues as to what's hot and what's not. They attend to advertising for symbols of adulthood, but pay only scant attention to warnings (Fletcher et al., 1995). "Teens are also more susceptible to the images of romance, success, sophistication, popularity, and adventure which advertising suggests they could achieve through the consumption of cigarettes" (Nichter & Cartwright, 1991, p. 242). Even brief cigarette ad exposures in lab settings can result in more favorable thoughts about smokers, enhance attitudes, increase awareness and change brand preferences of the young (Hoek, Gendall, & Stockdale, 1993; Pechmann & Ratneshwar, 1994).

This is consistent with consumer behavior knowledge as reflected in textbooks and journals. "Teenagers have become increasingly aware of new products and brands. They are natural 'triers'" (Loudon & Della Bitta, 1993, p. 151). They have "a lot of uncertainty about the self, and the need to belong and to find one's unique identity... (so) teens actively search for cues from their peers and from advertising for the right way to look and behave... (becoming) interested in many different products" that can express their needs for "experimentation, belonging, independence, responsibility, and approval from others" (Solomon, 1994, pp. 503–504). By high school, possessions and "badge products" like cigarettes are used as instruments for defining and controlling relations between people (Stacey, 1982).

As a 1974 RJR memo states: "To some extent young smokers 'wear' their cigarette and it becomes an important part of the 'I' they wish to be, along with their clothing and the way they style their hair" (Schwartz, 1996, p. A3). One starter brand in Canada, according to the R. J. Reynolds affiliate who marketed it, was popular with "very young starter smokers... because it provides them with an instant badge of masculinity, appeals to their rebellious nature and establishes their position amongst their peers" (Pollay & Lavack, 1993, pp. 268–269). Adults, in contrast, are not caught up in the processes of identity experimentation and formation. They are not as searching of their environment for consumption items symbolic of aspirational identities.

The image and badge aspects of brands are especially important to ethnic minorities. "While this is of utmost importance when marketing cigarettes in general, we feel it assumes even more importance when marketing cigarettes to blacks. Because blacks in general tend to be more insecure, for obvious reasons, it is critical that the public cigarette badge they adopt be one that supports what they are looking for in terms of psychological reassurance" (Reeves, 1979, p. 3). Thus, the Newport name has the virtue of connoting "quality and class," because of associations with status symbols such as Newport Beach and the Newport Jazz Festivals.

### Youths Are Persuasion-Coping Novices

The young, as consumers, tend to be less experienced in counterarguing against advertising and selling tactics, as well as more brand-conscious than older consumers (Brucks, Armstrong, & Goldberg, 1988; McNeal, 1992). They are also less experienced as shoppers, with fewer experiences of salesmen and persuasion tactics. Friestad and Wright (1994, p. 7) note that "novices in coping with advertising or selling encounters may recognize only simple, superficial patterns in these events and have little proficiency with self-regulatory processes... (and) coping strategies." Adults, with their longer histories, particularly as smokers, have less interest in, and greater resistance to, the temptations and appeals of most new brands and/or ad campaigns.

### Cigarette Addictiveness and Brand Loyalty Make Adults Proverbial "Old Dogs"

Cigarettes enjoy phenomenally high brand loyalty, the highest of all consumer products (e.g., Alsop, 1989). A relatively low rate of brand switching is the norm, usually 10 percent or less (Cohen, 1990, p. 239; FTC, 1985; Gardner, 1984; Siegel et al., 1996). Some of this nominal switching occurs only within brand families (e.g. from Brand X milds to Brand X lights), and is of little net consequence to the firm's sales or net profit. The high brand loyalty that naturally results from nicotine "satisfaction" of addictive physiological needs makes it very difficult and expensive to convert competitors' customers to your brands. Also, the bulk of the brand switching is the behavior of older, health-concerned or symptomatic smokers who are trading down, typically within a brand family, to products with lower tar and nicotine labeling, in the mistaken belief that those products are safe(r), a belief fostered by years of advertising.

## Youths Are Strategically More Attractive Than Adults

The trade of these older customers offers firms very little future and net present value, compared with the value inherent in attracting young starters, the bulk of whom will be brand-loyal (Tye, Warner, & Glantz, 1987). "This is a time when brand loyalties may be formed that could last well into adulthood" (Loudon & Della Bitta, 1993, p. 152, citing Moschis & Moore, 1981). The young are a "perpetually new market... thus a marketer must not neglect young consumers who come 'on stream' if the company's brand is to have continued success in the older-age market" (Loudon & Della Bitta, 1993, p. 155). Teens are a strategically important target audience, because brand loyalty is often developed during this time and this creates a "barrier-to-entry for other brands not chosen during these pivotal years" (Solomon, 1994, p. 504).

The death and quitting rates among aging smokers means that sales would drop rapidly were it not for a continuing influx of new starters. This strategic situation has been obvious to the industry for some time. R. J. Reynolds' research and development officers wrote in 1973: "Realistically, if our Company is to survive and prosper, over the long term, we must get our share of the youth market" (Schwartz, 1995). Contemporary corporate documents echo this idea, stating that "young smokers represent the major opportunity group for the cigarette industry," and "if the last ten years have taught us anything, it is that the industry is dominated by the companies who respond most effectively to the needs of younger smokers" (Pollay & Lavack, 1993, p. 267).

## Teens Are Three Times More Responsive Than Adults to Cigarette Ads

The latest research (Pollay et al., 1996) uses state-of-the-art techniques to analyze market share as a function of relative advertising, also known as *share of voice*. This measures the impact of cigarette brand advertising on realized market shares, allowing for both current and historical effects of advertising for nine major brands over twenty years. The results, which are robust under many alternative assumptions, show that brand choices among teenagers are significantly related to relative cigarette advertising. Moreover, the relationship between brand choices and brand advertising is significantly stronger among teenagers than among adults by a factor of about three. The greater advertising sensitivity among teenagers is in part due to *scale* (i.e., high fractions of teens concentrated on highly advertised brands), and in part due to *dynamics* (i.e., teen purchase patterns being more responsive to changes in advertising intensity). Further, the impact of advertising on brand choices among youth apparently cannot be dismissed as an inappropriate attribution (i.e., teenagers actually imitating adult brand choices rather than responding to advertising). Even when this aspect is factored into the analysis, the result remains consistent.

Greater advertising sensitivity among youth is consistent with earlier observations that brand choices of youth are highly concentrated on the most heavily advertised brands (CDC, 1992,

1994). California's Operation Storefront also found that "heavy advertising in stores exactly matches the brand preferences of children who smoke... but the ad prevalence does not match adult smoker preferences" (Hilts, 1995, p. B10). "Young people know advertising better, appreciate brand-stretching advertising more," and their ideal self-image matches the images offered by cigarette brands (Rombouts & Fauconnier, 1988; see also Aitken et al., 1987). A recent study (Pierce & Gilpin, 1995a, 1995b; Pierce, Lee, & Gilpin, 1994) reported data indicating that smoking rates among young women increased sharply in the late 1960s, coincidental with the launch of Virginia Slims and other nominally "female" brands.

## Industry Apologists Typically Offer Weak Research, or None at All

The so-called "experts" that the industry gets to testify in courts and before legislative groups almost always offer opinions that are conspicuously ignorant of true corporate activity. Instead they opine based upon simplistic theorizing and conclusions. Martin told a court that cigarette ads can be of no appreciable import, no matter what their content or character, insulting the competencies of many advertising agencies, and judging their diverse efforts as all failing to alter public perceptions of the product, either individually or collectively. Perhaps the most simplistic and common position used to exculpate the industry is the "mature market" theory, discussed above, typically asserted with no corroborating evidence, perhaps because there is none to be had.

The industry has long relied on Boddewyn to argue that cigarette advertising doesn't influence children, but the survey methodology and logic reported in Boddewyn (1987) is totally inadequate, biased, and superficial. This research was sponsored by the international tobacco industry lobbying organization, conducted by a British contract research firm, and published by an American advocacy organization, not by a peer-reviewed scholarly journal or scientific body. Its conclusion is based solely on a self-report question asking children to select, from a list of thirteen offered reasons, only the most important reason for smoking their first cigarette. This question is, to my knowledge, without precedent in either academic research or trade practice as the sole means of validly assessing advertising's role and effects. Not surprisingly, few choose "I had seen advertising" as the most compelling reason, since to do so requires that advertising's influence be consciously appreciated, willingly admitted to, and predominant among all of the prompted reasons, rather than just a contributing factor. One wonders how many might have agreed or disagreed with a statement like "advertising makes cigarettes seem attractive." While the apologists for the cigarette industry have ignored this grievous weakness, they dramatically raise their critical methodological standards when encountering results threatening their tobacco clients' economic or legal interests (e.g., Boddewyn, 1989). Martin (1993), for example, took the initiative to canvas researchers with a detailed questionnaire soliciting criticism of Pierce et al. (1991), who had found the cartoon Camel well known to the very young, while never commenting on the fallaciousness of Boddewyn's data and conclusions, and his client's political use of same....

## Advertising Experts and Trade Journals Doubt the Industry's Stance

Many ad executives, when confronted with the pioneering Surgeon General's Report, admitted that cigarette advertising influenced minors. John Orr Young, whose agency, Young & Rubicam, had cigarette experience, said that: "Advertising agencies are retained by cigaret (sic) manufacturers to create demand for cigarets among both adults and eager youngsters. The earlier the teenage-boy or girl gets the habit, the bigger the national sales volume" ("Agency would refuse," 1964a). Another leading advertising executive, the president of Mc-Manus, Johns, & Adams felt that "There is no doubt that all forms of advertising played a part in popularizing the cigaret (sic)" ("Make cigarets," 1964b).

Emerson Foote, a founder of Foote, Cone, and Belding, and later CEO of McCann-Erikson, bluntly debunked the industry claims that its advertising affects only brand switching and has no effect whatsoever on recruitment. "I don't think anyone really believes this... I suspect that creating a positive climate of social acceptability for smoking, which encourages new smokers to join the market, is of greater importance to the industry.... In recent years the cigarette industry has been artfully maintaining that cigarette advertising has nothing to do with total sales. Take my word for it, this is complete and utter nonsense" (Foote, 1981).

More currently, one advertising CEO comments generally that cigarette advertising is "even sicker than war. If you were to choose the ultimate insanity of our society, I'd put cigarette advertising at the top" (Horovitz, 1996). Another wrote about the cartoon Camel: "Those of us in the marketing business know exactly what he's up to; we should be the first to denounce him" (DesRoches, 1994). A Philip Morris executive adds, "You don't have to be a brain surgeon to see what's going on. Just look at the ads. It's ludicrous for them to deny that a cartoon character like Joe Camel isn't attractive to kids" (Ecanbarger, 1993). This cartoon campaign has been described as "one of the most egregious examples in recent history of tobacco advertising targeted at children," encouraging even *Advertising Age* editors to urge that it be dropped (Cohen, 1994, p. 12).

## The Industry's Latest Position Is Illogical and Ludicrous

The industry and its spokespersons would now have us believe that they have no influence at all on smoking onset, but that both their intent and the effect is exclusively on brand choice among existing smokers, now apparently admitted to include minors. When Pollay et al. (1996) reported on the impact of advertising on teens, a coalition of advertising groups, the Freedom to Advertise Coalition, said it "proves what we have been saying all along —that tobacco advertising is geared to influence market share among those people who already smoke" (Stolberg, 1996). This is saying that the firms' intentions and abilities are such that "we don't encourage children to smoke, only to switch brands." This has been satirized in editorial cartoons as a denial that cigarette advertisers entice kids to start smoking, because their marketing is aimed precisely at the second cigarette they smoke, not the first.

Research shows that the very young are aware of cigarette icons and associate these with both the product and brand. We also know that teens who have started smoking are substantially more affected by cigarette advertising than are adult smokers. Are the ones having their attitudes shaped at an early age all destined to make the perverse decision, from the advertisers' view, not to become smokers? Are the only ones who start smoking those who have had no awareness of, or attraction to, cigarette advertising they were exposed to while growing up (if, indeed, there can even be such a group of people)? Are those who start smoking, presumably despite their blindness and/or numbness to prior cigarette promotion, supposed to become instantly hypersensitive to it? Are we to believe that the children who have ignored advertising throughout their formative years suddenly are the only ones impacted by it?

As the perceptions, attitudes, and beliefs governing brand choice are influenced by cigarette advertising, it is totally implausible that those same brand perceptions, attitudes, and beliefs have no influence whatsoever on the temptation to start smoking. It is impossible to advertise a specific brand without also simultaneously advertising cigarettes as a product class. A Philip Morris marketing vice president, famous for managing Marlboro's success, once said, "A cigarette company's ads are not just competing with ads for other brands. You are competing with every other advertiser in America for a share of the consumer's mind" (Whiteside, 1974, p. 133). Advertising that makes a cigarette brand attractive inevitably also makes cigarette smoking attractive, at the very least the smoking of that brand. There is no known way to advertise so that only brand switching, but not product interest, is affected.

## CONCLUSION

Creating the illusion of controversy is a worn-out tactic, and ought to be treated with incredulous cynicism by scholars and policymakers. In fact, there seems to be far less controversy about the role of advertising than a strong convergence of diverse streams of research and analysis. Strategic analysis indicates that new users are far more attractive to firms than the few, frail and fickle brand switchers. Historical analysis documents the industry's long-standing strategic interest in youth. Analysis of contemporary corporate documents shows this to be an intensifying interest, for it is among minors where virtually all starting of smoking occurs, and starting now occurs at younger ages than ever before. Content analyses of advertising show that cigarette advertising imagery is largely pictures of health and images of independence, known by the industry to resonate with adolescent needs for autonomy and freedom from authority. Behavioral analyses show that cigarette advertising constitutes a psychosocial risk factor. Not only is teen smoking behavior related to past and present advertising, but also this relationship is about three times stronger among teens than among adults. Meta-analysis has shown cigarette advertising elasticity to be positive.

This has important public policy implications. Whether intended or not, cigarette advertising is significantly related to youth smoking behavior. To the extent that advertising influences the use of cigarettes among a consumer group to whom their sale is illegal, the government has a legitimate interest in regulating cigarette advertising. Convergent analyses and results suggest that regulating cigarette advertising may be an effective policy intervention to influence smoking behavior among adolescents. This should at least address advertising whose character is likely to appeal to the young, and placement in media where exposure to the young is inevitable. The authors of the Institute of Medicine's literature review recommend that this be done at federal, state, and local levels, although this would require repealing current pre-emptive federal legislation (Bonnie & Lynch, 1994). For more on legislative options with respect to tobacco advertising, see Arbogast (1986), Blum and Myers (1993), Burns (1994), and Pytte (1990).

Given the many various analyses and diversity of evidence, it seems an inescapable conclusion that cigarette advertising plays a meaningful role in influencing the perceptions, attitudes, and smoking behavior of youth. It also seems appropriate for scholars to react to assertions that there are no such effects on youth with disbelief, and to suspect industry sponsorship as a likely basis for such assertions.

# NO

Jacob Sullum

## COWBOYS, CAMELS, AND KIDS

On January 1, 1971, the Marlboro Man rode across the television screen one last time. At midnight a congressional ban on broadcast advertising of cigarettes went into effect, and the smoking cowboy was banished to the frozen land of billboards and print ads. With the deadline looming, bleary-eyed, hung-over viewers across the country woke to a final burst of cigarette celebration. "Philip Morris went on a $1.25-million ad binge New Year's Day on the Dick Cavett, Johnny Carson and Merv Griffin shows," *The New York Times* reported. "There was a surfeit of cigarette ads during the screening of the bowl games." And then they were gone. American TV viewers would no longer be confronted by happy smokers frolicking on the beach or by hapless smokers losing the tips of their extra-long cigarettes between cymbals and elevator doors. They would no longer have to choose between good grammar and good taste.

This was widely considered an important victory for consumers. The *Times* wondered whether the ad ban was "a signal that the voice of the consumer, battling back, can now really make itself heard in Washington." A *New Yorker* article tracing the chain of events that led to the ban concluded, "To an increasing degree, citizens of the consumer state seem to be perceiving their ability to turn upon their manipulators, to place widespread abuses of commercial privilege under the prohibition of laws that genuinely do protect the public, and, in effect, to give back to the people a sense of controlling their own lives."

As these comments suggest, supporters of the ban viewed advertising not as a form of communication but as a mysterious force that seduces people into acting against their interests. This was a common view then and now, popularized by social critics such as Vance Packard and John Kenneth Galbraith. In *The Affluent Society* (1958), Galbraith argued that manufacturers produce goods and then apply "ruthless psychological pressures" through advertising to create demand for them. In *The Hidden Persuaders* (1957), Packard described advertising as an increasingly precise method of manipulation that can circumvent the conscious mind, influencing consumers without their awareness. He reinforced his portrait of Madison Avenue guile with the

From Jacob Sullum, "Cowboys, Camels, and Kids," *Reason* (April 1998). Copyright © 1998 by The Reason Foundation, 3415 S. Sepulveda Boulevard., Suite 400, Los Angeles, CA 90034. www.reason.com. Reprinted by permission.

pseudoscientific concept of subliminal messages: seen but not seen, invisibly shaping attitudes and actions. The impact of such ideas can be seen in the controversy over tobacco advertising. The federal court that upheld the ban on broadcast ads for cigarettes quoted approvingly from another ruling that referred to "the subliminal impact of this pervasive propaganda."

Eliminating TV and radio commercials for cigarettes, of course, did not eliminate criticism of tobacco advertising. In 1985 the American Cancer Society, which decades earlier had called for an end to cigarette ads through "voluntary self-regulation," endorsed a government ban on all forms of tobacco advertising and promotion. The American Medical Association, the American Public Health Association, the American Heart Association, and the American Lung Association also began advocating a ban. Beginning in the mid-'80s, members of Congress introduced legislation that would have prohibited tobacco advertising, limited it to "tombstone" messages (black text on a white background), or reduced its tax deductibility. None of these bills got far.

In the '90s, since Congress did not seem inclined to impose further censorship on the tobacco companies, David Kessler, commissioner of the Food and Drug Administration, decided to do it by bureaucratic fiat. Reversing the FDA's longstanding position, he declared that the agency had jurisdiction over tobacco products. In August 1996 the FDA issued regulations aimed at imposing sweeping restrictions on the advertising and promotion of cigarettes and smokeless tobacco. Among other things, the regulations prohibited promotional items such as hats, T-shirts, and lighters; forbade brand-name sponsorship of sport-

ing events; banned outdoor advertising within 1,000 feet of a playground, elementary school, or high school; and imposed a tombstone format on all other outdoor signs, all indoor signs in locations accessible to minors, and all print ads except those in publications with a negligible audience under the age of 18.

The tobacco companies challenged the regulations in federal court, and in April 1997 U.S. District Judge William L. Osteen ruled that the FDA had no statutory authority to regulate the advertising and promotion of "restricted devices," the category in which the agency had placed cigarettes and smokeless tobacco. Under the nationwide liability settlement proposed last summer, however, the tobacco companies agreed not only to the FDA rules but to additional restrictions, including bans on outdoor ads, on the use of human or cartoon figures, on Internet advertising, and on product placement in movies, TV shows, or video games. Congress is considering that proposal now, and any legislation that emerges will dramatically change the way tobacco companies promote their products. Not content to wait, cities across the country, including New York, Chicago, and San Francisco, are imposing their own limits on cigarette signs and billboards. Elsewhere, the European Union plans to ban almost all forms of tobacco advertising by 2006.

These restrictions are based on the premise that fewer ads will mean fewer smokers—in particular, that teenagers will be less inclined to smoke if they are not exposed to so many images of rugged cowboys and pretty women with cigarettes. As a PTA official put it in 1967, "The constant seduction of cigarette advertising... gives children the idea that cigarettes are associated with all they hold dear—beauty, popularity, sex, athletic success." For three decades the debate over tobacco advertising has been driven by such concerns. Yet there is remarkably little evidence that people smoke because of messages from tobacco companies. The ready acceptance of this claim reflects a widespread view of advertising as a kind of magic that casts a spell on consumers and leads them astray.

Today's critics of capitalism continue to elaborate on the theme that Vance Packard and John Kenneth Galbraith got so much mileage out of in the '50s and '60s. Alan Thein Durning of the anti-growth Worldwatch Institute describes the "salient characteristics" of advertising this way: "It preys on the weaknesses of its host. It creates an insatiable hunger. And it leads to debilitating over-consumption. In the biological realm, things of that nature are called parasites." When combined with appeals to protect children, this perception of advertising as insidious and overpowering tends to squelch any lingering concerns about free speech.

## Busting Joe Camel's Hump

In 1988, R. J. Reynolds gave the anti-smoking movement an emblem for the corrupting influence of tobacco advertising. Introduced with the slogan "smooth character," Joe Camel was a cartoon version of the dromedary (known as Old Joe) that has appeared on packages of Camel cigarettes since 1913. Print ads and billboards depicted Joe Camel shooting pool in a tuxedo, hanging out at a nightclub, playing in a blues band, sitting on a motorcycle in a leather jacket and shades. He was portrayed as cool, hip, and popular —in short, he was like a lot of other models in a lot of other cigarette ads, except he

was a cartoon animal instead of a flesh-and-blood human being. Even in that respect he was hardly revolutionary. More than a century before the debut of Joe Camel, historian Jordan Goodman notes, the manufacture of Bull Durham smoking tobacco ran newspaper ads throughout the country depicting the Durham Bull "in anthropomorphic situations, alternating between scenes in which the bull was jovial and boisterous and those where he was serious and determined."

But Joe Camel, it is safe to say, generated more outrage than any other cartoon character in history. Critics of the ad campaign said the use of a cartoon was clearly designed to appeal to children. *Washington Post* columnist Courtland Milloy said "packaging a cartoon camel as a 'smooth character' is as dangerous as putting rat poison in a candy wrapper." In response to such criticism, R. J. Reynolds noted that Snoopy sold life insurance and the Pink Panther pitched fiberglass insulation, yet no one assumed those ads were aimed at kids.

The controversy intensified in 1991, when *The Journal of the American Medical Association* published three articles purporting to show that Joe Camel was indeed a menace to the youth of America. The heavily promoted studies generated an enormous amount of press coverage, under headlines such as "Camels for Kids" (*Time*), "I'd Toddle a Mile for a Camel" (*Newsweek*), "Joe Camel Is Also Pied Piper, Research Finds" (*The Wall Street Journal*), and "Study: Camel Cartoon Sends Kids Smoke Signals" (*Boston Herald*). Dozens of editorialists and columnists condemned Joe Camel, and many said he should be banned from advertising.

In March 1992 the Coalition on Smoking or Health, a joint project of the American Cancer Society, the American Heart Association, and the American Lung Association, asked the Federal Trade Commission to prohibit further use of the smooth character. Surgeon General Antonia Novello and the American Medical Association also called for an end to the campaign. In August 1993 the FTC's staff backed the coalition's petition, and a month later 27 state attorneys general added their support. In June 1994, by a 3-to-2 vote, the FTC decided not to proceed against Joe, finding that the record did not show he had increased smoking among minors. (During the first five years of the campaign, in fact, teenage smoking actually declined, starting to rise only in 1993.) In March 1997, after several members of Congress asked the FTC to reexamine the issue, the commission's staff again urged a ban, citing new evidence that R. J. Reynolds had targeted underage smokers. This time the commission, with two new members appointed by the Clinton administration, decided to seek an order instructing RJR not only to keep Joe out of children's sight but to conduct a "public education campaign" aimed at deterring underage smoking.

The two dissenting commissioners were not impressed by the new evidence, which failed to show that Joe Camel had actually encouraged kids to smoke. One wrote, "As was true three years ago, intuition and concern for children's health are not the equivalent of—and should not be substituted for—evidence sufficient to find reason to believe that there is likely causal connection between the Joe Camel advertising campaign and smoking by children." But the FTC's action turned out to be doubly irrelevant. R. J. Reynolds, along with its competitors, agreed to stop using cartoon characters as part of the proposed nationwide settlement, and last July it announced that it was discontinuing the "smooth character" campaign, replacing it with one that makes more subtle use of camels.

Although the *JAMA* articles were widely cited by Joe's enemies, including the FTC and President Clinton, they proved much less than the uproar would lead one to believe. In the first study, researchers led by Paul M. Fischer, a professor of family medicine at the Medical College of Georgia, asked preschoolers to match brand logos to pictures of products. Overall, about half the kids correctly matched Joe Camel with a cigarette. Among the 6-year-olds, the share was 91 percent, about the same as the percentage who correctly matched the Disney Channel logo to a picture of Mickey Mouse.

But recognizing Joe Camel is not tantamount to smoking, any more than recognizing the logos for Ford and Chevrolet (which most of the kids also did) is tantamount to driving. The researchers seemed to assume that familiarity breeds affection, but that is not necessarily the case. A subsequent study, funded by R. J. Reynolds and published in the Fall 1995 *Journal of Marketing*, confirmed that recognition of Joe Camel rises with age and that most 6-year-olds correctly associate him with cigarettes. Yet 85 percent of the kids in this study had a negative attitude toward cigarettes, and the dislike rose with both age and recognition ability. Among the 6-year-olds, less than 4 percent expressed a positive attitude toward cigarettes.

### Animal Magnetism

In the second *JAMA* study, Joseph R. DiFranza, researcher at the University of

Massachusetts Medical School, led a team that showed Joe Camel ads to samples of high school students and adults. They found that the teenagers were more likely to recognize Joe Camel, to recall the ads, and to evaluate them positively than the adults, whose average age was about 40. Since R. J. Reynolds contended that the Joe Camel campaign was aimed at young adults, these results were hardly surprising. Based on such comparisons, it is impossible to distinguish between an ad aimed at 16-year-olds and an ad aimed at 18-year-olds (or 21-year-olds).

DiFranza et al.'s most striking claim was that the Joe Camel campaign had caused a huge shift in brand preferences. Using data from seven surveys conducted in three states between 1976 and 1988, they estimated that 0.5 percent of underage smokers preferred Camels before the campaign began. By comparison, 33 percent of the teenage smokers in their study, conducted during 1990 and 1991, said they smoked Camels—a *66-fold* increase. "Our data demonstrate than in just 3 years Camel's Old Joe cartoon character had an astounding influence on children's smoking behavior," the researchers wrote. But the pre-1989 surveys and the *JAMA* study were not comparable, and neither used random samples of the national population, so it's doubtful that the results are representative of American teenagers in general. Data from the Centers for Disease Control and Prevention's Teenage Attitudes and Practices Survey, which does use a nationwide sample, suggest a much less dramatic (though still sizable) shift toward Camels. In 1993, 13.3 percent of the TAPS respondents said they usually bought Camels, compared to 8.1 percent in 1989.

The third *JAMA* article presented data from a 1990 California telephone survey. The researchers, led by John P. Pierce, head of the University of California at San Diego's Cancer Prevention and Control Program, reported that teenagers were more likely than adults to identify Marlboro or Camel as the most advertised brand. The survey also found that Marlboro's market share increased with age until 24, when it started to decline gradually. Camel, on the other hand, was considerably more popular among teenagers than among young adults. Comparing the California data to the results of a national survey conducted in 1986, Pierce et al. concluded that the market shares for both Marlboro and Camel had increased among adults (the 1986 survey did not include minors). Camel's increase was bigger, particularly among adults under the age of 30 (i.e., the segment R. J. Reynolds claimed to be targeting).

Taken together, these studies suggested that 1) most children know Joe Camel has something to do with cigarettes and 2) the Joe Camel campaign helped increase the brand's market share, especially among young smokers. Since most smokers pick up the habit before they turn 18, it seems likely that the tobacco companies would take an interest in the brand choices of teenagers, and that inference is supported by internal documents. In 1974, for example, Philip Morris hired the Roper Organization to interview young smokers about their brand choices, and more than a third of the 1,879 respondents were described as 18 or younger. "To ensure increased and longer-term growth for Camel filter," said a 1975 RJR memo, "the brand must increase its share penetration among the 14–24 age groups, which have a new set of more liberal values and which represent tomorrow's cigarette business." Last year, as part of an agreement settling state lawsuits, the Liggett Group said tobacco companies have deliberately targeted underage smokers.

The other companies continued to deny that charge. R. J. Reynolds maintained that Joe Camel was aimed at 18-to-24-year-olds, although the company had no way of assuring that he would not also appeal to people younger than 18. In response, David Kessler told ABC's Peter Jennings, "Tell me how you design an advertising campaign that affects only 18-year-olds." Which is sort of the point. If cigarette companies have to avoid any ad that might catch the eye or tickle the fancy of a 16-year-old, they might as well not advertise at all (which would suit Kessler fine). In any case, the important question is whether advertising encourages teenagers to smoke, not whether it steers them toward Camels instead of Marlboros.

In each of the Joe Camel studies, the researchers' conclusions (and the subsequent press coverage) went beyond what the data indicated. Fischer et al., whose comparison between Joe Camel and Mickey Mouse got the most attention, were relatively cautious: "Given the serious health consequences of smoking, the exposure of children to environmental tobacco advertising may represent an important health risk and should be studied further." DiFranza et al. said, "A total ban of tobacco advertising and promotions, as part of an effort to protect children from the dangers of tobacco, can be based on sound scientific reasoning." Pierce et al. flatly concluded that "[c]igarette advertising encourages youth to smoke and should be banned." These are all statements of opinion that

have little to do with what the studies actually showed.

Information that came to light in a lawsuit challenging the Joe Camel campaign (a case that R. J. Reynolds settled for $10 million in September) suggests that at least some of the researchers may have prejudged the issue. In a letter he wrote to a coauthor before the research began, DiFranza complained that he had not been able to give reporters "proof that the tobacco companies are advertising to children. I can't point to any one piece of evidence as a smoking gun and say 'here, this proves it.' Well I have an idea for a project that will give us a couple of smoking guns to bring to the national media." He explained, "I am proposing a quick and easy project that should produce... evidence that RJR is going after kids with their Camel ads." Toward the end of the letter, he said, "There, the paper is all ready, now all we need is some data."

## Switching Arguments

Neither DiFranza's "smoking gun" nor the other studies provided any evidence about the impact of advertising on a teenager's propensity to smoke, which is the crux of the issue. When critics complain that advertising encourages people to smoke, the tobacco companies reply that it encourages smokers to buy particular brands. Strictly speaking, these claims are not mutually exclusive. In principle, advertising can promote an industry's overall sales as well as drum up business for a specific company. An ad for a Compaq portable computer might encourage people to buy a Compaq (the company certainly hopes so), or it might get them thinking about laptops generally. But the tobacco companies argue that the U.S. market for cigarettes is mature, meaning that the product is universally familiar, like toothpaste or deodorant, and attempts to boost overall consumption are no longer cost-effective. Indeed, with smoking rates declining, the tobacco companies are fighting for pieces of a shrinking pie. Tobacco's opponents say this trend makes cigarette manufacturers all the more desperate to maintain their profits; they need advertising like the Joe Camel campaign to attract replacements for smokers who quit or die.

Advocates of an advertising ban contend that brand competition does not adequately explain the industry's spending on advertising and promotion, which totals about $5 billion a year. In 1995, the most recent year for which the Federal Trade Commission has reported figures, coupons, customer premiums (lighters, key chains, clothing, etc.), and allowances to distributors accounted for about 80 percent of this money. Cigarette companies spent about $900 million on newspaper, magazine, outdoor, transit, direct-mail, and point-of-sale advertising.

According to a widely cited article published in the Winter 1987 *Journal of Public Health Policy*, "A simple calculation shows that brand-switching, alone, could never justify the enormous advertising and promotional expenditures of the tobacco companies." Anti-smoking activist Joe B. Tye and his co-authors started with an estimate, based on marketing research, that about 10 percent of smokers switch brands each year. Then they calculated that the industry's spending on advertising and promotion in 1983 amounted to nearly as much per switcher as a typical smoker would have spent on cigarettes that year. They also noted that, since each cigarette maker produces various brands,

smokers who switch are not necessarily taking their business to another company.

"Thus," the authors concluded, "advertising and promotion can be considered economically rational only if they perform a defensive function—retaining company brand loyalty that would otherwise be lost to competitors who promote their products—of if they attract new entrants to the smoking marketplace, or discourage smokers from quitting." If defending market share were the only aim, Tye et al. added, the tobacco companies should support a ban on advertising and promotion, which would eliminate the threat from competitors. On the other hand, "If advertising and promotion increase cigarette consumption, then less than two million new or retained smokers—5.5 percent of smokers who start each year or try to quit (most failing)—alone would justify the annual promotional expenditure."

There are several flaws in this argument. To begin with, the estimate for the number of brand switchers does not include people who usually smoke, say, Benson & Hedges but occasionally smoke Camels. Based on its own marketing surveys, R. J. Reynolds reports that about 70 percent of smokers have a second-choice brand that they smoke now and then. About 25 percent regularly buy more than one brand each month. Even smokers who don't have a second favorite sometimes try other brands because of coupons, premiums, and promotional offers.

Another problem is that, in estimating the value of brand switchers, Tye et al. did not take into account the continuing revenue from a new customer; they considered only the money he spends on cigarettes in one year. By contrast, when they estimated the gain from getting someone to start smoking or keeping a smoker who otherwise would have quit, they used the net present value of the additional profit over a 20-year period, which they calculated as $1,085, more than three times a year's revenue.

Most important, Tye el al. did not acknowledge that tobacco companies could be competing for new smokers without actually creating them. Although the companies deny that they target minors in any way, building brand loyalty among teenagers is still not the same thing as making them into smokers.

Tye et al. considered the industry's opposition to an advertising ban prima facie evidence that tobacco advertising increases total consumption. But the tobacco companies might also have opposed a ban because it would help delegitimize the industry, opening the way to other kinds of regulation and defeats in product liability suits. Furthermore, a company's attitude toward restrictions on advertising (and brand competition in general) depends on its market position. Philip Morris and R. J. Reynolds, the market leaders, might well be less worried about an advertising ban than their competitors. Tellingly, these were the companies that spearheaded the settlement talks, and they included dramatic restrictions on advertising and promotion in their opening offer.

In any case, it is not clearly foolish for the tobacco companies to spend so much money on advertising and promotion, even without the hope of market expansion. More evidence is necessary to support the claim that tobacco advertising increases consumption. Broadly speaking, there are three ways of investigating this issue. You can look at the historical relationship between changes in advertising and changes in smoking. You can com-

pare smoking trends in places with different levels of advertising. And you can ask people questions in the hope that their answers will suggest how advertising influences attitudes and behavior. None of these approaches has yielded consistent or definitive results. Each has limitations that leave plenty of room for interpretation. The state of the research was aptly, if unintentionally, summed up by the subtitle of a 1994 article in the *International Journal of Advertising* that made the case for a causal link: "The Evidence Is There for Those Who Wish to See It."

### Does Life Imitate Ads?
Some analyses of historical data have found a small, statistically significant association between increases in advertising and increases in smoking; others have not. In a 1993 overview of the evidence, Michael Schudson, professor of communication and sociology at the University of California at San Diego, wrote, "In terms of a general relationship between cigarette advertising and cigarette smoking, the available econometric evidence is equivocal and the kind of materials available to produce the evidence leave much to be desired." This sort of research is open to challenge on technical grounds, such as the time period chosen and the methods for measuring advertising and consumption. There is also the possibility that advertising goes up in response to a rise in consumption, rather than the reverse. Industry critics often cite the increases in smoking by women that occurred in the 1920s and the late '60s to early '70s as evidence of advertising's power. "Yet in both cases," Schudson noted, "the advertising campaign followed rather than preceded the behavior it supposedly engendered." In other words, the tobacco companies

changed their marketing in response to a trend that was already under way.

International comparisons have also produced mixed results. There is no consistent relationship between restrictions on advertising and smoking rates among adults or minors. In some countries where advertising is severely restricted, such as Sweden, smoking rates are relatively low. In others, such as Norway, they are relatively high. Sometimes smoking drops after advertising is banned; sometimes it doesn't. It is hard to say what such findings mean. Countries where smoking is already declining may be more intolerant of the habit and therefore more likely to ban advertising. Alternatively, a rise in smoking might help build support for a ban. Furthermore, advertising bans are typically accompanied by other measures, such as tobacco tax increases and restrictions on smoking in public, that could be expected to reduce cigarette purchases. The one conclusion it seems safe to draw is that many factors other than advertising affect tobacco consumption.

The best way to resolve the issue of advertising's impact on smoking would be a controlled experiment: Take two groups of randomly selected babies; expose one to cigarette advertising but otherwise treat them identically. After 18 years or so, compare smoking rates. Since such a study would be impractical, social scientists have had to make do with less tidy methods, generally involving interviews, questionnaires, or survey data. This kind of research indicates that the most important factors influencing whether a teenager will smoke are the behavior of his peers, his perceptions of the risks and benefits of smoking, and the presence of smokers in his home. Exposure to advertising does not independently predict the decision to smoke, and smokers themselves rarely cite advertising as an important influence on their behavior.

Critics of the industry have been quick to seize upon studies indicating that teenage smokers disproportionately prefer the most advertised cigarette brands. But such research suggests only that advertising has an impact on brand preferences, which the tobacco companies have conceded all along. Several studies have found that teenagers who smoke (or who say they might) are more apt to recall cigarette advertising and to view it favorable. Such findings do not necessarily mean that advertising makes adolescents more likely to smoke. It is just as plausible to suppose that teenagers pay more attention to cigarette ads after they start smoking, or that teenagers who are inclined to smoke for other reasons are also more likely to have a positive view of cigarette ads.

In reporting on research in this area, the mainstream press tends to ignore such alternative interpretations. Consider the coverage of a 1995 study published in the *Journal of the National Cancer Institute*. The study, co-authored by John Pierce, found that teenagers who scored high on a "receptivity" index—which included "recognition of advertising messages, having a favorite advertisement, naming a brand [they] might buy, owning a tobacco-related promotional item, and willingness to use a tobacco-related promotional item"—were more likely to say they could not rule out smoking in the near future. Such "receptivity" was more strongly associated with an inclination to smoke than was smoking among parents and peers.

According to *The New York Times*, these results meant that "[t]obacco advertising is a stronger factor than peer pressure in encouraging children under 18 to smoke." Similarly, *The Boston Globe* reported that the study showed "cigarette advertising has more influence on whether adolescents later start smoking than does having friends or family members who smoke." The Associated Press went even further: "Of all the influences that can draw children into a lifelong habit of smoking, cigarette advertising is the most persuasive." In reality, the study showed only that teenagers who like smoking-related messages and merchandise are more receptive to the idea of smoking—not exactly a startling finding.

A study reported last December in *Archives of Pediatric and Adolescent Medicine* received similar treatment. The researchers surveyed about 1,200 students in grades six through 12 and found that kids who owned cigarette promotional items such as jackets and backpacks were four times as likely to smoke as those who did not. "Tobacco Gear a Big Draw for Kids," announced the headline in *The Boston Globe*. The story began, "If tobacco manufacturers hope to promote smoking by producing clothing or accessories emblazoned with cigarette logos, research by Dartmouth Medical School suggests that the tactic works well." Under the headline, "Study: Logos Foster Smoking," *Newsday* reported that "children who own cigarette promotional items... are far more likely to smoke."

Yet as the researchers themselves conceded, "The finding of an association between CPI [cigarette promotional item] ownership and being a smoker could easily be an expression of an adolescent who acquired these items after having made the decision to become a smoker." Later in the article, they wrote, "Our study and others published to date are subject to the usual limitations inherent in cross-sectional studies, in that we are unable to infer a direction between the exposure (ownership of a CPI) and smoking behavior, limiting our ability to invoke a causal relationship between CPI ownership and smoking." Translation: We would like to say that promotional items make kids smoke, but our study doesn't show that. This shortcoming did not stop the authors from concluding that "all CPI distribution should end immediately."

**Marginal Effects**
Overall, the evidence that advertising plays an important role in getting people to smoke is not very convincing. In 1991 the economist Thomas Schelling, former director of Harvard's Institute for the Study of Smoking Behavior and Policy, said: "I've never seen a genuine study of the subject. Most of the discussion that I hear—even the serious discussion —is about as profound as saying, 'If I were a teenage black girl, that ad would make me smoke.' I just find it altogether unpersuasive. I've been very skeptical that advertising is important in either getting people to smoke or keeping people smoking. It's primarily brand competition." The 1989 surgeon general's report conceded that "[t]here is no scientifically rigorous study available to the public that provides a definitive answer to the basic question of whether advertising and promotion increase the level of tobacco consumption. Given the complexity of the issue, none is likely to be forthcoming in the foreseeable future." The 1994 surgeon general's report, which focused on underage smoking, also acknowledged the "lack of definitive literature."

It's possible, of course, that tobacco advertising has an effect that simply cannot be measured. The 1989 surgeon general's report concluded that, while "the extent of the influence of advertising and promotion on the level of consumption is unknown and possibly unknowable," the weight of the evidence "makes it more likely than not that advertising and promotional activities do stimulate cigarette consumption." The 1994 report, based on suggestive evidence, said "cigarette advertising appears to increase young people's risk of smoking." Similarly, Michael Schudson—who says "[a]dvertising typically attempts little and achieves still less"—argues that cigarette advertising "normally has only slight effect in persuading people to change their attitudes or behaviors." But he adds, "It is reasonable to believe that some teens become smokers or become smokers earlier or become smokers with less guilt or become heavier smokers because of advertising."

Serious critics of tobacco advertising do not subscribe to a simple stimulus-and-response theory in which kids exposed to Joe Camel automatically become smokers. They believe the effects of advertising are subtle and indirect. They argue that the very existence of cigarette ads suggests "it really couldn't be all that bad, or they wouldn't be allowed to advertise," as Elizabeth Whelan of the American Council on Science and Health puts it. They say advertising imagery reinforces the notion, communicated by peers and other role models, that smoking is cool. They say dependence on advertising revenue from tobacco companies discourages magazines from running articles about the health consequences of smoking. They do not claim such effects are sufficient, by themselves, to make people smoke. Rather, they argue that at the margin—say, for an ambivalent teenager whose friends smoke—the influence of advertising may be decisive.

Stated this way, the hypothesis that tobacco advertising increases consumption is impossible to falsify. "Fundamentally," writes Jean J. Boddewyn, a professor of marketing at Baruch College, "one cannot prove that advertising does *not* cause or influence smoking, because one cannot scientifically prove a negative." So despite the lack of evidence that advertising has a substantial impact on smoking rates, tobacco's opponents can argue that we should play it safe and ban the ads—just in case.

The problem with this line of reasoning is that banning tobacco advertising can be considered erring on the side of caution only if we attach little or no value to freedom of speech. If cigarette ads are a bad influence on kids, that is something for parents and other concerned adults to counter with information and exhortation. They might even consider a serious effort to enforce laws against cigarette sales to minors. But since we clearly are not helpless to resist the persuasive powers of Philip Morris et al.—all of us see the ads, but only some of us smoke—it is hard to square an advertising ban with a presumption against censorship. Surely a nation that proudly allows racist fulminations, communist propaganda, flag burning, nude dancing, pornography, and sacrilegious art can safely tolerate Marlboro caps and Joe Camel T-shirts.

# POSTSCRIPT

## Does Tobacco Advertising Influence Teens to Smoke?

According to an article in the *American Journal of Public Health* (November 1996), exposure to a variety of tobacco promotions may make teens more likely to smoke. Researcher David Altman and colleagues from the Bowman Gray School of Medicine in North Carolina contend that cigarette advertising has a cumulative effect on teens. Those who have been exposed to the most promotion are the most likely to use tobacco products.

Tobacco companies counter that cigarette advertising does not cause children, teenagers, or young adults to begin smoking. Their position on advertising is that it influences brand choices among current adult smokers. The R. J. Reynolds Tobacco Company maintains that Joe Camel, their popular logo, was not designed to turn children into smokers. However, sales of Camel cigarettes rose from $6 million to $476 million after the introduction of the Joe Camel ads, while Camel's share of the youth market rose from 0.5 percent to 32.8 percent. In reports issued before the introduction of Joe Camel, consultants advised the company that the cartoon character would attract kids, but R. J. Reynolds officials maintained that they made sure "Joe Camel did not appeal to kids." See "Behind the Smoke Screen," *Newsweek* (June 1, 1998).

Because of studies relating cigarette advertising and teen smoking, the government has been investigating ways to reduce the impact of the tobacco industry. While many are in favor of banning cigarette advertising in any form, the tobacco industry claims its right to free speech has been affected. Some argue that antismoking forces are targeting adults as well as children with the restriction of smoking in public places, increased taxation, a proposed ban on cigarette vending machines, and restrictions on advertising. Jacob Sullum states that adult smokers are the real target, not teens. Sullum maintains that the government is trying to dictate behavior to adults. See "Child's Ploy," *National Review* (April 6, 1998) and *For Your Own Good: The Anti-Smoking Crusade and the Tyranny of Public Health* (Free Press, 1997). Barbara Dority, in "The Rights of Joe Camel and the Marlboro Man," *The Humanist* (January/February 1997) states that she supports free speech and that the government should stay out of regulating personal behaviors. Other articles that discuss smoking and advertising include "Can Pols Really Stop Teens from Smoking?" *U.S. News and World Report* (June 1, 1998); "Child's Play," *Marketing Tools* (April 1998); "Tobacco Promotions Have Addictive Power to Persuade Teens," *Brown University Digest of Addiction* (April 1997); and "Last Drag," *Across the Board* (March 1996).

# ISSUE 9

## Should Moderate Use of Alcohol Be Recommended?

**YES: Dave Shiflett,** from "Here's to Your Health," *The American Spectator* (October 1996)

**NO: Meir J. Stampfer, Eric B. Rimm, and Diana Chapman Walsh,** from "Alcohol, the Heart, and Public Policy," *American Journal of Public Health* (June 1993)

### ISSUE SUMMARY

**YES:** Writer Dave Shiflett contends that for years the antidrinking establishment has insisted that even moderate drinking is bad for health despite the fact that science indicates otherwise.

**NO:** Physicians Meir J. Stampfer and Eric B. Rimm and professor Diana Chapman Walsh argue that encouraging the use of alcohol, even in moderation, could lead to an increase in its consumption, with potentially dangerous results.

Moderate drinking has been associated with many positive health effects, including a reduction of heart disease, overall longevity, better circulation, and less stress. More than 100 studies have found that alcohol reduces the risk of coronary heart disease and that moderate drinkers live longer, healthier lives than nondrinkers. Alcohol reduces the risk of heart problems due to its apparent ability to elevate levels of HDLs (the "good" cholesterol) and to prevent blood clots from forming. The studies all found these results among individuals who consumed a moderate amount of alcohol, or fewer than two drinks per day.

Moderate alcohol consumption appears to offer health benefits, but excessive usage—over two drinks per day—increases the risk of cancer, cirrhosis of the liver, and other health problems, and leads to alcoholism. Alcoholism is a factor in automobile fatalities, family dysfunction, and crime. Should moderate consumption be recommended to reduce heart disease if it could lead to excessive drinking?

A core of this debate is the definition of moderate consumption. Moderation is two or fewer drinks per day to a researcher but may be considerably more to actual drinkers. Some individuals abstain from drinking all week and have several drinks on Friday night. Are they drinking moderately? An additional issue is how much does a person need to drink to achieve the benefits of alcohol? Should alcohol be promoted at the expense of other activities that promote a healthy heart, such as exercise and smoking cessation? And what about individuals such as pregnant women who should not drink at all?

Beyond two drinks a day, alcohol has direct adverse effects on the heart. With as many as four drinks a day, men are less likely to die of heart disease than a nondrinker, but these men are at increased risk of death from other illnesses. Specifically, they have a greater probability of dying from cancer of the esophagus and stomach as well as from cirrhosis of the liver and from being involved in automobile accidents. In France, where the average citizen drinks eight to ten times as much wine as Americans, the rates of cirrhosis of the liver, accidents, and suicides are higher than in the United States. Women are also at risk—studies have shown that alcohol increases the risk of breast cancer. For many women, the hazards of drinking outweigh the benefits.

Promoting alcohol in moderation to reduce heart disease may help save lives. On the other hand, researchers agree that no one should start drinking for the express purpose of reducing this risk. The potential for alcohol abuse is too high, and there are much safer and healthier ways to protect the heart. For instance, although alcohol boosts HDLs, exercising and losing excess weight raise them even more. Exercise, in addition to elevating HDLs, also reduces the risk of diabetes, lowers blood pressure, and improves circulation. Exercise does not carry the health risks of alcohol.

In the following articles, Dave Shiflett asserts that science has indicated that moderate drinking is beneficial, but government busybodies keep insisting that it is harmful. Meir J. Stampfer, Eric B. Rimm, and Diana Chapman Walsh argue that the benefits of moderate drinking over abstinence are unclear. They are against promoting the message that moderate consumption is beneficial because of the ambiguity of the concept of "moderate" and the potential for alcohol abuse.

# YES

**Dave Shiflett**

## HERE'S TO YOUR HEALTH

*Said Aristotle unto Plato,*
*"Have another sweet potato?"*
*Said Plato unto Aristotle,*
*"Thank you, I prefer the bottle."*

—Owen Wister

Were America's students still burdened with the duty of rote memorization, we can nevertheless be assured they wouldn't be asked to learn a ditty so dangerous as Mr. Wister's. Quite the contrary. Anyone who spouted such sentiments in a contemporary classroom might find that the rules against washing out young mouths with soap can be lifted on special occasions.

Consider the case of poor Shannon Eierman, a 16-year-old honor student and all-county softball player at Atholton (Md.) High School. On a school ski trip to Vermont in February of this year [1996], Eierman walked into the room of some friends and discovered they were drinking beer. Hoping to avoid trouble, she grabbed two beers and began pouring them out.

Too late. Chaperones suddenly appeared; soon a dozen or so of the youngsters had been relieved of their ski passes and forced to write detailed accounts of their transgressions. Seven of the guilty, including Eierman, were suspended from school, she for five days. Shannon was also forced to attend an alcohol treatment program and was banned from extracurricular activities for two quarters—a punishment that may have cost her a sports scholarship.

It could have been worse. Shannon had actually received the minimum punishment under Howard County's "zero tolerance" program. As the *Washington Post* reported, "Last year, Howard officials provoked an uproar when they suspended students who drank a glass of wine with dinner in France on a school trip."

For a generation steeped in mescaline, marijuana, and tequila shooters, the baby boomers take a fanatically harsh stance on beer drinking by their children—harsher, indeed, than the stiff old Puritans who proclaimed drink a "gift from God." Students who bring even a non-alcoholic beer to a Fairfax

County (Va.) school face suspension, even though those concoctions' alcohol content is only .5 percent (By way of comparison, one study indicates that after three days in the refrigerator, Dole pineapple juice becomes .04 percent alcohol.)

And nationwide, alcohol education campaigns have not shied from comparing booze use to cocaine snorting. Indeed, one poster, featuring a bottle of beer tipped by a hypodermic needle, carries this message: "Beer contains alcohol. Alcohol is a drug. Alcohol is the number one drug problem in the country. Not marijuana. Not cocaine. Alcohol. Talk to your kids about alcohol."

In fidelity to Uncle Sam's auntish predilections, the latest edition of the official United States nutritional guidelines warns that drinking can lead to high blood pressure, cancer, "accidents, violence, suicides, birth defects, and overall mortality." Yet the guidelines also declare, in a stunning turnaround, that "moderate drinking is associated with lower risk for Coronary Heart Disease in some individuals." This is a significant change from earlier statements that alcohol had "no benefit" and suggestions to avoid any level of drinking whatsoever. It also gives rise to an amusing paradox: While the federal government says moderate alcohol intake can prolong life, public schools and the government-funded "anti-abuse" apparatus treat alcohol like rat poison. All of which raises at least two interesting questions: What does the scientific evidence tell us, and what effect does this evidence have on public policy?

* * *

There is nothing new about health claims for alcohol. Among the most extravagant were made on behalf of distilled spirits by one Hieronymous Brunschwig, who practiced medicine in fifteenth-century Germany:

> It eases diseases coming of cold. It comforts the heart. It heals all old and new sores on the head. It causes a good color in a person. It heals baldness and causes the hair well to grow, and kills lice and fleas. It cures lethargy.... It eases the pain in the teeth, and causes sweet breath. It heals the canker in the mouth, in the teeth, in the lips, and in the tongue. It causes the heavy tongue to become light and well-speaking. It heals the short breath. It causes good digestion and appetite for to eat, and takes away all belching. It draws the wind out of the body.

Nowadays the claims are not quite so grandiose, yet the idea is the same: Moderate drinking is good for most people. A March 1996 article in the *British Medical Journal* offered this overview: "The inverse association between moderate alcohol consumption and coronary heart disease is well established. Evidence for a causal interpretation comes from over 60 ecological, case-control, and cohort studies."

Indeed, anyone requesting similar evidence will have it delivered by the truckload. The Harvard Medical School analyzed 200 studies and found that moderate drinking is associated with as much as a 45 percent reduced risk of heart disease. The Honolulu Heart Study put the decrease at 50 percent. When "60 Minutes" did a story on the subject, it broadcast this hearty endorsement by Dr. Curtis Ellison of the Boston School of Medicine: "I think the data are now so convincing that the total mortality rates are lower among moderate drinkers. It seems quite clear that we should not do anything that would decrease moderate drinkers in the population."

So convinced is the British government of the benefits of moderate drinking that it actually suggests that older abstainers abandon their teetotaling. The UK guidelines, called "Sensible Drinking," make these recommendations for men:

- The health benefit from drinking relates to men aged over 40 and the major part of this can be obtained at levels as low as one unit a day with the maximum health advantage lying between one and two units a day.
- Regular consumption of between three and four units a day by men of all ages will not accrue significant health risks.
- Consistently drinking four or more units a day is not advised as a sensible drinking level because of the progressive health risk it carries.

Because women tend to be lighter than men, and because their bodies contain a lower proportion of water which results in higher tissue concentration of alcohol, their guidelines are somewhat more stringent:

- The health benefit from drinking for women relates to post-menopausal women and the major part of this can be obtained at levels as low as one unit a day, with the maximum health advantage lying between one and two units a day.
- Regular consumption of between two and three units a day by women of all ages will not accrue any significant health risk.
- Consistently drinking three or more units a day is not advised as a sensible drinking level because of the progressive health risk it carries.

The good news doesn't stop there. In what will probably be a shock to Americans of both sexes, the UK guidelines even dismiss the idea that pregnant women should abstain: "In the light of the evidence received, our conclusion is that, to minimize risk to the developing fetus, women who are trying to become pregnant or are at any stage of pregnancy, should not drink more than 1 or 2 units of alcohol once or twice a week, and should avoid episodes of intoxication."

From reduction in cholesterol gallstones to lower rates of Ischaemic stroke, "Sensible Drinking" finds many benefits to moderate tippling, including this stunner: "Drinking in the range of 7 units to 40 units a week lowers the risk of [Coronary Heart Disease] by between 30% and 50%." (A British drink is somewhat smaller than an American drink: about 9–10 grams of alcohol vs. 12–14 grams.)

American advocates of healthy drinking have been singing the same song for many years, though not under government auspices. Lewis Perdue, author of *The French Paradox and Beyond* and publisher of *Healthy Drinking* magazine, notes a 1991 Harvard study which found that male doctors who drank on average one-half to one drink per day had 21 percent less coronary artery disease than abstainers, or a relative risk of .79 for the drinkers compared to 1.00 for abstainers. "The relative risk," Perdue crows, "continued to drop with increased consumption. Men who consumed one to one and a half drinks per day reduced their Coronary Artery Disease risk by 32 percent, three to four and a half per day reduced it by 43 percent, and those drinking more than four and a half drinks per day reduced their risk by 59 percent."

Perdue admits that there are tradeoffs, even for those who favor moderate drinking. "The World Health Association's statistics for 1989 showed that the U.S. death rate from cirrhosis was 17 per 100,000 while cardiovascular disease killed 464 per 100,000. By contrast, the same study shows France with almost double the cirrhosis rate—31 per 100,000 —but with cardiovascular rates at only 310 per 100,000. Using these figures, it is not hard to see that if the U.S. rates were normalized with those of France, 14 more people per 100,000 would die of cirrhosis, but 154 fewer people would die of cardiovascular disease, a net savings of 140 people per 100,000 population who would live longer in order to die of something else."

\* \* \*

While there is solid scientific consensus on the benefits of moderate drinking, don't expect a quick change in American attitudes about alcohol, or national policies. The chief reason is that American society has had an uneven relationship with alcohol. Sometimes they love it. Other times they can't pour it down the gutters quickly enough. Contemporary policies tend to reflect the latter passion.

David Hanson, a professor of sociology at SUNY-Potsdam and author of *Preventing Alcohol Abuse,* writes that while beer drinking even by the very young was common early in our history, an increasing concern with public drunkenness led to social crackdowns of a somewhat Muslim nature starting in the early nineteenth century. By the 1830's, a temperance movement had taken hold that pushed for total abstinence; by 1855, thirteen of the then forty states and territories had instituted prohibition.

If those were tough days for bartenders, they were terrific for the writers of tracts. The Women's Christian Temper-

ance Union, Hanson reports, pumped out over 1 billion pages of anti-alcohol propaganda between 1865 and 1925. When the Anti-Saloon League began publishing operations in 1909, it quickly rose to a level of 250 million book pages per month. Among the warnings:

- "The majority of beer drinkers die from dropsy."
- "It turns the blood to water."
- "A cat or dog may be killed by causing it to drink a small quantity of alcohol. A boy once drank whisky from a flask he had found, and died in a few hours ..."
- "When alcohol is constantly used, it may slowly change the muscles of the heart into fat.... It is sometimes so soft that a finger could easily be pushed through its walls."

Today's tract writers work for lobbying organizations, federal agencies, and other special interest groups, but their end goal —"no use" of alcohol—remains the same. Not surprisingly, extremism in the defense of abstinence is not considered a vice. In one of its official publications, the federal Center for Substance Abuse Prevention (CSAP), which supports anti-drinking programs throughout the country, was generous to the point of praise about the work of Artfux, a group that (illegally) defaces alcohol-advertising billboards: "While Artfux recognized that the billboards were private property, these artists viewed their actions as the lesser of two evils.... Furthermore, Artfux contended that they were providing health information that was hidden from the public by the alcohol and tobacco industries."

This sort of vandalism is not so lightly brushed aside when it is aimed at abortion providers and the like, but is indicative of the fanaticism that animates some workers in the prohibitionist vineyard. The more dedicated drys have indeed taken it upon themselves to teach Americans to be alcophobic, as reflected in a CSAP monograph: "One of the main points of this volume is that an essential ingredient for success is the creation of an environment in which substance use, regardless of the form it takes, is defined clearly and consistently as unacceptable." Similar desires are found in pamphlets from the tax-supported Marin Institute.

To achieve this "no use" goal, these activists advocate bans on advertising and increases in alcohol excise taxes which, as public policy analyst Doug Bandow has pointed out, results in an unethical and illegal phenomenon: "Taxpayers, most of whom drink alcohol, are underwriting what amounts to a prohibitionist campaign."

* * *

The new nutritional guidelines were not well received in the dry community. The Center for Science in the Public Interest, which is not interested in the science of moderation, greeted the guidelines with a wagging finger: "Providing information about the scientific evidence, and drawing conclusions about its utility for the general population, are two different issues. . . . One thing [governments] should not do is provide generalized recommendations. They should give as much attention to what the findings don't say, which is, 'Who won't benefit? And who will be harmed?'"

The same spirit holds forth among those who design and implement alcohol "awareness" programs in the public schools. When asked if the guidelines will affect school alcohol education policies, Bill Modzeleski, director of the Department of Education's Safe and Drug Free Schools program, which supports programs in 97 percent of the nation's school districts, said, "Probably not. For our population, alcohol is an illegal substance." He thoroughly disagrees with the idea that children are receiving mixed messages from the government on drinking, with schools saying alcohol is bad and the guidelines saying it can prolong life. "Our population doesn't drink for its health effects," he says.

Nor do the youngsters listen to health warnings. "Many students are heavily into binge drinking," Modzeleski says. Drinking remains "pretty steady" and has been "high right along." Maryland officials say that 70.1 percent of seniors in Shannon Eierman's school district reported having a drink within the past twelve months, and nationwide surveys reflect similar consumption patterns.

Schools will, of course, accommodate some of their charges' "inappropriate" behaviors, even to the point of showing them how to don condoms (probably not a revelation to many). Perhaps young tipplers should argue that they're going to drink anyway, so the schools should provide cab fare. In any event, the practice has been to reject any curriculum suggesting there is such a thing as responsible drinking. Instead, students are taught that drinking alcohol in any amount is yet another form of drug use, which has caused more than one family unnecessary friction at the cocktail hour.

* * *

Children are not the only Americans shielded from the moderate drinking message. While the latest health guidelines carry a reasoned message, few Americans are familiar with them. In the one place such a message would be seen by the greatest number of interested parties—the labels on alcoholic beverages—the good news about moderation suffers blackout.

Currently, the Bureau of Alcohol, Tobacco and Firearms, which oversees the labeling process, is considering three attempts to add health messages to the bottles which, by law, must continue to carry the Surgeon General's warnings about alcohol-related health and safety problems. The mildest proposal comes from the Wine Institute, which has petitioned to force labels to suggest that drinkers write off for the nutritional guidelines. The Competitive Enterprise Institute (CEI) is campaigning for a label that reads, "There is significant evidence that moderate consumption of alcoholic beverages may reduce the risk of heart disease." These will not strike many consumers as excessive claims, but ATF is in no hurry to allow changes on bottle labels. Paternalism comes first.

"The Wine Institute and others want to put forth a positive attitude about their product," says the highly personable Bill Earle, deputy associate director for regulatory programs at ATF. "They want to move up to the next level. But we're going to be very cautious. A short message could be misleading if it only communicates partial information. Remember, the dietary guide lines refer to good and bad effects of drink."

Because the bottles already contain a health warning, a suggestion of benefits could balance the picture. Yet Earle responds, "Our position with the industry is that the best place to conduct dialogue is in the free press, not necessarily in labeling or advertising by wine companies." In the meantime, he notes, "Dietary guidelines disconnected the language of 'alcohol and other drugs,' which HHS and others have used for years. That's a subtle but telling observation about the changing view."

Such subtlety is not good enough for CEI's Ben Lieberman, who says his organization is prepared to sue the bureau for not responding in a timely manner to its petition, which was delivered over a year ago. While fully understandable, CEI should not think that it is being singled out for the glacier treatment. Coors Brewing Company was forced to wage a court battle over the course of eight years to be allowed to include the strength of beers on its labels. The case ended last year when the Supreme Court ruled 9–0 to allow brewers to disclose the information, thus overcoming a 1935 law that was enacted after Prohibition's repeal.

That victory was not without its ironies, including the fact that not all beer manufacturers initially supported the change. "We think it is suicidal to market a product based on its alcohol content," said August A. Busch IV, vice-president of Anheuser-Busch. Strangely enough, all alcoholic beverages except beer are required to disclose their alcoholic content on their labels.

Ultimately the push to cut alcohol consumption is built on the belief that some 10 percent of American adults have what are called "drinking problems"—a figure that, like every statistic associated with alcohol, is questioned by specialists.

Researcher Joseph E. Josephson, writing in a publication for the Columbia University School of Public Health, has questioned the very idea that there is a large number of problem drinkers in America: "An objective assessment of government statistics on alcohol-related problems, many of them compiled in the Third Report to the U.S. Congress on Alcohol and Health in 1978, indicates that there is little sound basis for claims that there are upwards of 10 million problem drinkers (including alcoholics) in the adult population and that their number is increasing; that there are 1.5 to 2.25 million problem drinkers among women; that there are over 3 million problem drinkers among youth; that the heavy consumption of alcohol by pregnant women leads consistently to a cluster of birth defects... [and] that half of all motor vehicle accident fatalities are alcohol-related.... These and other claims about the extent and consequences of alcohol use and abuse—some of them fanciful, others as yet to be supported to research—are part of the 'numbers game' which besets discussion of alcohol-related problems and policy."

Epidemiologist Harold A. Mulford, writing in the *Encyclopedic Handbook of Alcoholism*, made a similar charge:

NIAAA's [National Institute on Alcohol Abuse and Alcoholism] legislatively mandated reports to Congress contain the official prevalence and distribution data for the nation. They are the most publicized prevalence and distribution conclusions and the ones most often cited by politicians and program policy makers. Their official character, however, is not to be confused with scientific validity. Whether by design or not, the reports to Congress likely reflect a contemporary fact of life. The welfare, perhaps even the survival, of NIAAA depends on (1) the apparent magnitude of the alcohol problem, and (2) whether it is made to appear that a disease (rather than a moral or social problem) is being attacked.

Similar skepticism showed up in a ruling this year by the Supreme Court of Louisiana, which affirmed a lower court's ruling that the state's 21-year-old drinking age was unconstitutional. Among other things, the court cited earlier research by Professor Robert Gramling of the University of Southwestern Louisiana, which stated that "there is a lack of empirical evidence to support the assumption that raising the drinking age to 21 years old will result in less alcohol consumption by eighteen to twenty year olds. Dr. Gramling's affidavit further states his research strongly suggests that greater quantities of alcohol may be consumed by eighteen to twenty year olds where the drinking age is raised to twenty one. Finally, Dr. Gramling concludes raising the legal drinking age in 1986 did not significantly change the alcohol consumption of eighteen to twenty year olds in Louisiana."

The court added that "our review of the evidence reveals the State's own statistics clearly show that, in Louisiana, persons between the ages of twenty-one and twenty-three are involved in significantly higher numbers of alcohol related injury and fatality accidents than eighteen to twenty year olds." Louisiana has been warned that lowering the drinking age will cost it federal highway funds.

In recent years the government has undertaken a number of questionable public-safety campaigns, from banning lawn darts (which killed three people over the course of seventeen years) to targeting college coeds with AIDS prevention messages. And while some people should avoid drinking, alcohol's health benefits are no longer a matter of scientific debate. These benefits, presented reasonably, could do much more to enhance the lives of most Americans than all the cod liver oil-type admonitions foisted upon us by our surgeon generals. Plato would no doubt agree.

# NO

## Meir J. Stampfer, Eric B. Rimm, and Diana Chapman Walsh

## ALCOHOL, THE HEART, AND PUBLIC POLICY

Light to moderate drinkers have substantially lower rates of cardiovascular mortality and mortality from all causes than do nondrinkers or heavy drinkers. This finding has been observed repeatedly in several dozen epidemiological studies using a variety of designs. Recent research has added further persuasive evidence to support a causal interpretation of this association.

In epidemiological studies, classification of moderate alcohol consumption ranges from half a drink per day (or less) in some studies up to six drinks a day in others. A 5-oz glass of wine, a 12-oz can of beer, or a shot (1.5 oz) of spirits contains about 13 g to 15 g of alcohol. We consider moderate drinking to be one to two drinks per day for a man and perhaps somewhat less for a woman. For most individuals, this is a safe definition. However, tolerance to alcohol depends on age, sex, body size, and cultural situation; therefore, no single global definition of "moderate" can be made. History of past consumption, rate of consumption, and proximity to meals also alter metabolism of alcohol.

In widely disparate populations, from across Europe and North America to Australia and Thailand, a consistent 20% to 40% reduction in coronary disease has been reported among moderate drinkers. This association is not in dispute. Although a causal interpretation is most plausible, a few investigators have advocated the alternative explanation that the comparison group of nondrinkers is at higher risk of coronary disease because that category includes covert alcohol abusers and those who quit drinking because of ill health.

Work from our group and from others strongly refutes these theories. We compared estimated average alcohol intake from our questionnaire with actual intake from 14 days of diet records. We found, in both men and women, a correlation of approximately .9 between alcohol consumption estimated from the questionnaire and that measure from diet records. Furthermore, we found highly significant correlations between reported alcohol intake and high-density lipoprotein cholesterol in both groups.

From Meir J. Stampfer, Eric B. Rimm, and Diana Chapman Walsh, "Alcohol, the Heart, and Public Policy," *American Journal of Public Health* (June 1993). Copyright © 1993 by The American Public Health Association. Reprinted by permission. References omitted.

For the heaviest alcohol users, a questionnaire or interview may not provide valid information. However, alcohol abusers are far less likely than others to participate in epidemiological studies and therefore the purported presence of heavy drinkers in the nondrinker category is an untenable explanation for the inverse association.

In large and detailed studies, one also may compare moderate alcohol consumption with very light consumption. In our analyses of 87,000 nurses and 51,000 male health professionals we found a significant inverse association with increasing alcohol consumption even with total abstainers excluded. In our two large cohorts we also tested the second, related, noncausal explanation, that men and women with preexisting disease abstain from alcohol. If true, this would tend to produce an artifactual association between abstinence and higher risk of coronary disease.

In most prospective studies, participants with diagnosed coronary disease are excluded at the start of follow-up. However, those with risk factors such as diabetes, hypertension, or hypercholesterolemia are usually not excluded. As expected, we did find a higher prevalence of these conditions among the abstainers in our cohorts. However, in alternative analyses excluding participants with those risk factors, we still found a strong inverse association between alcohol and coronary disease.

Other prospective studies have reported similar findings. Although Shaper originally did not find a similar association after excluding men with preexisting disease in the British Regional Heart Study, with additional follow-up a reduction in ischemic heart disease was found even among men free of existing disease.

Overall mortality was not reduced, but this could be explained in part by the categorization of those reporting from one half up to six drinks per day as "moderate" drinkers. Further, in this population of 7,735 men, the strong correlation between drinking and smoking makes it difficult to obtain precise estimates of the independent effect of drinking. The data from 276,802 men enrolled in the American Cancer Society prospective study provide much more convincing evidence. They show a maximal reduction in total mortality at one to two drinks per day among all participants, both before and after excluding those who were ill at baseline.

In the Kaiser-Permanente study of over 120,000 persons, Klatsky and Armstrong reported reduced coronary mortality among drinkers compared with lifelong nondrinkers. This important finding tends to refute the hypothesis that the protective effect is an artifact caused by the inclusion in the nondrinker group of moderate drinkers who quit because of disease. Similarly, in our cohorts, we excluded men and women with a marked decrease in alcohol intake over the previous 10 years; in those analyses the substantial reduction in risk among the moderate drinkers remained apparent.

Recently, attention has focused on the possible differences in the effect of different alcoholic beverages, particularly the purported special benefits of red wine. The epidemiological evidence suggests that all alcoholic beverages are similarly protective. Some studies find wine more protective; others, beer or spirits. For example, in the Health Professionals Follow-Up Study, men consuming two drinks per day of spirits were at slightly lower risk than those who consumed alcohol from other sources. In the Nurses'

Health Study, wine was found to be a bit more protective, and in an earlier prospective study, Yano et al. reported the lowest risk for moderate beer drinkers. Frankel et al. reported on specific components of red wine that may act as antioxidants to reduce atherosclerosis. However, in a recent update from the large Kaiser cohort, Klatsky and Armstrong found that white wine drinkers had a slight advantage over red wine drinkers, though both groups were at reduced risk compared with nondrinkers.

The best documented mechanism of the cardioprotective effect of alcohol is that it raises the concentration of high-density lipoprotein (HDL). At one time, it was believed that alcohol raised only the HDL-3 subfraction and that only the HDL-2 subfraction was protective. Both of these beliefs are incorrect. Alcohol increases both subfractions, but it raises HDL-3 more than it does HDL-2. Both subfractions are associated with decreased risk, and fractionating high-density lipoprotein provides little or no additional information about risk beyond that derived from total high-density lipoprotein.

Other mechanisms are likely. Alcohol intake decreases platelet aggregability and causes a marked short-term increase in tissue-type plasminogen activator. Both effects point toward an acute reduction of clot formation and hence a decrease in risk. These mechanisms are consistent with a recent case-control study that found a short-term protective effect of alcohol consumption in addition to a benefit of habitual moderate intake.

A protective effect of moderate alcohol consumption is well established from epidemiological data and plausible biological mechanisms. What are the public health implications of this finding? In a 1979 editorial, Castelli concluded that although two drinks per day appear to be protective, "with 17 million alcoholics in this country we perhaps have a message for which this country is not yet ready."

Is this a message for which the country ought to ready itself? If the medical and health establishments were to advocate regular drinking of small amounts of alcohol, would the risk of increased problem drinking outweigh the benefit of healthier hearts? Whose risk would increase and who would benefit? Can clinicians correctly identify patients from whom such advice would be contraindicated?

People—and not only alcoholics—often experience unpleasantness, and occasionally very much worse, as a result of their drinking. What we see far less clearly is how various factors combine to produce these bad outcomes—what the risk (and protective) factors are that explain why in some circumstances some people get into trouble with alcohol whereas others escape. Roughly half of American men who qualify as heavy drinkers never experience problems in connection with their alcohol use. Of those whose episodic abuse does lead to serious trouble, about half are not habitual heavy drinkers.

Studies have identified markers of substance abuse in adolescents: early trial and initiation; strong peer influences; nonconformity and rebelliousness; low achievement in school; lack of family limit-setting, involvement, and support. Among adults, being male, being younger than 30 years, having lower income, being in the working class, and coming from a family with a history of alcoholism increase the risk of heavy drinking, alcohol abuse, and alcoholism. Paradoxically, some of the same high-risk groups have higher proportions of abstainers and would, as a consequence, be particular targets of the pro-drinking message. Numerous theories —genetic, metabolic, psychological, social, cultural, and addiction-based—have been advanced to explain the onset and uneven course of problem drinking, alcohol abuse, or alcoholism. But no theory or combination of theories adequately explains what many scholars now believe are diverse phenomena. Meanwhile, numerous studies have demonstrated that physicians frequently miss the diagnosis even of severe alcoholism.

In the United States, less than 10% of the population reports drinking more than two drinks per day, the cutoff for "heavy drinking" in national survey research. This means that "moderate" drinkers, because of their much greater numbers, probably account for well over half of all alcohol problems, a finding that led researchers at the Institute of Medicine to observe in a groundbreaking report that "if all the clinically diagnosed alcoholics were to stop drinking tomorrow, a substantial fraction of what we understand as alcohol problems would still remain." The statement heralded a conceptual watershed in the way the world thinks about alcohol control, diverting the focus from treating alcoholics toward what was termed a new "public health" approach. Two key assumptions behind that approach are especially pertinent here.

First, public health thinking implies a systems approach, the object of which is to mobilize a range of change strategies—education, moral suasion, and formal rules and laws—in an integrated program of controls aimed at host, agent, and environment. In this approach, a united front and the absence of mixed messages become very important, because the hope is to create a constancy of messages and policies. The possibility that a daily dose of alcohol might be cardioprotective is a perturbation that threatens to complicate or dilute messages designed to alert drinkers to risks.

The second important assumption behind the public health approach to alcohol control is that it seeks to move the whole consumption curve toward lower per capita consumption overall. The hope is that alcohol problems will, as a consequence, abate. Again, the emergence of scientific evidence that alcohol may be salutary seems to fly in the face of this goal. It suggests that health risks increase at both tails of the consumption curve, so that wholesale shifting of the curve could put a subgroup of underconsumers at risk for heart disease.

Should we therefore promote the consumption of small amounts of alcohol? In theory, this would increase the "social availability" of alcohol—the perception among the public that drinking is normative. We simply do not know what the effect might be on overall consumption rates and on alcohol-related problems. But we do have fairly robust evidence that problems decrease with reductions in the physical and economic availability of alcoholic beverages. Problem indicators decline when sales of alcohol are sharply curtailed or prohibited and increase again when restrictions on access are relaxed. Raising the taxes on alcohol reduces consumption, even among heavy drinkers, and at least some associated injuries and deaths. Increasing the minimum legal drinking age seems to reduce highway crashes.

The public health response to alcohol abuse is far from optimal. Both the reach and the range of alcohol treatment strategies need to be expanded. We need more inventive strategies to get people with nascent problems to notice them earlier and avail themselves of low-intensity interventions and supports, which must be made more diverse.

We also need to develop innovative programs to reach people where they study, live, and work and through the mass media. The focus of such efforts should be to change public awareness and behavior concerning alcohol-associated risk. The messages should promote norms that would presumably be protective against alcohol problems:

- It is always acceptable to decline a drink.
- It is never acceptable to become really intoxicated.
- It is never acceptable to drink in situations in which alcohol is associated with significant risk—during pregnancy, while taking medications, before driving a car or using other dangerous machinery, at work, or while engaged in other pursuits that demand coordination and full possession of one's faculties.

It is impossible to predict with confidence what the public health impact might be of an effort to promote the regular consumption of small amounts of alcohol. Large longitudinal studies would be required before we could safely say who might be at risk of progressing to heavier or hazardous drinking. Resources for such research have not been available. Comprehensive cost-benefit analyses are needed to sort out the benefits and risks to individuals and to society. Research is needed, too, to clarify whether the protective effect of alcohol is general or whether the message should apply only to a subgroup. Even with better risk-factor models, we would still be hard pressed to foresee situations, which unfortunately are not uncommon, in which episodes of alcohol abuse among usually moderate drinkers might result in the injury or death of the drinker or someone else.

If a prodrinking campaign were to be mounted, it should certainly seek to avoid communicating the message to certain groups: anyone with a family history of alcoholism, people younger than age 21, and pregnant women. It should also address all risk factors for cardiovascular disease, since the others—such as smoking and hypertension—can be reduced by individuals without putting the health of others at risk. But our society is so lacking in effective social controls on alcohol abuse and pays such a heavy price for its inadequate response that, although a policy opposing moderate alcohol consumption may be inadvisable, the thought of a public policy promoting alcohol consumption runs strongly against the grain, however much it might capture at lease some hearts.

# POSTSCRIPT

## Should Moderate Use of Alcohol Be Recommended?

A recent article in the *Journal of the American Medical Association* estimates that although excessive drinking causes more than 100,000 deaths a year, if Americans stopped drinking altogether, an additional 81,000 people a year would die of heart disease. Alcohol's potential health benefits may have an impact on public policy issues, including excise taxes and advertising. Alcohol producers currently enjoy major influence on Capitol Hill. According to the Center for Responsive Politics, a Washington-based campaign watchdog group, the contributions from the alcohol industry were nearly $4.4 million in 1994.

Alcohol trade groups have promoted positive information about the benefits of moderate drinking to government agencies, the media, and trade groups with good results. The National Institute on Alcohol Abuse and Alcoholism is spending $2 million to study the health effects of moderate alcohol consumption. In 1995 the Department of Agriculture revised the alcohol section of its dietary guidelines for Americans to state, "Current evidence suggests that moderate drinking, defined as up to two drinks a day for men and one for women, is associated with a lower risk of coronary heart disease in some individuals." The guidelines still claim that heavy drinking can increase the risk of health problems and even moderate consumption poses a risk for pregnant women and alcoholics, but alcohol use is indirectly being promoted. Some trade groups are even suing the government to allow alcohol advertisements and labels to carry information about the potential health benefits of drinking.

Although the positive effects of moderate drinking have been demonstrated, there are many issues to be considered. Alcohol in moderation can be beneficial for some people because it reduces their risk of cardiovascular disease. For others, alcohol, even in moderation, can be a health risk. If alcohol is promoted as a healthful beverage, will abstainers be inclined to take up drinking? And will individuals predisposed to alcoholism become alcoholic? For an overview of addiction to drugs and alcohol, see "How We Get Addicted," *Time* (May 5, 1997) and "What Is Addiction?" *Consumer Reports on Health* (April 1996). For additional readings on the benefits and risks of alcohol consumption, see "Drink to Your Heart's Content" and "Alcoholism: Character or Genetics?" *Insight* (March 3, 1997); "The Hazards of Alcohol," *Current Health* (January 1996); "Alcohol: Spirit of Health?" *Consumer Reports on Health* (April 1996); and "Uncorking the Facts About Alcohol and Your Health," *Tufts University Diet and Nutrition Letter* (August 1995).

# ISSUE 10

## Is Marijuana Dangerous and Addictive?

**YES: Eric A. Voth,** from "Should Marijuana Be Legalized as a Medicine? No, It's Dangerous and Addictive," *The World & I* (June 1994)

**NO: Ethan A. Nadelmann,** from "Reefer Madness 1997: The New Bag of Scare Tactics," *Rolling Stone* (February 20, 1997)

### ISSUE SUMMARY

**YES:** Eric A. Voth, medical director of Chemical Dependency Services at St. Francis Hospital in Topeka, Kansas, argues that marijuana produces many adverse effects and that its effectiveness as a medicine is supported only by anecdotes.

**NO:** Ethan A. Nadelmann, director of the Lindesmith Center, a New York drug policy research institute, asserts that government officials continue to promote the myth that marijuana is harmful and leads to the use of hard drugs. He states that the war on marijuana is being fought for purely political, not health, reasons.

At one time there were no laws in the United States regulating the use or sale of drugs, including marijuana. Rather than by legislation, their use was regulated by religious teaching and social custom. As society grew more complex and more heterogeneous, the need for more formal regulation of drug sales, production, and use developed.

Attempts at regulating patent medications through legislation began in the early 1900s. In 1920 Congress, under pressure from temperance organizations, passed an amendment prohibiting the manufacture and sale of all alcoholic beverages. From 1920 until 1933, the demand for alcohol was met by organized crime, who either manufactured it illicitly or smuggled it into the United States. The government's inability to enforce the law and increasing violence finally led to the repeal of Prohibition in 1933.

Many years later, in the 1960s, drug usage again began to worry many Americans. Heroin abuse had become epidemic in urban areas, and many middle-class young adults had begun to experiment with marijuana and LSD by the end of the decade. Cocaine also became popular first among the middle class and later among inner-city residents. Today, crack houses, babies born with drug addictions, and drug-related crimes and shootings are the images of a new epidemic of drug abuse.

Many of those who believe illicit drugs are a major problem in America, however, are usually referring to hard drugs, such as cocaine and heroin. Soft drugs like marijuana, though not legal, are not often perceived as a major threat to the safety and well-being of citizens. Millions of Americans have tried marijuana and did not become addicted. The drug has also been used illegally by those suffering from AIDS, glaucoma, and cancer to alleviate their symptoms and to stimulate their appetites. Should marijuana be legalized as a medicine, or is it too addictive and dangerous? In California, Proposition 215 passed in the November 1996 ballot. A similar measure passed in Arizona. These initiatives convinced voters to relax current laws against marijuana use for medical and humane reasons.

Opponents of these recent measures argue that marijuana use has been steadily rising among teenagers and that this may lead to experimentation with hard drugs. There is concern that if marijuana is legal via a doctor's prescription, the drug will be more readily available. There is also concern that the health benefits of smoking marijuana are overrated. For instance, among glaucoma sufferers, in order to achieve benefits from the drug, patients would literally have to be stoned all the time. Marijuana appears to be beneficial for combating the weight loss and wasting associated with AIDS and some cancers because it stimulates the appetite and controlls nausea. There are, however, legal, effective prescription drugs on the market that stimulate the appetite and control nausea. Unfortunately, the efficacy of marijuana is unclear because, as an illicit drug, studies to adequately test it have been thwarted by drug control agencies.

Although marijuana's effectiveness in treating the symptoms of disease is unclear, is it actually dangerous and addictive? Scientists claim that the drug can negatively affect cognition and motor function. It can also have an impact on short-term memory and can interfere with perception and learning. Physical health effects include lung damage. Until recently, scientists had little evidence that marijuana was actually addictive. Whereas heavy users did not seem to experience actual withdrawal symptoms, studies with laboratory animals given large doses of THC, the active ingredient in marijuana, suffered withdrawal symptoms similar to those of rodents withdrawing from opiates.

Not all researchers agree, however, that marijuana is dangerous and addictive. The absence of well-designed, long-term studies on the effects of marijuana use further complicates the issue, as does the current potency of the drug. Growers have become more skilled about developing strains of marijuana with high concentrations of THC. Today's varieties may be 3 to 5 times more potent than the pot used in the 1960s. Much of the data are unclear, but what is known is that young users of the drug are likely to have problems learning. In addition, some users are at risk for developing dependence.

In the following selections, Eric A. Voth argues that marijuana causes many physical and psychological effects, including potential addiction. Ethan A. Nadelmann states that there are no proven studies to support the view that marijuana is more dangerous than previously thought or that it is a gateway to more dangerous drugs.

# YES

Eric A. Voth

## SHOULD MARIJUANA BE LEGALIZED AS A MEDICINE? NO, IT'S DANGEROUS AND ADDICTIVE

To best understand the problems associated with legalizing marijuana, it is useful to examine drug legalization in general and then to discuss the specific pitfalls of legal marijuana.

Advocates generally argue that crime would decrease under legalization, that dealers would be driven out of the market by lower prices, that legalization works in other countries, that government would benefit from the sales tax on drugs, that Prohibition did not work, and that the "war on drugs" has failed.

Examining currently legal drugs provides an insight as to the possible effect of legalizing other drugs. First, alcohol is responsible for approximately 100,000 deaths every year and 11 million cases of alcoholism. Virtually every bodily system is adversely affected by alcoholism. While Prohibition was an unfortunately violent time, many of the hardships of that era were really the result of the Depression. Prohibition did decrease the rate of alcohol consumption; alcohol-related deaths climbed steadily after Prohibition was repealed.

Tobacco use is responsible for 400,000 premature deaths per year. It causes emphysema, chronic bronchitis, heart disease, lung cancer, head and neck cancers, vascular disease, and hypertension, to name a few disorders. The taxes on tobacco come nowhere close to paying for the health problems caused by the drug.

The argument that legalization would decrease crime exemplifies a great lack of understanding of drug abuse. Most drug-associated crime is committed to acquire drugs or under the influence of drugs. The Netherlands has often been heralded by the drug culture as a country where decriminalization has worked. In fact, drug-related holdups and shootings have increased 60 percent and 40 percent, respectively, since decriminalization. This has caused the government to start enforcing the drug laws more strictly.

Because of its powerful drug lobby, the Netherlands has never been able to mount a taxation campaign against its legal drugs. We suffer a similar phenomenon in the United States in that the tobacco lobby has successfully defeated most taxation initiatives against tobacco.

The argument that drug dealers would be driven out of the market by lower prices ignores the fact that legalization will probably result in as many as 250,000 to over two million new addicts. Broader markets, even with lower prices, certainly will not drive dealers out of the market. Our overburdened medical system will not be able to handle the drastic increase in the number of addicts.

## MEDICAL MARIJUANA

Richard Cowan, national director of the National Organization for the Reform of Marijuana Laws (NORML), has stated that acceptance of medicinal uses of marijuana is pivotal for its legalization.

In 1972, the drug culture petitioned the Drug Enforcement Administration (DEA) to reschedule marijuana from a Schedule I drug (unable to be prescribed, high potential for abuse, not currently accepted for medicinal use, unsafe) to a Schedule II drug (high potential for abuse, currently accepted for medical use, potential for abuse, but prescribable).

This rescheduling petition was initiated by NORML, the Alliance for Cannabis Therapeutics (ACT), and the Cannabis Corporation of America. Of note is the fact that none of these drug-culture organizations has a recognized medical or scientific background, nor do they represent any accredited medical entity.

After substantial legal maneuvering by the drug culture, the DEA carefully documented the case against the rescheduling of marijuana and denied the petition. To examine the potential for therapeutic uses of marijuana, the DEA turned to testimony from nationally recognized experts who rejected the medical use of marijuana (published in the *Federal Register*, December 29, 1989, and March 26, 1992).

In the face of this expert testimony, the drug lobby could only produce anecdotes and the testimony of a handful of physicians with limited or absent clinical experience with marijuana. (Marijuana has not been accepted as a medicine by the AMA, the National Multiple Sclerosis Society, the American Glaucoma Society, the American Academy of Ophthalmology, and the American Cancer Society.)

The drug culture organizations appealed the DEA's decision. Recently, the U.S. Court of Appeals for the District of Columbia denied their petition to reschedule marijuana. This important decision also sets forth the new guideline that only rigorous scientific standards can satisfy the requirement of "currently accepted medical use." These preconditions are:

1. The drug has a known and reproducible chemistry;
2. Adequate safety studies;
3. Adequate and well-controlled studies proving efficacy; and
4. Qualified experts accept the drug.

In addition, the decision stated, "The administrator reasonably accorded more weight to the opinions of the experts than to the laymen and doctors on which the petitioners relied."

In his 1993 book *Marihuana: The Forbidden Medicine*, the psychiatrist Dr. Lester

Grinspoon assembled a group of anecdotes to justify the rescheduling of marijuana. Similar to the promarijuana lobby during rescheduling hearings, Grinspoon asserts that marijuana should be used to help relieve nausea (during cancer chemotherapy), glaucoma, wasting in AIDS, depression, menstrual cramps, pain, and virtually unlimited ailments. His anecdotes have no controls, no standardization of dose, no quality control, and no independent medical evaluation for efficacy or toxicity.

## ONLY ANECDOTES PROVE ITS EFFICACY

The historical uses of marijuana in such cultures as India, Asia, the Middle East, South Africa, and South America are cited by Grinspoon as evidence of appropriate medical uses of the drug. One of Grinspoon's references is an 1860 assertion that marijuana had supposed beneficial effects "without interfering with the actions of the internal organs" (this is inaccurate). Let us not forget that medicine in earlier years was fraught with potions and remedies. Many of these were absolutely useless or even harmful to unsuspecting subjects. This is when our current FDA [Food and Drug Administration] and drug scheduling processes evolved, which should not be undermined.

The medical marijuana campaign gained momentum in February 1990, when a student project, initiated by Rick Doblin, published interpretations of a questionnaire that he had sent to oncologists. Doblin is closely associated with the Multidisciplinary Association for Psychedelic Studies, a drug-culture lobbying organization. This group strongly supports the legalization and medical uses of the street drugs LSD and MDMA (Ecstasy). Doblins' staff sponsor at Harvard, Mark Kleiman, voiced his support for the legalization of marijuana in his recent book *Against Excess*. Neither author has a medical background, nor do they disclose their intrinsic bias toward the legalization of marijuana.

By manipulation of the statistics, the authors contend that 48 percent of their respondents would prescribe marijuana if legal and 54 percent feel it should be available by prescription. But the researchers fail to relate that the respondents account for only 9 percent of practicing oncologists. Only 6 percent of those surveyed feel that marijuana was effective in 50 percent or more of their patients.

Only 18 percent of the surveyed group believe marijuana to be safe and efficacious. Five percent of those surveyed favor making marijuana available by prescription. These numbers become less significant if compared to the number of all practicing oncologists. Furthermore, this survey was conducted before the release for use of the medication ondansetron (Zofran®), which is extremely effective to relieve the nausea associated with chemotherapy.

Unfortunately, the "results" of this unscientific but well-publicized study incorrectly give the impression that oncologists want marijuana available as medicine. But researchers neither asked if the oncologists had systematically examined their patients for negative effects of marijuana use nor if the oncologists were familiar with the myriad of health consequences of marijuana use. Furthermore, they did not ask oncologists if their attitudes about marijuana were affected by their own current or past marijuana use.

Contrary to the findings of Doblin and Kleiman, Dr. Richard Schwartz determined through a survey of practicing oncologists that THC (the major active ingredient of marijuana) ranked ninth in their preference for the treatment of mild nausea and sixth for the treatment of severe nausea. Only 6 percent had prescribed THC (by prescription or marijuana) for more than 50 patients. It was found that nausea was relieved in only 50 percent of the patients who received THC and that 25 percent had adverse side effects.

## COMPLICATIONS OF MARIJUANA USE

According to the 1992 National Household Survey on Drug Abuse, 48 percent of young adults have used marijuana and 11 percent continue to use it. In 1992, 8.2 percent of young adults age 26 to 34 admitted having used marijuana in the last month, a figure that was up from 7.0 percent in 1991. Marijuana remains the most frequently used illegal drug. The chronic use of marijuana has now been demonstrated to lead to higher utilization of the health-care system, a long-suspected phenomenon.

Mental, affective, and behavioral changes are the most easily recognized consequences of marijuana use. Concentration, motor coordination, and memory are adversely impacted. For example, the ability to perform complex tasks such as flying is impaired even 24 hours after the acute intoxication phase. The association of marijuana use with trauma and intoxicated motor vehicle operation is also well established.

Memory is impaired for several months after cessation of use. After chronic use, marijuana addicts admit that their motivation to succeed lessens. Several biochemical models have demonstrated abnormal changes in brain cells, brain blood flow, and brain waves. Pathologic behavior such as psychosis is also associated with marijuana use. The more chronic the use, as would be necessary for treating diseases such as glaucoma, the higher the risk of mental problems.

Despite arguments from the drug culture to the contrary, marijuana is addictive. This addiction has been well described by users. It consists of both a physical dependence (tolerance and subsequent withdrawal) and a psychological habituation. Strangely, in the course of the rescheduling hearings, prodrug organizations admitted that "marijuana has a high potential for abuse and that abuse of the marijuana plant may lead to severe psychological or physical dependence," points that they now publicly deny. Unlike those addicted to many other drugs, the marijuana addict is exceptionally slow to recognize the addiction.

The gateway effect of marijuana is also well established in research. Use of alcohol, tobacco, and marijuana are major risk factors for subsequent addiction and more extensive drug use.

Smoked marijuana contains double to triple the concentrations of tar, carbon monoxide, and carcinogens found in cigarette smoke. Marijuana adversely impairs lung function by causing abnormalities in the cells lining the airways of the upper and lower respiratory tract and in the airspaces deep within the lung. It has been linked to head and neck cancer.

Contaminants of marijuana smoke include certain forms of bacteria and fungi. Users with impaired immunity are at particular risk for disease and infection when they inhale these substances.

Adverse effects of marijuana on the unborn were suspected after studies in Rhesus monkeys demonstrated spontaneous abortion. When exposed to marijuana during gestation, humans demonstrate changes in size and weight as well as neurologic abnormalities. A very alarming association also exists between maternal marijuana use and certain forms of cancer in offspring. Additionally, hormonal function in both male and female children is disrupted.

One of the earliest findings was the negative effect of marijuana on various immune functions, including cellular immunity and pulmonary immunity. Impaired ability to fight infection is now documented in humans who use marijuana. They have been shown to exhibit an inability to fight herpes infections and a blunted response to therapy for genital warts. The potential for these complications exists in all forms of administration of marijuana.

It should be clear that use of the drug bears substantial health risks. In populations at high risk for infection and immune suppression (AIDS and cancer chemotherapy patients), the risks are unacceptable.

## SUMMARY

The unfortunate reality is that the drug culture is exploiting the unwitting public and the suffering of patients with chronic illnesses for its own benefit. Under the false and dangerous claims that smoking marijuana is a harmless recreational activity and that it offers significant benefits to those suffering from a variety of tragic ailments, the drug culture seeks to use bogus information to gain public acceptance for the legalization of marijuana.

# NO                    Ethan A. Nadelmann

## REEFER MADNESS 1997: THE NEW BAG OF SCARE TACTICS

"The war on drugs is really a war on marijuana," says professor Lynn Zimmer, a sociologist at Queens College, in New York, who is widely regarded as one of the nation's leading analysts of drug policy. Marijuana, says Zimmer, is the leading justification for drug testing in the workplace, the main target of anti-drug efforts in the schools and the media, and the principal preoccupation of drug warriors in and out of government today. The drug warriors' tactics include—along with arrests, seizures, incarceration and the intimidation of doctors who would prescribe pot for the terminally ill—a more sinister approach. Spokesmen are quoted by journalists and appear on the evening news and on talk shows, making frightening claims about marijuana's harmful effects, spinning unproven theories and, in some cases, distorting the known truth in an effort to demonize even casual users of pot.

It's no wonder that the warriors find themselves in a quandary. They're essentially fighting a war against the 70 million Americans who have tried marijuana, including half of all Americans aged 18–35 and more than a quarter of everyone older than 35. Polls have indicated that a fourth of all adult Americans favor legalizing pot, which, after alcohol, tobacco and caffeine, is the fourth most popular psychoactive drug in the world.

"You can't scare middle-class parents with a war on heroin and cocaine," says Zimmer. "These drugs are too removed, too remote. Marijuana brings it home."

Bill Clinton's administration, desperate not to appear soft on drugs, has indulged in its share of scare tactics. Clinton's newly appointed drug czar, Gen. Barry McCaffrey, has set the tone for the federal government's new stance, threatening sanctions against medical doctors in California and Arizona (RS 750/751), where citizens voted in November to allow the medicinal use of cannabis. More typical, however, is the approach taken by Secretary of Health and Human Services Donna Shalala, who disingenuously told reporters last December [1996], "All available research has concluded that marijuana is dangerous to our health."

Is pot dangerous? Is there any scientific research to back up Shalala's claim? There are, of course, reasons to be concerned about marijuana. It is, like alcohol, a powerful psychoactive drug. Used irresponsibly, it contributes to accidents on the roads and in the workplace. During the period of intoxication, short-term memory is impaired. Heavy pot smokers face some of the same risks as cigarette smokers. And some people become dependent upon marijuana, using it as a crutch to avoid dealing with relationships and responsibilities.

Among kids, especially, it is the daily use of marijuana, not experimental or occasional use, that merits concern. According to the latest annual survey of drug use among high-school students, the percentage of eighth-graders who admit to daily pot smoking increased from 0.2 percent in 1991 to 1.5 percent in 1996. Among 10th-graders, there was an increase from 0.8 percent to 3.5 percent; among seniors, an increase from 2 percent to nearly 5 percent. Of course, smoking marijuana every day would contribute to a teenager's problems in school and socially, but more likely it is an indicator of something else that is basically wrong.

On the other hand, there is ample evidence that the majority of the 70 million Americans who have tried marijuana are doing just fine. Since the early 1970s, the government has funded studies that have ended up proving that pot is not harmful, then disavowed the findings. In 1988, following an extensive review of the scientific evidence on marijuana, the Drug Enforcement Administration's own administrative-law judge, Francis Young, concluded that marijuana "in its natural form is one of the safest therapeutically active substances known to man." Virtually every independent commission assigned to examine the evidence on marijuana and marijuana policy —including the Shafer Commission appointed by President Richard Nixon, a National Academy of Sciences committee in the early 1980s, and numerous others both in the U.S. and abroad—have concluded that marijuana poses fewer dangers to individuals and society than either alcohol or tobacco and should be decriminalized.

And there is little reason to expect anything different from the Clinton administration's January [1997] announcement that it will spend $1 million to review all the evidence on the medical benefits of marijuana. The problem is that no Congress or president has ever had the guts to follow through on the recommendations of independent commissions assigned to balance the risks and harms of marijuana with the risks and harms of marijuana policies. It's still impossible, for instance, for any government official to speak out publicly about the difference between responsible and irresponsible use of marijuana, as they would with alcohol. All marijuana use is defined as drug abuse—notwithstanding extensive evidence that most marijuana users suffer little if any harm. That position may be intellectually and scientifically indefensible, but those in government regard it as politically and legally obligatory.

So the government resorts to scare tactics and misinformation, relying increasingly on three claims: that today's marijuana is much more potent than the version that kids' parents smoked a decade or two ago; that new research has shown the drug to be more dangerous to our health than previously thought; and that marijuana use is a gateway to more dangerous drugs.

Are these claims true? Is today's marijuana much more potent? Is marijuana much more dangerous than previously believed? Is marijuana a "gateway drug"?

Most marijuana researchers depend on government grants to finance their studies. This poses two problems. First, the government tends to encourage and fund only those research proposals that seek to identify harmful effects of marijuana. There are few incentives to investigate the benefits of marijuana, medicinal or otherwise, and little interest in determining either the safety margins of occasional use or ways of reducing the harms of marijuana use. Studies that identify marijuana as harmful are well publicized by the governments' public-affairs officers. Findings that fail to confirm any harms are ignored.

Second, few marijuana researchers dare publicly challenge the government's anti-marijuana campaign. Scientists know that the grant-review process can be both scientifically objective and politically subjective. If too many studies fail to identify and emphasize the harms of marijuana, subsequent research proposals may not fare well in grant competitions. It takes a lot of courage for a scientist—dependent upon government grants for his or her livelihood—to raise questions about government policies and statements regarding marijuana. Not many scientists are that brave.

Fortunately, there are a few researchers who maintain their independence. Zimmer, the sociologist at Queens College, and Dr. John P. Morgan, a physician and pharmacologist who teaches at the City University Medical School, in New York, don't rely on government funding. They have recently completed a book, *Marijuana Myths, Marijuana Facts: A Review of the Scientific Evidence*, that systematically analyzes and dissects hundreds of studies on marijuana, including virtually all of those cited by government officials and other anti-drug crusaders to justify the war on marijuana. The result is the most comprehensive and objective review of the scientific evidence on marijuana since the National Institute of Medicine's report in 1982—one that both debunks many of the myths propagated by drug warriors and tells the truth about what is actually known of marijuana's harms and margins of safety. What follows is drawn largely from their work.

## THE POTENCY QUESTION

No claim has taken hold so well as the charge that marijuana is much more potent than in the past. "If people ... confessing to marijuana use in the late '60s ... sucked in on one of today's marijuana cigarettes, they'd fall down backward," said William Bennett, President George Bush's first drug czar, in 1990. "Marijuana is 40 times more potent today ... than 10, 15, 20 years ago," another drug czar, Lee Brown, claimed, in 1995. And from the ranking Democrat of the Senate Judiciary Committee, Joseph Biden, in 1996: "It's like comparing buckshot in a shot-gun shell to a laser-guided missile."

Is any of this true? No. Although high-potency marijuana may be more available today than previously, the pharmacological experience of smoking marijuana today is the same as in the 1960s and 1970s. The only data on marijuana potency over time comes from the government-funded Potency Monitoring Project at the University of Mississippi. Since 1981, the average THC (tetrahydrocannabinol, marijuana's principal psychoactive chemical) content of PMP samples—all of which come from drug seizures by U.S. police agencies—has fluctuated between 2.28 percent and 3.82 percent. The project's findings during the 1970s were substantially lower, possibly because the samples were improperly stored (which can cause degradation of THC) and partly due to an overdependence on low-grade Mexican "kilobricks." Independent analyses of marijuana during the 1970s, which included samples from sources other than police agencies, reported much higher THC levels, ranging from 2 percent to 5 percent, with some samples as high as 14 percent.

Marijuana of less than 0.5 percent potency has almost no psychoactivity; in fact, in laboratory studies, subjects are often unable to distinguish a placebo from marijuana with less than 1 percent THC. It's not very likely that marijuana would have become so popular during the 1970s if the average THC content had been so low. Today, some regular marijuana users may have access to expensive, high-potency marijuana, often grown indoors under artificial light by small-scale, low-volume growers. But the potency of the "commercial grade" marijuana smoked by most Americans is not much different than it was 10, 15 or 20 years ago.

Even if marijuana potency had increased, that would not mean the drug has necessarily become more dangerous. It is impossible to consume a lethal dose of marijuana, regardless of its THC content. And in laboratory studies, smokers often fail to distinguish variations in potency of up to 100 percent. Increases of 200 percent to 300 percent in potency result in only 35 percent to 40 percent increases in smokers' "subjective high" ratings. "Bad trips" and other adverse psychoactive reactions typically have little to do with marijuana potency. Moreover, when potency increases, smokers tend to smoke less, thus causing less damage to their lungs.

The bottom line is this: If parents want to know what their kids are smoking today, they need only recall their own experiences. Neither marijuana nor the experience of smoking marijuana has changed much.

## SEX, HEALTH AND MEMORY

Claims of increased THC potency aside, much of the new war on marijuana relies on claims of new scientific research that shows marijuana to be far more dangerous than previously thought.

There are tons of anecdotal reports that marijuana enhances sex. And there are repeated claims that marijuana interferes with male and female sex hormones, can cause infertility, and produces feminine characteristics in males and masculine characteristics in females. Speaking at Framingham High School, in Massachusetts, in late 1994, President Clinton spoke about "the danger of using marijuana, especially to young women, and what might happen to their childbearing capacity in the future."

What's the truth? Some animal studies indicate that high doses of THC diminish the production of some sex hormones and may impair reproduction. In human studies, however, scientists typically find no impact on sex-hormone levels. In the few studies that do show some impact, such as lower sperm counts and sperm motility, the effects are modest, temporary and of no apparent consequence for reproductive capacity. A real-life example: Jamaica's Rastafarians, who smoke large amounts of the sacred herb, appear to have no problem making babies.

In 1972, a letter to the *New England Journal of Medicine* described three cases of breast enlargement in men who had smoked marijuana. In 1980, a letter to the *Journal of Pediatrics* described a 16-year-old marijuana smoker who had failed to progress to puberty. Both reports received substantial publicity, but neither has been confirmed through research. But studies involving larger numbers of marijuana users and non-users have found no evidence that marijuana distorts or delays sexual development, masculinizes females or feminizes males. There may be good reasons for telling kids not to smoke marijuana, but the president's warnings were based on myth, not fact.

Now that thousands of people with AIDS are smoking marijuana to stimulate their appetites and promote weight gain, opponents keep insisting that marijuana's damaging effects on the immune system negate any potential benefits. Here again, the claims are based almost entirely on studies in which laboratory animals are given extremely large doses of THC. There's no evidence that marijuana users have higher rates of infectious disease than non-users. That's not to say that there are no dangers. For people with compromised immune systems, smoking can cause lung infections. There is also a risk for AIDS patients that they will contract a pulmonary disease called aspergillosis caused by fungal spores sometimes found on improperly stored marijuana. One solution to this problem would be careful screening of marijuana supplies, a role for the government or pharmaceutical companies. And that is another reason to prescribe legal, controlled marijuana to more than the

eight Americans who are now entitled to receive it.

Everyone knows that marijuana—like other psychoactive drugs consumed in sufficient doses—screws up short-term memory. Kids who get high (or drunk) before going to class are less likely to learn what their teachers are trying to teach them. Their minds are more likely to wander. People under the influence of marijuana can remember things they learned previously, but their capacity to learn and recall new information is diminished. Although some find marijuana useful for problem solving and creative tasks, there is little question that marijuana is not conducive to learning in school and other highly structured environments.

The question of whether marijuana use permanently impairs memory and other cognitive functions is a separate issue. During the '70s, the U.S. government funded three comprehensive field studies in Jamaica, Greece and Costa Rica, in which long-term heavy cannabis users and non-users were subjected to a battery of standardized tests of their cognitive functions. The researchers found virtually no differences between the two groups.

More recently, two studies funded by the National Institute on Drug Abuse reported evidence of cognitive harm in high-dose marijuana users. The first, published in *Psychopharmacology*, in 1993, found that heavy marijuana users—who reported seven or more uses per week for an average of 6.5 years—scored lower than non-users on math and verbal tests. But the researchers also found that "intermediate" users—those smoking marijuana five to six times per week—were indistinguishable from non-users.

The second study, published in the *Journal of the American Medical Association,* in 1996, found differences between daily marijuana users and those who smoked fewer than 10 times per month, but the differences were minor. The light smokers performed slightly better on two memory tests and one card-sorting test—while no differences were found on tests of attention, verbal fluency and complex drawing.

What we know now, based on existing research, is that if heavy marijuana use produces cognitive impairment, it is relatively minor—and may have little or no practical significance.

**Gateway Drugs?**
The "gateway theory," formerly known as the "steppingstone hypothesis," has long been a staple of anti-marijuana campaigns. Marijuana use, it is claimed, leads inexorably to the use of more dangerous drugs like cocaine, heroin and LSD. If we can stop kids from trying marijuana, we can win the drug war.

The most recent, and oft-repeated, version of the gateway theory—an analysis conducted by the National Center on Addiction and Substance Abuse at Columbia University—asserts that youthful marijuana users are 85 times more likely than non-users to use cocaine. To obtain this figure, the proportion of marijuana users who had ever tried cocaine (17 percent) was divided by the proportion of cocaine users who had never used marijuana (0.2 percent). The "risk factor" is large not because so many marijuana users experiment with cocaine—only a minority actually do—but because people who use cocaine, a relatively unpopular drug, are likely to have also used the more popular drug marijuana. Similarly, marijuana users are more likely than non-users to have had previous experience with legal drugs like alcohol, tobacco and caffeine.

Alcohol, tobacco and caffeine do not cause people to use marijuana. And marijuana does not cause people to use cocaine, heroin or LSD. There is no pharmacological basis for the gateway theory, since marijuana does not change brain chemistry in a way that causes drug-seeking, drug-taking behavior. In fact, there is no theory here at all—just a description of the typical sequence in which people who use many drugs begin by using ones that are more common.

The relationship between marijuana use and the use of other drugs is constantly changing. In some societies, marijuana use follows, rather than precedes, use of heroin and other drugs. Among American high-school seniors, the proportion of marijuana users who have tried cocaine decreased from a high of 33 percent, in 1986, to 14 percent, in 1995. Americans who smoke pot may be more likely to try other illegal drugs than those who don't smoke it. But for a large majority of marijuana users, marijuana is a terminus rather than a gateway drug.

"Now we're putting the research into the hands of parents," Donna Shalala claimed at a recent press conference, renewing the government's war against marijuana. But if it's the truth that Shalala wants to distribute, Zimmer and Morgan's *Marijuana Myths, Marijuana Facts* is a better source.

# POSTSCRIPT

## Is Marijuana Dangerous and Addictive?

Recent initiatives in California and Arizona that bring marijuana closer to being legal are making many people nervous. The propositions in those states would allow the drug to be prescribed by physicians for medicinal purposes. The majority of Americans are against making marijuana completely legal. A compromise would be to decriminalize marijuana, making it neither strictly legal nor illegal. If decriminalized, there would be no penalty for personal or medical use or possession, although there would continue to be criminal penalties for sale for profit and distribution to minors. Marijuana has been decriminalized in a few states, but it is illegal in most of the country.

Decriminalization appeals to attorney Peter Riga, in "The Drug War Is a Crime: Let's Try Decriminalization," *Commonweal* (July 16, 1993); editor Marcia Angell, in "Alcohol and Other Drugs: Toward a More Rational and Consistent Policy," *The New England Journal of Medicine* (August 25, 1994); and journalist Robert Hough, in "Reefer Sadness," *Toronto Globe and Mail* (November 9, 1991). Eric Schlosser, in "Reefer Madness," *The Atlantic Monthly* (August 1994), argues that there are far too many people in jail for marijuana offenses.

In early 1992 the Drug Enforcement Administration published a document claiming that the federal government was justified in its continued prohibition of marijuana for medicinal purposes. The report indicated that too many questions surrounded the effectiveness of medicinal marijuana. See "Medical Marijuana: To Prescribe or Not to Prescribe, That Is the Question," *Journal of Addictive Diseases* (vol. 14, 1995). The effectiveness of marijuana as therapy for cancer and AIDS patients continues to be debated, but the Center on Addiction and Substance Abuse of Columbia University maintains that recent research suggests that the drug is addictive and can wreck the lives of users, particularly teenagers. They argue that legalizing marijuana would undermine the impact of drug education and increase usage.

Other articles that debate the safety and legality of marijuana include "Does Heavy Marijuana Use Impair Human Cognition?" *JAMA* (February 21, 1996); "The Return of Reefer Madness," *The Progressive* (May 1996); "Smoke Alarm," *Reason* (May 1996); "Pot Luck," *National Review* (November 11, 1996); "The Battle for Medical Marijuana," *The Nation* (January 6, 1997); "Federal Foolishness and Marijuana," *The New England Journal of Medicine* (January 30, 1997); "The War Over Weed," *Newsweek* (February 3, 1997); "Prescription Drugs," *Reason* (February 1997); "Marijuana: Useful Medicine or Dangerous Drug?" *Consumers' Research Magazine* (May 1997); and "Moving Marijuana," *Reason* (May 1998).

# On the Internet . . .

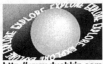

http://www.dushkin.com

## University of Maryland/Women's Studies
This site provides a wealth of resources related to women's physical and emotional well-being. Links to topics such as body image, comfort (or discomfort) with sexuality, and personal relationships are given.
*http://www.inform.umd.edu/EdRes/Topic/WomensStudies/*

## The Men's Issues Page
The Men's Issues Page has an alphabetical subject index of men's issues, including fatherhood, physical health, and related topics. This site addresses a variety of men's health, social, and psychological concerns.
*http://www.vix.com/pub/men/index.html*

## National Alliance of Breast Cancer Organizations
The National Alliance of Breast Cancer Organizations' Web site supplies information on breast cancer and the latest listings for treatment and other research opportunities.
*http://www.nabco.org*

## Body Health Resources Corporation
This site is a multimedia AIDS and HIV information resource. It includes basic AIDS information, treatment details, and advice on quality of life.
*http://www.thebody.com/index.shtml*

# PART 4

## Sexuality and Gender Issues

*Few issues could be of greater controversy than those concerning gender and sexuality. Recent generations of Americans have rejected "traditional" sexual roles and values, which has resulted in a significant increase in babies born out of wedlock, the spread of sexually transmitted diseases, and a rise in legal abortions. This section debates the health risks of breast implants, the alleged gender gap in health care, late-term abortions, drug therapy for menopausal women, and the issue of confidentiality for people with AIDS.*

■ Are Silicone Breast Implants a Health Risk to Women?

■ Does Health Care Delivery and Research Benefit Men at the Expense of Women?

■ Should Confidentiality Remain a Priority for People With AIDS?

■ Should Partial-Birth Abortion Be Banned?

■ Will Most Postmenopausal Women Benefit from Estrogen Replacement Therapy?

# ISSUE 11

## Are Silicone Breast Implants a Health Risk to Women?

**YES: Jennifer Washburn,** from "Reality Check: Can 400,000 Women Be Wrong?" *Ms.* (March/April 1996)

**NO: Michael Fumento,** from "A Confederacy of Boobs," *Reason* (October 1995)

### ISSUE SUMMARY

**YES:** Reporter Jennifer Washburn challenges two studies that claim silicone gel implants do no harm and finds that over 10 percent of the women who received implants are ill.

**NO:** Journalist Michael Fumento argues that special interests and the press have conspired to ban implants despite the fact that no scientific study has linked them to cancer or other diseases.

From 1979 to 1992, the peak years for breast implant surgery in the United States, nearly 150,000 women had their breasts enlarged or reconstructed. By 1994 breast augmentation was the third most common cosmetic operation in America, despite the 1992 ban by the Food and Drug Administration (FDA). Overall, approximately 1 million women have had the surgery. Because of health concerns, the FDA banned silicone gel, which was replaced with implants filled with sterile salt water. Initially, silicone appeared to be a perfect substance to enlarge breasts (or other body parts); but it became apparent that injecting any foreign substance into the body causes an inflammatory response. When silicone was initially used to enlarge breasts, it was injected directly into the body, but this caused pain and infection. Dow Corning, in 1962, developed a silicone-filled prosthesis that adhered to the chest muscles. The device prevented the silicone from migrating to other body parts, reducing the risk of inflammation.

In 1992 Dr. David Kessler, the FDA director, banned silicone breast implants after responding to mounting concerns that they caused autoimmune and connective tissue damage and disease. The autoimmune disorders included cancer, lupus, rheumatoid arthritis, scleroderma, and polymyalgia. The ban resulted in a flood of lawsuits, as women by the thousands sued the manufacturers of the implants. Juries sympathetic to the women's plight awarded huge damages. In April 1994, in a class action settlement, the major manufacturers agreed to pay over $4 billion to women with breast implants, $1 billion of which was set aside for the attorneys.

Do breast implants actually cause these diseases? Interestingly, there were almost no reliable scientific studies published by the time of the 1992 ban. Since then, several have been published. In investigations conducted by the Mayo Clinic and Harvard University, no connection was found between implants and connective tissue disease. As other studies are added to the evidence, however, absolute proof of the relationship between implants and autoimmune disease is lacking, though some women did experience surgical complications (as with any surgery, complications, including infection and hemorrhage, can occur). In addition, some women experienced scar tissue formation around the breasts and, in some cases, the implant ruptured, releasing silicone gel into the surrounding tissues and flattening the breast.

How, then, in the absence of proof from well-designed studies, did the idea of autoimmune disease risk develop in the first place, and why did women with implants win in court? Probably from a mixture of anecdotes and speculation. As isolated reports became the basis of litigation and as the publicity in the media grew, more women came forward with similar symptoms. Since the ban, women with implants who have these symptoms are more likely to come to light because of the heightened awareness of the situation. This extra attention may increase the impression that there is a *proven* link even if there is not. Also, some physicians who are sympathetic and believe in a relationship between implants and disease tend to draw these women to their practices. As a result, studying these women does not answer the question of whether or not implants actually increase the risk of autoimmune disease.

Many scientific organizations, including the American Medical Association, the FDA advisory panel on General and Plastic Surgery Devices, and committees commissioned by the British, Canadian, and French governments, have all agreed that there is no proof that silicone implants cause autoimmune diseases or systemwide harm. Why, then, were the courts, the media, and the public so certain that breast implants are dangerous?

According to Dr. Marcia Angell, executive editor of *The New England Journal of Medicine*, the answer to this question is in the way science, the public, and the law regard evidence. As our society becomes more dependent on science and technology, there are bound to be further misconceptions about scientific evidence that could become a danger to the public. In the following selections, Jennifer Washburn disagrees. She asserts that the major studies disputing a relationship between implants and autoimmune disease are full of holes and should be discounted. Michael Fumento agrees with Angell. He states that the attack and litigation involving silicone breast implants is nothing more than a campaign of misinformation.

# YES

Jennifer Washburn

# REALITY CHECK: CAN 400,000
# WOMEN BE WRONG?

In September 1993, Charlotte Mahlum, a waitress from Elko, Nevada, and the mother of two children, sued the Dow Corning Corporation and one of its parent companies, the Dow Chemical Company, alleging that silicone breast implants manufactured by Dow Corning had made her sick. Mahlum, 44 years old, had had the implants put in after a double mastectomy in 1985. Six years later, she developed joint and muscle aches, full-body rashes, and chronic fatigue. Soon afterward, she began to suffer tremors and seizures, and was diagnosed with axonal polyneuropathy, a condition that prevents brain signals from reaching the outermost nerves. At times she suffered fits of uncontrollable shaking, and she eventually lost control of her bowels.

When Mahlum had her implants taken out in 1993, silicone breast implants had been off the market for a year (for all but mastectomy patients), removed by the Food and Drug Administration (FDA), whose commissioner, David Kessler, said at the time, "We know more about the life span of automobile tires than we do about the longevity of breast implants." When Mahlum's surgeon opened up her chest, he discovered that one implant had ruptured, but he was unable to remove all of the gel that had seeped into surrounding tissue. Today, Charlotte Mahlum is still extremely ill.

In May 1995, Dow Corning declared bankruptcy, placing itself beyond the reach of the trial courts. The bankruptcy was announced days after the collapse of the Breast Implant Global Settlement, in which implant manufacturers had agreed to compensate the members of a class action suit who claimed to have—or feared the development of—illnesses associated with silicone implants. At least 400,000 women had signed up for the suit, and their numbers were growing.

Mahlum proceeded with her case against Dow Chemical, which owns 50 percent of Dow Corning's stock. Although Dow Chemical never manufactured silicone breast implants, it performed much of the original research and testing on liquid silicone, which makes up 80 to 85 percent of the gel used in Dow Corning implants. On October 30, 1995, a Nevada jury ruled in Mahlum's favor, awarding $14.1 million to her and her husband, $10 million of it in punitive damages. It was one of the highest awards ever granted in a breast implant case. Dow Chemical plans to appeal this ruling.

Although the Mahlum jury had reviewed internal documents that showed that both companies knew liquid silicone was dangerous inside the body, the verdict outraged implant manufacturers, who insist that there is no proven link between silicone implants and disease. It also sparked an outpouring of criticism in the media. "It's the judges' fault," blasted a Wall Street Journal editorial, lamenting that breast implant companies are "paying billions in damages despite a mountain of evidence they didn't do anything wrong." Even advocates of legal reform got into the act, insisting that the case proved that the U.S. legal system is in desperate need of fixing.

More than 100,000 of the approximately one million U.S. women who have received silicone breast implants are currently ill. But the companies and many commentators insist that the autoimmune diseases thousands of women suffer from don't exist. For proof they point to two studies published in the New England Journal of Medicine. The first, by the Mayo Clinic, appeared in 1994. The second came out a year later, reporting on research performed by Harvard University and Brigham and Women's Hospital, which is affiliated with Harvard's medical school. Both say there is no link between silicone breast implants and autoimmune diseases. The studies have been held up as proof that lawyers like Mahlum's are using "junk science" to win large awards at the expense of innocent corporations.

Is that true? Or could two such respected institutions as the Mayo Clinic and Harvard University actually be guilty of practicing shoddy science themselves? Ms. [magazine] has found, through speaking with doctors, researchers, plaintiffs' lawyers, and the two institutions as well, that there is a great deal wrong with these studies.

Although plastic surgeons have been promising their patients that silicone breast implants are perfectly safe ever since the products became available in 1963, implants were put on the market without long-term testing. But that doesn't mean that no testing was done at all. In a letter to the New York Times, Fredric Ellis and Ernest Hornsby, lawyers for Charlotte Mahlum, stated that "Dow Chemical found out in the 1960s that liquid silicone affected the immune system and central nervous system and could even be effective as an insecticide. Instead of disclosing this research to the scientific community, Dow Chemical concealed the results and entered into secret development agreements with Dow Corning to develop silicone as a drug and as an insecticide." When Dow Corning did report the results of research, it was often far from truthful. In a 1973 article in Medical Instrumentation, Dow reported on a study of four dogs that had been implanted with miniature silicone breast implants. The article only reported the six-month results—that the dogs had suffered some inflammation, but no other adverse effects—since Dow said the results at the end of the study's full two years were the same. But in fact, lawyers for a woman who was suing Dow proved in court that after two years, one dog had died and the others suffered from severe chronic inflammation, thyroiditis, autoimmune response, and spots on the spleen.

Doctors soon began seeing the effects of Dow's decision not to fully disclose the results of silicone testing. Women came to them describing debilitating pain, often in the chest and shoulder. As we now know, within two to four years of receiving a silicone implant, nearly 70 percent of patients suffer capsular contracture, a hardening of the scar tissue around the implant, which squeezes the implant into a hard disk. But as painful and disfiguring as capsular contracture can be, it is not nearly as serious as the danger women face when silicone enters their bodies, either through leakage or implant rupture. In its early literature, Dow Corning said that the implants would last a lifetime, but in reality, many don't make it past 15 years. A study published in *Annals of Plastic Surgery* in 1994 reported that among women surveyed who had implants for five years or less, 93 percent of the implants were intact. But only 30 percent of implants that were six to 15 years old remained intact. And in 1995, the same journal reported on a study of 300 breast implant patients: 71.3 percent of them had experienced rupture or severe silicone leakage.

Dow Corning knew that gel could leak from its implants and that they had a high rupture rate. In a 1983 company memo, a researcher points out that the safety of implants is based upon the assumption that "ruptures do not occur or are removed quickly when they do occur by additional surgery. Experience has shown this latter assumption to not be accurate... some physicians have noted ruptures... that may go undetected for unknown time periods."

Yet Dow Corning failed to investigate the long-term health consequences of liquid silicone leaking into the body. Other researchers have, and although their research is still in progress, there are some things we do know. Doctors have found proof that silicone can travel to internal organs and can settle there. Dr. Douglas Shanklin, a professor of medicine at the University of Tennessee, who has been studying what he believes to be silicone-related disorders for ten years, says he recently saw an implant patient with silicone fluid in her brain and spinal fluid. This woman cannot feel where her feet and hands are, has lost her memory, and cannot keep her balance because her nerve sensors are impaired. "They have been grounded out, just like an electrical wire," says Dr. Shanklin.

\* \* \*

According to Shanklin, silicone leaking into the body causes a "cellular immune reaction," which shows up initially as inflammation. "The body's immune system is trying to get rid of this stuff, but it can't. We can't metabolize silicone." Our immune system doesn't know that and keeps on fighting. "Eventually, after 10, 12, or 14 years, this primary attack... is exhausted. Then the body begins attacking its own cell tissue and organs," resulting in autoimmune disease, says Shanklin. Traditional autoimmune, or connective tissue, diseases include rheumatoid arthritis and lupus.

But Dr. Shanklin and the majority of doctors treating women with implants have found that the women primarily suffer not from traditional autoimmune diseases, but from a specific constellation of problems—including joint pains, skin rashes, numbness, and fatigue—that medicine has never before seen grouped together in this way. Rather than analyze and define what this new syndrome might be, most large-scale studies have concentrated on looking for previously identified diseases—and have rarely found them.

The Harvard/Brigham study, also known as the "Nurses' Study," and the Mayo Clinic study should have changed all that. Considering how much was riding on this research, it is surprising to discover that both studies are full of holes—thanks to problems in design as well as to conflicts of interest.

\* \* \*

Neither the Mayo nor the Harvard/Brigham study focused on "atypical" symptoms. The Mayo Clinic looked at 14 isolated symptoms, although researchers believe it is the clustering of these symptoms that indicates silicone disease. The researchers relied on information on medical charts, where symptoms like skin rashes are less likely to have been noted than are firm disease diagnoses. Women in the study were never examined or interviewed by Mayo's researchers, and no attempt was made to inquire about symptoms that weren't on the charts.

The Harvard/Brigham study claims to have looked at a broad range of atypical symptoms, but only women who reported being diagnosed with a *traditional* connective-tissue disease were given the questionnaire on atypical symptoms. Many women who are severely ill would inevitably have been excluded with this method. (The final count included only 32 women with implants *and* connective tissue disease.) During questioning under oath, the study's authors admitted that, despite earlier claims, they had, in fact, only examined traditional diseases.

"We're dealing with atypical disorders. Anyone who read the literature going back to the 1970s would have known that you need to look beyond classical diseases," says Dr. Gary Solomon, who is the associate director of rheumatology at the

Hospital for Joint Diseases Orthopaedic Institute in New York City. "It is frankly disturbing that these medical studies did not consider this. One can only suspect that this was intentional."

Critics also say that the studies look at too few women to find an increased risk of even the traditional diseases that they were looking for. The Mayo Clinic studied the health records of 749 women with implants (and 1,498 controls). The Harvard researchers chose 1,183 women with implants (876 of them silicone) for their study. But since a traditional autoimmune disease like scleroderma —a fibrotic thickening of skin and vital organs—occurs in only .02 to .04 percent of the population, "to detect even a doubling of the baseline rate of scleroderma, you would need to have at least 30,000 women in your study," explains Dr. Solomon.

And neither study considered a long enough "latency period." Doctors estimate that the average length of time it takes for a woman with implants to begin showing symptoms of illness is eight to ten years. In the Mayo study, women were tracked for a mean of 7.8 years after implantation. The Harvard researchers interviewed women who had had implants for a mean of 9.9 years, but they included women whose implants were only 30 days old. (Even more astonishing, the researchers included one woman who said she'd had her silicone implants nearly 40 years, even though the first implants were not available until 1963—29 years before the study began.) "This is not unlike R. J. Reynolds funding a study that examines people in their thirties, and finding no increased risk of lung cancer," says Dr. Shanna Swan, an epidemiologist at the University of California at Berkeley's School of Public Health. Many doctors believe it may take decades for the full effects of silicone poisoning to appear.

* * *

Both studies have also been plagued with conflict of interest charges. Dr. Matthew Liang, for instance, a coauthor of the Harvard study, was paid $2,525 by law firms representing Dow Corning and other manufacturers, for consulting work. Meanwhile, the Mayo study was funded by the National Institutes of Health (NIH) and the Plastic Surgery Educational Foundation (PSEF), which receives funding from implant manufacturers. Part of the $174,000 that PSEF gave the Mayo Clinic came from Dow Corning and two other manufacturers, McGhan Medical and Bristol-Meyers Squibb. The companies say this isn't a problem, that they have "no input on what research the foundation chooses to fund." But documents show that they do influence which studies get money, and sometimes they oversee research. In an August 31, 1990, letter to Abt Associates, a research firm that was hoping to study atypical diseases, foundation president Barrett Noone wrote: "The manufacturer's group in general and Dow Corning in specific were disinclined to behave in a collaborative manner.... My colleagues and I are disappointed by their decision not to fund your study." On November 24, 1992, the vice president for research and development at Mentor Corporation, also an implant manufacturer, wrote to the foundation concerning a different study, one the company *did* want to fund: "We are in direct contact with these authors and discussing the various aspects of these study plan[s]. As the protocols are finalized, these authors will directly send the final protocol to your organization."

Dow Corning may have had an even more direct hand in the Harvard study. Three months before a questionnaire was sent to participants, researcher Dr. Jorge Sanchez Guerrero provided a copy of the questionnaire to Dow Corning epidemiologists. At press time, Matthew Liang had refused to release information to the courts that could reveal whether the questionnaire was altered to suit Dow Corning.

Given the problems with these studies, is there any research that can clarify the relation between silicone implants and disease? There are, in fact, hundreds of peer-reviewed medical studies that have found that silicone breast implants and their components are dangerous to human health. But these studies, like those of Harvard and Mayo, are not definitive. Nevertheless, they point to areas for concern. At an NIH workshop a year ago, several studies showed evidence of autoimmune problems linked to silicone. One, by Dr. Michael Potter of the National Cancer Institute, found that after being injected with silicone gel, as many as 80 per cent of mice developed the equivalent of multiple myeloma, a rare cancer that attacks immune system cells.

Another study (not presented at the NIH workshop) that has caused concern is one led by Dr. Shanklin at the University of Tennessee, and a colleague, Dr. David Smalley. Their research indicates that children born to symptomatic women with silicone implants sometimes have the same silicone-specific cellular immune activity as their mothers—i.e., their bodies are fighting a foreign substance that appears to be silicone.

The NIH is finally putting together a large-scale investigation of "atypical disease symptoms," using 18,000 women, 13,000 of whom have implants. In addition, a "Silicone-Related Syndrome Study Group" has been created by members of the American College of Rheumatology (ACR) to define and describe the diseases that some women with implants are suffering from. (The ACR itself is caught in a battle over silicone. At the college's annual meeting in October 1995, its directors announced that implants do not cause rheumatic diseases, claiming that the courts that had ruled in favor of women with implants were relying on "anecdotal evidence." Members of the ACR were furious and demanded that the directors retract their statement, pointing out that 16 out of 18 studies presented at the conference indicated links between implants and certain diseases.)

Some doctors are pinning their hopes on Harvard's "Women's Health Cohort Study," of nearly 400,000 women, but others worry that Dow Corning has also funded this study—to the tune of its full $6.8 million. As it turns out, interim findings from the cohort study (that were leaked to the press in 1995) indicate a 45 to 49 percent increased risk of rheumatoid arthritis among women with silicone implants. Despite these findings, which admittedly could change when the data are fully analyzed, Matthew Liang publicly insists that implants are safe.

\* \* \*

Meanwhile, claiming that Americans sue each other too much, the Republican Congress seeks to make it more difficult for the women who have yet to go to court to win their cases against silicone implant manufacturers. Advocates claim they are trying to curb a litigation explosion that is burdening the courts. Yet, according to the National Center for State Courts, tort suits (cases concerning injury or damages) are just 9 percent of all state court filings, and product liability suits are only 4 percent of that. To many analysts, today's tort reform is another case of corporations using their political clout to escape potential liability. And liability is certainly a big issue for both Dow Chemical and Dow Corning.

The Manhattan Institute, a conservative think tank and long-time lobbyer for tort reform, held a conference in Washington last June, featuring Dow Corning's CEO, Richard Hazleton, who took the opportunity to deliver Dow's wish list on reform. First came the "exclusion of biomaterials suppliers from litigation brought against medical device manufacturers." Dow, of course, is a supplier to many implant manufacturers. Next was a cap on punitive damages; under the cap proposed by the Republicans, Charlotte Mahlum—who will be sick for the rest of her life—would not have received much more than $250,000.

Despite Dow's obvious interest in legal reform, much of the media has bought into the company's analysis of the implant crisis. Marcia Angell, the executive editor of the *New England Journal of Medicine,* wrote an article in *The New Republic* last year in which she blasted "rapacious attorneys," "well-paid doctors who stretch the science and ethical limits of their profession," and "healthy women" for "responding to the lure of big financial awards."

The *New York Times* also promotes this interpretation. Gina Kolata, a *Times* science reporter, pronounced the Harvard study "so compelling... that some leading rheumatologists contend that the issue of whether implants cause these diseases can now be considered closed." What about the women who have been diagnosed with illnesses? Kolata told *Ms.*

that some of them might be responding to "the power of suggestion."

We have been down this road before. Women in real pain going to doctors and being told that it is all in their heads. Women being encouraged to use medical devices that don't function properly and being told these devices are perfectly safe when they aren't. What we haven't had before, certainly not on this scale, is tens of thousands of women who were perfectly healthy being given something that has jeopardized their health. At the same time, women who are in the midst of fighting one devastating disease—breast cancer—are being asked to risk other illnesses. And the time bomb is still ticking. Only about 300,000 women have passed the latency period (half of all women who have received breast implants got them after 1988). There are approximately 700,000 more women who, if they are not sick yet, must wait and watch to see if they will be.

# NO

## Michael Fumento

# A CONFEDERACY OF BOOBS

"Not only are they abusing the judicial system, but they are emotionally abusing the women." That's what one silicone breast implant recipient told the *Boston Herald* following the decision of Dow Corning to file for bankruptcy. Dow Corning had contributed about half of a $4.2 billion settlement—the biggest ever—for women claiming to suffer various illnesses from their implants.

[In 1995], however, it became clear that there were far more women trying to get a piece of the pie than there were slices. Plaintiffs' attorneys were saying that $74 billion might be needed to satisfy just the first set of claims against the companies. Rather than close its doors forever, Dow Corning chose to try to limit its losses.

Financially, it's unclear where the bankruptcy leaves implant claimants. But what has become more and more certain since the settlement was reached back in 1993 is that while both the judicial system and silicone implant recipients have been terribly abused, the villain isn't Dow Corning or any other implant maker.

Indeed, women with breast implants have been nothing more than pawns in a bizarre game involving lawyers, feminists, headline hounds, and super-inflated bureaucratic egos. The stakes, however, go beyond the physical and mental health of women with implants to include the future health of millions of Americans who will need insertable medical devices. Indeed, the multimillion-dollar awards against silicone implant manufacturers have already triggered a wave of suits against medical implants made of solid silicone and even some containing no silicone at all.

"We have great concerns that any medical device with silicone in it will not survive," says Elizabeth Connell, a professor of gynecology and obstetrics at Emory University and head of two Food and Drug Administration [FDA] silicone breast implant panels that unsuccessfully recommended leaving the devices on the market. Since June 1992, most uses of silicone breast implants have been banned by the FDA. Annually, some 1.5 million patients receive silicone eye lenses; another 670,000 get artificial silicone joints. All told, about 7.5 million medical devices are implanted in Americans each year. Many of these devices—such as pacemakers, heart valves, and shunts which draw fluid off the brain—are life savers.

Hence, the misinformed campaign against silicone breast implants raises issues that go far beyond the not insignificant question of whether women should be able to change their appearance as they see fit. A strange alliance of diverse interests, including FDA bureaucrats interested in broadening their powers, feminists who equate boob jobs with mutilation, and reporters more interested in good copy than relevant medical research, worked together to take implants off the market. The anti-implant campaign is nothing less than a case study in how medical public policy is often driven by anecdotal rather than epidemiological evidence, formulated by ideologues who have little regard for what individuals might value, and discussed in a consistently one-sided manner.

The use of silicone implants to enlarge the size of the breast dates back to 1963. Somewhere around one million American women have received them. Implants may be used either for "augmentation"— making a healthy breast or pair of breasts larger—or to replace a breast removed during mastectomy. It appears that about 60 percent of breast implants have been used for augmentation.

While there has been mention of possible disease caused by implants as far back as 1978, the kick-off point of the scare that ultimately prompted the FDA to ban silicone implants may have been the airing of an implant feature on CBS's *Face to Face with Connie Chung* in 1990. Chung's graphic imagery—she called silicone gel "an ooze of slimy gelatin that could be poisoning" women —spurred one stampede of women to

have their implants removed and another to file suits against implant makers.

As Chung herself later put it, the show "unleashed a torrent of protests and investigations around the country." Soon, women were bombarded with such stories as "Toxic Breasts," "The Hazards of Silicone," and "Time Bombs in the Breasts." The height of hysteria may have been reached when, after the FDA moratorium, two women removed their own implants with razor blades. They said they had no success in getting doctors to remove them.

A new front opened up in December 1991, when a California jury awarded a Marin County woman, Mariann Hopkins, $7.3 million from Dow Corning. She alleged aches, pains, and fatigue caused by her implants without citing any illness more specific than autoimmune disease, a catchall phrase for a variety of connective-tissue diseases such as rheumatoid arthritis, scleroderma, lupus, Sjogren's Syndrome, fibromyalgia, and Raynaud's Disease.

In January 1992, the FDA declared a voluntary (but strongly recommended) moratorium on the sale and use of silicone breast implants pending review of additional information, saying, "physicians should cease using them and manufacturers should stop shipping them." Four months later, the FDA essentially converted this to a ban, although the agency did allow continued use of the implants for women who had suffered mastectomies and permitted a small number of women who wanted implants for cosmetic purposes to enroll in long-term studies.

\* \* \*

Like many health scares, the one over silicone implants is primarily American.

Only a few countries besides the United States forbid the devices within their borders. One is Canada, even though the Canadian Independent Advisory Committee review showed no causal link between silicone breast implants and serious illness. While most countries haven't even seriously considered removing silicone implants from use, some, such as the United Kingdom, have reviewed the evidence and affirmatively stated that implants should remain available. In June 1994, the 20-member European Committee on Quality Assurance and Medical Devices in Plastic Surgery declared it "does not support any restriction on the use of silicone-gel filled implants."

Because of the ban in the United States, American women have gone to other countries, including the United Kingdom, Mexico, France, and Germany, to get implants. One popular package mixing implantation in an English hospital with a trip to Shakespeare's birthplace is called "Boobs n' Bard." Having to go abroad for implants, of course, prices some women out of the market. Women who do travel for implants face different problems: If something goes wrong with the surgery, the doctor is thousands of miles away. And malpractice suits are difficult to pursue in much of the world and virtually impossible in South and Central America.

The FDA seriously considered pulling saline-filled implants off the market as well. But in late 1994, it decided to allow their continued use pending approval applications due in 1998. Silicone is generally preferred to saline because it gives the breast a more natural feel. To keep saline-filled breasts from swishing like a waterbed, it is necessary to pack them tight with the solution. In breasts that are quite small to begin with, wrinkles or ripples in the implant surface are more easily visible through the skin and the breast may not move or hang as naturally as it would with silicone implants.

Whatever goes into the implant of the future, the silicone implants of today are in the bodies of a million or more women who need to know what risk, if any, these devices pose.

There are two ways that women can be exposed to silicone from an implant. One is when microscopic droplets of silicone fluid "bleed" through the envelope of a gel-filled implant. "Low-bleed" implants have been available since the early 1980s and have reduced the amount of silicone that escapes from the implant. In any event, because scar tissue quickly forms around the implant, the gel usually goes no further than one or two millimeters beyond the implant wall.

The other way women can be exposed is through rupture. According to the FDA, about 4 percent to 6 percent of silicone implants have ruptured, though studies in progress indicate this figure is probably too low.

Nonetheless, again the scar "capsule" that invariably grows around the implant tends to hold any silicone even if it breaks, which explains why so many ruptures are outwardly undetectable. While the gel has gone beyond the pouch, it still usually remains in place, although it has been found in the lymphatic system of some women.

That implants can cause physical problems is beyond doubt. It has long been known, for instance, that the scar capsule can harden and constrict, sometimes painfully so. This hardening can make necessary follow-up treatment to remove the scar tissue. Makers of later model implants claim to have reduced this problem, but it's too early to say what success they may have had.

But when critics warn of the dangers of silicone implants, this usually minor problem is seldom what they're talking about. According to Jack Fisher, a San Diego plastic surgeon and outspoken defender of implants, more than 50 symptoms are alleged to be caused by implants, including memory loss, dry mouth, cancer, bladder problems, difficulty swallowing, joint pain, decreased sex drive, and a host of autoimmune diseases. Some have referred to this broad constellation of symptoms as "silicone-gel syndrome." But if it is a syndrome it appears the proper definition would have to be any illness that any woman with implants ever contracts.

To sympathetic observers, such a wide array of symptoms must seem alarming. But a general rule of epidemiology is that the more diverse the symptoms allegedly related to a single cause are, the less likely it is that the suspected cause is real. This basic precept is, in a sense, the mirror image of snake-oil cures that promise to remedy all sorts of unrelated symptoms. Many of the most commonly cited symptoms of silicone exposure—such as fatigue, headaches, and difficulty swallowing—can be brought on by suggestion. As a result, people who hear that implants may cause certain problems may then develop them. These are the same "side effects" described by participants in drug studies who are actually receiving placebos.

And, in fact, most of the evidence against implants is anecdotal: It is based on reports from women who are sick and have implants and claim the two conditions are related. Thus, if a woman with implants ever develops symptoms that doctors can't readily explain, everyone simply assumes that silicone is the cause. Sometimes this sort of reasoning is expressed in the very titles (of the implant scare articles. Consider the headline for the *San Francisco Chronicle's* article about Mariann Hopkins: "After Breast Implant, Horror Began."

While such a loose correlation may be appealing to people looking for quick and easy answers, it is essentially the same logical fallacy that blames black cats for inexplicable illness. Yet, in some cases, the silicone-gel symptoms actually predate the implants. Indeed, such a curious time frame appears to have been the case even in the first big implant settlement.

One of Mariann Hopkins's treating physicians testified that, although her diagnosis of mixed connective-tissue disease did not come until after the implants were put in, she had already displayed symptoms of connective-tissue disease as early as two years before receiving implants. The doctor even testified that another physician was so concerned that he subjected her to a battery of tests for one type of connective-tissue illness called systemic rheumatic disease. Those came back negative, but they were not tests specifically for mixed connective-tissue disease. Had they been and had they come back positive, it's unlikely Hopkins would have ever received the $7.3 million award.

But then again, the jury did not seem overly influenced by those most knowledgeable of Hopkins's medical history. At the time of trial, Hopkins was basically free of symptoms, thanks to a low dose of medicine. And none of Hopkins's treating physicians testified at the trial that they believed her illness to be related to the implants.

Instead, the jury made its finding on the basis of outside testimony that implants could cause such disease, testimony from professional anti-implant witnesses such as Tampa, Florida, physician Frank Vasey, who makes his living by treating women he says are sick from their implants.

Perhaps the most serious charge against silicone implants is also the weakest—that they may cause breast cancer. Although such influential groups as Sidney Wolfe's Public Citizen (founded by Ralph Nader) have made the claim, repeated studies have shown no such link. The only cancers ever plausibly attributed to silicone—in a study released over 40 years ago—were connective-tissue sarcomas that appeared in strains of rodents especially susceptible to cancer.

* * *

The simple truth is that no epidemiological studies have linked cancer in people to implants. The largest study is also the most recent: After looking at a group of almost 11,000 women from the Alberta, Canada, area, the Alberta Cancer Board concluded, "The incidence of breast cancer among the women who had breast augmentation could not be said to be either significantly higher or lower than that among the general population.

Polyurethane implants, which make up about 10 percent of implants currently in use, are a special case. Manufactured by Surgitek Inc., a subsidiary (of Bristol-Myers Squibb Co., these implants featured a gel-filled pouch with a layer of polyurethane foam coating the silicone envelope. The implants were a special target of Connie Chung's *Face to Face* report. Under such heat, Surgitek felt it had no choice but to remove them from the market in 1991. (Nevertheless, a *USA To-day* illustration in May 1995 accompanying an anti-implant editorial depicted a polyurethane-coated implant.)

The purpose of the foam was to reduce the chance of scar tissue contracting around the implant. But when the foam breaks down chemically, it produces a substance called 2-toluene diamine (TDA) that is considered a probable animal carcinogen and a possible human one. Although that would seem to be an obvious source of trouble, it turns out that, like all the other serious accusations against breast implants, the charges against polyurethane implants don't hold up under epidemiological scrutiny. The only difference is that in this case the FDA has admitted it.

In late June, Bristol-Myers Squibb concluded an FDA-solicited study to determine how much TDA really ended up in the system of women with polyurethane implants. The amount (when any was found at all) was so small that even assuming it is a *definite* human carcinogen—using the FDA's own rating system—the risk of cancer was one in a million. Since only about 110,000 women have had such implants, the FDA stated in a position paper, "FDA estimates it is unlikely that exposure to TDA will cause cancer in even one of the women with these implants." The agency added, "The health risk connected with surgical removal of the implants is far greater than the risk of developing cancer."

There's another, deeper irony in the whole polyurethane controversy, one the FDA obviously couldn't state: that a product designed to alleviate the only absolutely certain health problem clearly linked to implants was forced off the market because of worries over other unproven health effects.

Since silicone gel from implants is most commonly accused of causing autoimmune disease, or connective-tissue disease, it isn't surprising that a large number of studies on both animals and humans have looked for a link between silicone exposure and autoimmune/connective-tissue disease. When the British Department of Health undertook a review of these studies earlier this year, it found approximately 270 papers published after 1971 alone.

The animal studies, the department concluded, "provide no immunological reason for concern over the use of silicone gels in implants." The report went even further, however: "None of these studies demonstrated that the coexistence of connective-tissue disease with silicone breast implants is any more prevalent than would be expected by chance."

The largest study of connective-tissue disease to date appeared in the *New England Journal of Medicine* [in] June [1995]. Conducted by the Harvard School of Public Health and the Brigham and Women's Hospital in Boston, the study looked for evidence of 41 types of connective-tissue disease among 87,501 nurses, of whom 1,183 had implants.

* * *

The results were unambiguous. The researchers found no "association between silicone breast implants and connective-tissue diseases, defined according to a variety of standardized criteria." Already anticipating the charge that they knew would be forthcoming from plaintiffs' lawyers—that silicone implants cause a special kind of autoimmune disease that doesn't show up with standardized criteria—the authors added, "or signs or symptoms of these diseases." In fact, they reported that women with silicone implants were significantly less likely to relate symptoms of these diseases or to complain of symptoms or signs of illness resembling connective-tissue disease.

For many health professionals, the *NEJM* study, added on top of all the others, was the final piece of proof needed. "I think we have enough data to end the moratorium," George E. Erlich, a Philadelphia rheumatologist and head of the FDA arthritis advisory committee, told *The New York Times*. Erlich emphasized he was speaking for himself and not the FDA committee, but he added that the International League of the Associations of Rheumatology also agreed unanimously there was no evidence linking implants to connective-tissue disease. And long before that, the American College of Rheumatology had already issued its own statement, saying, "There is no convincing evidence that these implants cause any generalized disease."

If the evidence against silicone implants is so weak—and has always been so—why have they inspired such commotion and fear? The chief reason has to do with the federal bureaucrat whose various power-grabbing machinations would embarrass a villain from Central Casting: David Kessler, commissioner of the FDA.

In December 1991, Kessler called together a panel of physicians, self-styled consumer representatives, and the like to evaluate the evidence of potential harm caused by implants. The verdict of the panel, though by no means unanimous, was that the devices should remain on the market pending collection of further data from studies already underway.

That, however, did not please Kessler, who ordered FDA staffers to solicit case histories from doctors of implant recipients who later claimed to have suffered ills as a possible result. Since lawyers had already begun soliciting women with complaints and sending them on to specially chosen doctors, finding such case histories was probably not difficult. In any event, case histories reveal little because they don't allow for comparison groups. That's what the epidemiological studies were, but Kessler couldn't wait for them.

In January 1992, Kessler implemented the moratorium, citing the case studies as the reason (and glossing over the fact that he himself solicited them). The next month, he reconvened the panel to ply them with his new "evidence." The panel didn't budge and Kessler once again ignored its advice.

"We still saw no clear evidence of danger, though there were a number of unanswered questions," says Emory's Connell, who served as the chair of both panels. "We felt breast implants should stay available to women who, with informed consent, wanted to use them." Three and a half years after the first panel voted to recommend keeping the implants available, Connell says she would clearly do so again. "I think the difference is we could say it this time with a great deal more assurance."

"A whole new literature has been developed since that time," she explains. "We were operating on anecdotal evidence and case history. Now the evidence has been gathered by good people in well-designed studies so it's an entirely different situation."

So why did the FDA ban silicone implants despite the lack of evidence that they are harmful? Pressure came from repeated anecdotal reports in both print and television media. The moratorium that became a ban occurred after more than a year of intense media pressure, including Connie Chung's inflammatory show, which was repeated a year later.

Congressional pressure, in the form of the late Rep. Ted Weiss (D-N.Y.), also came down on the FDA. Weiss, who chaired the House committee with jurisdiction over the FDA, accused Dow Corning of possible misconduct in its effort to document the safety of silicone implants and called for both the Justice Department and the FDA to investigate the company. ([In] May [1995], the Justice Department dropped the investigation for lack of evidence.) He also accused the FDA of dragging its feet over the polyurethane-implant issue.

To be sure, there was pressure to keep implants available, too. It came from the American Medical Association, implant makers, plastic surgeons, and breast-cancer groups. But this was not the sort of public pressure that can embarrass an agency, and the breast cancer groups' objections were dealt with by allowing continued use of silicone implants for breast reconstruction following mastectomy.

The decision to ban implants was just the sort of thing one would expect from a regulatory body that puts so much emphasis on safety that it can't take anything else into account. *New England Journal of Medicine* Editor Marcia Angell has said that the FDA probably acted the way it did because implants are cosmetic and are therefore of only subjective worth. Such worth, says Angell, can't be plugged into Kessler's cost-benefit analysis.

In an *NEJM* editorial, Angell noted that nobody questions allowing the use of automobiles, even though they kill over 40,000 Americans a year, because we all have a common understanding of the worth of cars. "In the case of breast implants" though, wrote Angell, "the benefit has to do with the personal judgments about the quality of life, which are subjective and unique to each woman." But given "the difficulty of assessing the benefits, the FDA has acted as though there were none—at least when implants are used for augmentation." The result, said Angell, "is that [FDA Commissioner Kessler] may be holding breast implants to an impossibly high standard: Since there are no benefits, there should be no risks."

\* \* \*

The FDA's pseudo-scientific approach lends support to the more obviously ideological attack on breast implants from feminists. To many of the most vocal and influential feminists, a preference for big breasts represents female oppression. Susan K. Brownmiller, in her landmark 1984 book *Femininity*, opined that "[e]nlarging one's breasts to suit male fantasies" represents the exploitation of women. "Big breasts are one of many factors that have slowed women down in the competitive race of life," she said. "Symbolically, in the conservative Fifties, when American women were encouraged to stay at home, the heavily inflated bosom was celebrated and fetishized as the feminine ideal. In decades of spirited feminist activity such as the Twenties and the present when women advance into untraditional jobs, small, streamlined breasts are glorified in fashion."

If large breasts signal oppression, say these feminists, then the implants used to enlarge one's breasts are tools of oppression. Scarsdale psychologist Rita Freedman, writing in *Beauty Bound*, claims, "Having been taught that feminine beauty means having full, softly rounded breasts, women judge them-selves against this standard. Missing the mark, they put on padded bras or suffer silicone implants." Naomi Wolf, in her 1991 bestseller *The Beauty Myth*, states, "Breast surgery, in its mangling of erotic feeling, is a form of sexual mutilation."

Having gone this far with imagery, it's a small step to start blaming implants for physical ills. This is precisely what happened after anecdotes began to appear linking implants to disease. Susan Faludi, in her popular book *Backlash: The War Against Women*, wrote matter-of-factly that leaking implants "could cause toxicity, lupus, rheumatoid arthritis, and autoimmune diseases such as scleroderma."

To such polemicists, it doesn't matter that the evidence for negative effects was weak. It was just too fitting that something in their minds so harmful to women as a class should be harmful to them as individuals.

Two women on the FDA panel translated such thoughts into direct action. Vivian Snyder, the panel's "consumer representative," told Kessler in a letter that "[t]he federal government now has the power to deliver a profoundly important message to the American public involving basic values, concepts of beauty and health," adding, "it would really be wonderful if the FDA could address such attitude-impacting mental health issues as what is really healthy and normal and maybe even beautiful...."

The other panelist was *Beauty Bound* author Rita Freedman. She sent a letter to Kessler decrying that implants "perpetuate the myth of Barbie Doll's Body" and asked whether breast augmentation will become, "like rhinoplasty [nose surgery], a rite of passage for affluent teens."

Such feminist participation in the anti-implant crusade has proven ironic, since the FDA's virtual ban has denied what feminists have always proclaimed as their goal—a woman's right to choose for herself. Faludi herself acknowledges that at one time the leading feminist journal, *Ms.*, "deemed plastic surgery a way of 'reinventing yourself—a strategy for women who dare to take control of their lives.'"

Writing in *NEJM*, Angell says, "It is possible to deplore the pressures that women feel to conform to a stereotyped standard of beauty, while at the same time defending their right to make their own decisions." If anything, says Angell, the act of withdrawing implants could be viewed as sexist because "people are regularly permitted to take risks that are probably much greater than the likely risk from breast implants," citing cigarette smoking and excess alcohol consumption.

\* \* \*

When the FDA slapped the moratorium on implants, the impact went far beyond prohibiting a single surgical technique. "The widespread fear—and the multimillion-dollar lawsuits—have dated largely from the FDA's removal of breast implants from the market," says Angell.

One study comparing the attitudes of women with implants before and after the FDA moratorium found that after the moratorium the level of satisfaction dropped markedly, from 98 percent satisfied to 71–79 percent satisfied. The study authors said their findings were similar to those of the American Society for Plastic and Reconstructive Surgery in another poll.

As for prompting the "multimillion-dollar lawsuits," one need look no further for evidence than so many of the attorney advertisements soliciting silicone implant recipients. "THE FDA WARNS THAT SILICONE GEL-FILLED BREAST IMPLANTS PRESENT HEALTH RISKS" blared a typical ad of this sort in the Newark, New Jersey, *Star-Ledger*. Implant critics often cite money as the only concern of Dow Corning and other manufacturers. But few notice that the group which stands to gain the most from liability cases—trial lawyers—has a love of filthy lucre. In a single case involving three women complaining of implant-related illness, a jury in 1994 awarded $33.5 million, although the judgment was later reversed by an appeals court and then settled. Thirty-three percent of a multi million-dollar award—lawyers typically take a third off the top—can be a powerful incentive for a law firm.

It's hardly surprising, then, that the American Trial Lawyers Association conducts regular seminars for implant plaintiffs' attorneys. It does so using selected data provided by Sidney Wolfe of Public Citizen, the group most identified with criticism of implants. For $750, Public Citizen will also provide trial lawyers a list of medical experts and consultants, FDA reviews and FDA panel testimony, and a variety of other litigation documents. It will also refer clients to those lawyers.

Suing implant manufacturers has become a boom industry in the United States, with lawyers out to convince women that even though they may feel just fine they are really sick and must be properly compensated. With so much money to spread around, it also isn't difficult to get doctors to find patients.

"I get calls from women who say, 'I have implants. Where do I pick up the money?'" says Sandy Finestone of the Women's Implant Information Center in Irvine, California. The center disseminates information on implant safety. "You dangle $4 billion in front of them and it certainly gets their attention." Finestone has two polyurethane-coated implants that she makes clear will not be the subject of litigation.

Indeed, attorneys have not only ignored scientists, they've attacked them. After Mayo Clinic rheumatologist Sherine E. Gabriel published a study in *NEJM* in June 1994, a lawyer claiming to represent 2,000–3,000 implant recipients began filing legal demands against her. "The magnitude of the demands is staggering; the burden is staggering," she told *The New York Times*. "They want over 800 transcripts from researchers that were here, they want hundreds of data bases, dozens of file cabinets and the entire medical records of all Olmsted County [Michigan] women, whether or not they were in the study."

Not surprisingly, Gabriel says the demands have "severely compromised" her ability to do research and made colleagues of hers back off from doing their own implant research, for fear their findings would also infuriate plaintiffs' lawyers. "Some," she says, "determined that the price in terms of their own research careers is too high to pay."

The widespread association of silicone implants with various illnesses is largely the result of unsophisticated reporting on the topic. "The media may be portraying a closer link between implants and autoimmune disease that is actually merited because younger women tend to be more prone to autoimmune disease than other groups," explains David Leffell, associate professor of dermatology at the Yale School of Medicine. But the real question, says Leffell, is whether women with silicone implants are getting these diseases at levels higher than expected. All signs point to no.

With silicone implants, the media have managed to make news as much as report it. Clearly, they have had a significant impact on public perceptions, which then fueled both litigation and contributed to the FDA moratorium. This in turn fueled more litigation.

Whatever role sheer confusion—and ignorance of scientific data and principles—played on the part of the media, it is disturbing to realize that opportunities to present the other side were often ignored. In 1991, for instance, CBS reran the Connie Chung show that did so much to kick off the implant scare. But at the last minute, the network yanked a Dow Corning rebuttal to the program's charges. CBS didn't explain its decision. Apparently it felt its viewers would not benefit from an airing of both sides of the issue.

Unfortunately, the anti–silicone implant crusade has given women something very tangible to fear. Because of the negative publicity, as early as 1991 insurance companies were already denying or restricting medical coverage to women with implants. Now, because some doctors and lawyers have tied various illnesses to implants, women with implants who do eventually get any of those illnesses may find themselves without medical coverage. The founder of the Washington, D.C., chapter of the Y-ME National Breast Cancer Organization told a congressional panel, "In some instances, it is easier for a cancer patient to obtain insurance than one who has implants."

\* \* \*

In early June, even before the *NEJM* connective-tissue disease study, Y-ME Executive Director Sharon Green wrote to Kessler asking him to "make a public statement regarding the most recent epidemiological studies... to stop the current frenzy." The only statement he issued that month was a response to the *NEJM* study saying yet more evidence was needed.

Emory's Connell says the FDA's actions and the legal profession's high-tech ambulance chasing are "costing us not only what we [already] have but the chance for new and better products in the future. I think we're in a worse mess in American medicine than we've ever been in. Instead of leading the world, we're now a third-rate country in terms of our ability to develop new drugs and devices."

Indeed, J. Donald Hill, chairman of cardiovascular surgery at California Pacific Medical Center, worries that the anti-implant crusade will broaden into an attack against a wide variety of medical aids already on the market. The first device to go down the tubes may be the Norplant contraceptive, which after implantation into the arm releases a tiny amount of silicone into the system. While no suits have yet been filed, lawyers are encouraging women with the devices who have any sort of illness to contact them. Trial lawyer seminars are already being held, using some of the same instructors and same self-styled medical experts who torpedoed breast implants.

In a country so heavily dependent on science to improve the quality of our lives, to defend our shores, to feed our growing population, to prevent and cure illness, the resoundingly anti-scientific and successful crusade against silicone implants portends problems that right now cannot even be guessed.

# POSTSCRIPT

## Are Silicone Breast Implants a Health Risk to Women?

Why have so many women had silicone sacs surgically implanted in their chests? Some who have had breasts removed due to cancer have opted for breast reconstruction, but the most common reason has been that healthy women wished to achieve better body proportions. They often claim that the devices have enhanced their self-confidence and the quality of their lives. Overall, about 90 percent of these women are satisfied with their implants. Others, however, feel very strongly that women who have the implants have been victimized by society and men; that breast enlargement through surgery was something that had been thrust upon them by a society obsessed with unnatural ideas of female attractiveness. The editors of *Ms.*, in a March/April 1996 editorial, claim that the image of unnaturally large breasts as perfect begins in childhood when little girls play with Barbie dolls. "Keeping us in a constant state of insecurity about our looks not only fuels the multibillion-dollar beauty and fashion industries and the boom in cosmetic surgery, but it also helps maintain the status quo." To many feminists, a preference for large breasts represents female oppression. In her book *Femininity* (Fawcett, 1985), Susan K. Brownmiller contends that enlarging breasts to please male fantasies represents the exploitation of women.

For whatever reasons women opt for breast implants, the safety issue remains. Pathologist Nir Kossovsky believes silicone breast implants can negatively affect a woman's immune system and has testified in court to that effect. See "Silicone in the System," *Discover* (December 1995). Another publication that questions the safety of silicone implants is "How Silicone Ended Up in Women's Breasts," *Ms.* (March/April 1996). "Assessing Breast Implant Complications," *The New England Journal of Medicine* (March 1997) discusses a study that investigated 749 women who received implants between 1964 and 1991. Nearly 24 percent had had localized complications, including infection and scar tissue formation. The study did not assess autoimmune complications. In *Science on Trial: The Clash of Medical Evidence and the Law in the Breast Implant Case* (W. W. Norton, 1996), Marcia Angell discusses the lack of scientific rigor used in the breast implant litigation. Dr. Angell asserts that public opinion and media, not valid data, determined the outcome of the $4 billion lawsuit. She also maintains that although localized problems have occurred among women with implants, evidence does not show that systemic conditions, including cancer and autoimmune diseases, result from silicone breast implants.

# ISSUE 12

## Does Health Care Delivery and Research Benefit Men at the Expense of Women?

**YES: Leslie Laurence and Beth Weinhouse,** from *Outrageous Practices: The Alarming Truth About How Medicine Mistreats Women* (Fawcett Columbine, 1994)

**NO: Andrew G. Kadar,** from "The Sex-Bias Myth in Medicine," *The Atlantic Monthly* (August 1994)

### ISSUE SUMMARY

**YES:** Health and medical reporters Leslie Laurence and Beth Weinhouse assert that women have been excluded from most research on new drugs, medical treatments, and surgical techniques that are routinely offered to men.

**NO:** Physician Andrew G. Kadar argues that women actually receive more medical care and benefit more from medical research than men do, which explains why women generally live longer than men.

According to many researchers, women appear to respond differently from men to a varied array of medications and diseases. For instance, although heart disease is the leading killer of both men and women, women are less likely to survive heart attacks and heart surgery. Since the most influential studies of heart disease have studied only men, scientists and researchers are unable to explain the gender differences. Women activists claim that medical research has focused on men for too long and that it is now time to change this pattern.

Heart disease, the leading killer of both men and women, has long been considered a male condition by both physicians and the public. This is probably because men develop the affliction at an earlier age than women do. But women catch up after menopause. By age 65 about one-third of women have some form of heart disease, high blood pressure, or stroke.

As a result of this perception, doctors tended to ignore womens' complaints of chest pains and other symptoms of heart disease or considered them to be psychosomatic. When women *were* treated for heart disease, they were often treated less aggressively than men with similar symptoms.

In 1989 Harvard University reported that taking an aspirin tablet every other day could prevent heart disease based on a study involving 22,000 male physicians. The findings were generalized to include both men and women, and the final reports claimed that aspirin, which helps prevent blood clotting, would be useful to all adults. Dr. Suzanne Oparil, president of the American Heart Association, however, believes that aspirin might not be beneficial to women because they have generally faster rates of blood clotting than men.

Why were women excluded in the Harvard aspirin study or in other research that might help prevent their premature deaths or disabilities? The answer goes back to 1975, when the National Commission for the Protection of Human Subjects of Biomedical and Behavioral Research issued guidelines limiting research on pregnant women. This ban on using women stemmed from fears following the thalidomide crisis in the late 1950s.

In 1985 the National Institutes of Health (NIH) issued a statement urging researchers to include women in their studies. In 1990 it was reported, however, that women were still excluded in major federally funded clinical studies and that the NIH was not enforcing its policy of including women.

Things began to change, beginning with the 1991 launching of the *Women's Health Initiative*, a 14-year study of women's health. And in 1993 the FDA lifted its ban on using women in drug trials.

A relatively recent concern pertains to AIDS and HIV-related conditions. In particular, AIDS research has a proportionately higher number of men participating in drug and other scientific trials. What is known about HIV and AIDS seems to have been acquired from research on men only.

Despite concerns that health care and research in the United States benefit men at the expense of women, there is ample evidence to the contrary: Department of Health and Human Services studies show that women see their physicians more frequently, have more surgery, and are admitted to hospitals more often than men. Currently, two out of three medical dollars are spent by women.

Women have benefited from medical research involving high-tech procedures. Laparoscopic surgery and ultrasound are two advanced techniques that were first developed for use on women's bodies (these procedures were later adapted for men). Women's diseases have also been the recipient of research dollars. Breast cancer, the second leading cancer killer of women, has received more funding than any other tumor research. In 1993 the National Cancer Institute spent over $213 million dollars on breast cancer and $51 million dollars on prostate cancer. Although one-third more women die of breast cancer than men of prostate cancer, research into breast cancer received more than four times the funding of prostate cancer research.

In the following selections, Leslie Laurence and Beth Weinhouse argue that women have been shortchanged with regard to health care and medical research. Andrew G. Kadar disagrees, claiming that though it is often believed that women do not get the same consideration in medical care and research as men, the truth appears to be exactly the opposite.

# YES

Leslie Laurence and
Beth Weinhouse

## OUTRAGEOUS PRACTICES: THE ALARMING TRUTH ABOUT HOW MEDICINE MISTREATS WOMEN

There is unfortunately a clear path from the ignorant attitudes about women's bodies prevalent in the last century to the ignorant attitudes that exist today. A century ago physicians removed women's ovaries to treat a variety of unrelated complaints. They believed women's reproductive organs were responsible for almost everything that can and did go wrong with the human body. How much has changed? Recent medical students say that, during anatomy lectures on the female reproductive system, lecturers take pains to describe the female reproductive system as inefficient, badly designed, and prone to problems....

We may be horrified by the "ovariotomies" and "clitoridectomies" of the nineteenth century, but what of the hundreds of thousands of unnecessary hysterectomies being performed today?...

Nearly 550,000 hysterectomies are performed in the United States each year, making hysterectomy one of the most common operations of all. Yet the vast majority of these operations are elective, not lifesaving. When the American College of Obstetricians and Gynecologists recently announced its wish for ob-gyns to become the primary-care physicians for postmenopausal women, one woman doctor retorted, "If they want to do that, they're going to have to leave some organs in first."

How far have we really come from the days when women were told their psychological symptoms were due to physical problems and their reproductive organs were removed as a cure? Today women are frequently told that their very real physical symptoms—chest pains, menstrual problems, endometriosis, gastrointestinal pain—are psychological, and are handed a prescription for antidepressants or tranquilizers.

The medical textbooks of the 1800s may seem laughably ignorant today, but as recently as the 1970s physicians were being taught that morning sickness was caused by a woman's resentment at being a mother, PMS [premenstrual syndrome] was also a psychological disorder, and menopause represented the end of a woman's usefulness in life. And the doctors who were trained with those textbooks are still practicing medicine.

Instead of putting today's inequities in perspective, the examples of past abuses of women serve only to show that we haven't come as far as we thought....

## THE RESEARCH GAP

In June 1990, American women got a rude shock. For all the complaints women leveled against the health care system —most having to do with insensitive male doctors and dissatisfaction with gynecological and obstetric care—the majority of women still assumed that at least they were included in America's state-of-the-art medical research. But they were wrong. For at least the past several decades women in this country had been systematically excluded from the vast majority of research to develop new drugs, medical treatments, and surgical techniques.

It was on June 18, 1990, that the government's General Accounting Office (GAO) released its report of an audit of the National Institutes of Health (NIH). The audit found that although NIH had formulated a policy in 1986 for including women as research subjects, little had been done to implement or monitor that policy. In fact, most researchers applying for NIH grants were not even aware that they were supposed to include women, since the NIH grant-application book contained no mention of the policy. Because the 1986 policy urged rather than required attention to gender bias, most institutes, and most researchers, had simply decided to ignore it altogether or pay it only slight heed: "It used to be

enough for a researcher to say, 'Women and minorities will not be excluded from this study,' " explains one woman in NIH's Division of Research Grants. But not excluding women is very different from actively recruiting and including them....

The GAO found that women were being underrepresented in studies of diseases affecting both men and women. In the fifty applications reviewed, one-fifth made no mention of gender and over one-third said the subjects would include both sexes, but did not give percentages. Some all-male studies gave no rationale for their exclusivity. "The [NIH] may win the Nobel Prize, but I'd like to see them get the *Good Housekeeping* seal of approval," said Congresswoman Barbara Mikulski (D-Md.), voicing her hopes that the behemoth medical institution could be made more woman-friendly.

As if medical research were some kind of exclusive male club, some of the biggest and most important medical studies of recent years had failed to enroll a single woman:

- The Baltimore Longitudinal Study, one of the largest studies to examine the natural process of aging, began in 1958 and included no women for its first twenty years because, according to Gene Cohen, then deputy director of the National Institute on Aging (NIA), the facility in which the study was conducted had only one toilet. The study's 1984 report, entitled "Normal Human Aging," contained no data on women. (Currently 40 percent of the participants in this study are women ... although 60 percent of the population over age sixty-five is female.)
- The by-now-infamous Physicians' Health Study, which concluded in 1988

that taking an aspirin a day might reduce the risk of heart disease, included 22,000 men and no women.

• The 1982 Multiple Risk Factor Intervention Trial, known as Mr. Fit, a long-term study of lifestyle factors related to cholesterol and heart disease, included 13,000 men and no women. To this day no definitive answer exists on whether dietary change and exercise can benefit women in preventing heart disease.

• A Harvard School of Public Health study investigating the possible link between caffeine consumption and heart disease involved over 45,000 men and no women.

• Perhaps most unbelievably, a pilot project at Rockefeller University to study how obesity affected breast and uterine cancer was conducted solely on men. Said Congresswoman Olympia Snowe (R-Me.) upon hearing of this study, "Somehow, I find it hard to believe that the male-dominated medical community would tolerate a study of prostate cancer that used only women as research subjects." ...

*Protection or Paternalism?*

The objection to women's participation in health research that is most difficult to counter is the concern over exposing a fetus to a drug or treatment that might be dangerous, or at least has not been proven safe. Recent history makes it impossible to dismiss these fears. In the 1950s the drug thalidomide, given to European women to combat nausea during pregnancy, caused thousands of children to be born with severe deformities. In this country the drug diethylstilbestrol (DES) was widely prescribed to pregnant women during the 1940s and 1950s to prevent miscarriage, but has led to gynecological cancers and other medical problems in the offspring of the women who took it.

But in their effort to expose the fetus to "zero risk," scientists have shied away from including not just pregnant women in their studies, but any woman who could potentially become pregnant.

Translated into research practice, that meant that no woman between the ages of fifteen and fifty could participate in the earliest stages of new drug research unless she had been surgically sterilized or had a hysterectomy. (And since many studies have an upper age limit of sixty-five, that leaves a narrow window of opportunity for women to participate.) Exceptions were made only in the case of extremely severe or life-threatening illnesses.

While policies to protect unborn children seem to make sense on first reading, upon closer examination they represent protectionism run amok. An increasing number of studies are showing that exposure to chemicals and environmental toxins can affect *sperm*, yet no one is suggesting that men be excluded from research in order to protect their unborn children. When Proscar, a drug used to treat enlarged prostate glands, was found to cause birth defects in the offspring of male animals given the drug, men in the drug trials simply had to sign a consent form saying they would use condoms. Women weren't given the option of using contraception during the trial. By grouping together all women between the ages of fifteen and fifty as potentially pregnant, researchers were implying that women have no control over their reproductive lives. ...

# WOMEN'S HEARTS: THE
# DEADLY DIFFERENCE

Kathy O'Brien (not her real name), a forty-two-year-old smoker, had been experiencing chest pains on and off for about a year. Her father and two of her uncles had died of heart attacks when young. She went to a clinic in the rural area of northwest New Jersey where she lived, and there the local doctors told her she probably had gallstones. When the pain got worse, she went back to the clinic, where they told her she'd have to have a sonogram of her gallbladder. She left without having it done. Instead Kathy went home, collapsed from chest pain, and nearly died. She had suffered a massive heart attack and gone into cardiac arrest. Technically dead, she had to be defibrillated with electrical shocks on the way to the hospital. The following day she was transferred to a larger, teaching hospital, where doctors did an angiogram and found a blockage in a major blood vessel. After bypass surgery she recovered well. But why, wondered the cardiologists at the larger hospital, didn't anyone recognize heart disease in a heavy smoker with chest pain and a serious family history of death from heart attack?

Though it has been the leading cause of death in American women since 1908, heart disease is one of the best-kept secrets of women's health. It wasn't until 1964 that the American Heart Association [AHA] sponsored its first conference on women and heart disease. . . .

The real topic of this conference wasn't women and heart disease, however. It was how women could take care of their *husbands'* hearts. "Hearts and Husbands: The First Women's Conference on Coronary Heart Disease" explained to women the important role they played in keeping their spouses healthy. "The conference was a symposium on how to take care of your *man:* how to feed him and make sure he didn't get heart disease, and how to take care of him if he did," explains Mary Ann Malloy, M.D., a cardiologist at Loyola University Medical Center in Chicago, and head of the AHA's local Women and Heart Disease committee. The conference organizers prepared an educational pamphlet called "Eight Questions Wives Ask." There was no discussion at all of ways for women to recognize their own symptoms or to prevent the disease that was killing more of them than any other, no mention of how women could look after their own heart health. And no one objected, including women, because, for the medical profession and the public, heart disease was an exclusively male problem.

Both physicians and the public still harbor the misconception that women do not suffer from heart disease. Yet many more women die from cardiovascular disease—478,000 in 1993—than from all forms of cancer combined, which are responsible for 237,000 deaths. Although women seem to fear breast cancer more, only one in eight women will develop it (and not all of them will die of it), while one in two will develop cardiovascular disease. And for those who persist in thinking of heart disease as a male province, in 1992 (the most recent statistics available), more women than men died of cardiovascular disease. Among women, 46 percent of all deaths are due to cardiovascular disease; in men it's 40 percent. Because heart disease tends to be an illness of older, postmenopausal women, the incidence of heart disease, and the number of deaths, have been rising as women's life expectancies have increased. "Women didn't die of heart disease when the median age of death was the fifties or sixties," says Nanette K. Wenger, M.D., professor of medicine (cardiology) at Emory University School of Medicine in Atlanta.

Yet despite these ominous numbers, the vast majority of research into coronary artery disease, the type of heart disease that causes most heart attacks, has been done on middle-aged men. "We're very much in an infancy in terms of understanding heart disease in women," says Irma L. Mebane-Sims, Ph.D., an epidemiologist at the National Heart, Lung and Blood Institute. Compared with men's hearts, women's hearts are still largely a mystery....

### "IT'S ALL IN YOUR HEAD": MISUNDERSTANDING WOMEN'S COMPLAINTS

Just as the physical diseases of women are poorly understood, so, too, are a panoply of psychosomatic disorders, extremely controversial diagnoses in which emotional distresses are transferred into physical symptoms for which people then seek treatment. Somatization, as this process is known, has existed for centuries and is, to this day, remarkably common: Some 80 percent of healthy adults are believed to have psychogenic symptoms in any given week—for instance a stomachache that coincides with an important deadline or a headache that comes on after a fight with the boss....

Such a dynamic has a great bearing on women: they make up the majority of people suffering from such psychosomatic disorders as chronic fatigue syndrome, fibromyalgia, irritable bowel syndrome, and chronic pelvic pain (which can also be the result of an organic disorder such as endometriosis). The hidden scandal is that there is no shortage of doctors who will treat women's psychogenic complaints as if they're organic in origin, often leading to a chamber of medical horrors, including an array of unnecessary surgeries instead of the treatment women may really need: help in understanding the emotional reasons for their disease.

Of course women are willing participants in their mistreatment. Resisting psychological consultation, they embark on a medical odyssey, dragging their strange array of symptoms from specialist to specialist until they find someone who will give them the one thing they desperately need: a diagnosis. "These are very beleaguered patients," says Nortin Hadler, M.D., a North Carolina rheumatologist with a particular interest in somatization. "The worst thing to happen to any patient is not to be believed. You can't get better if you can't prove you're ill."

The corollary is that, because women suffer from psychosomatic illness disproportionately and express their medical problems in a more open and emotional style compared with men, their complaints frequently *aren't* listened to—even when they're directly related to an organic disease. "The perception among many physicians is that women tend to complain a lot, so you shouldn't pay too much attention to them," says Donna Stewart, head of women's health at Toronto Hospital, a teaching hospital affiliated with the University of Toronto. As a result, many of women's *legitimate* physical ailments are not attended to, sometimes with serious consequences....

## WOMEN AND DOCTORS: A TROUBLED RELATIONSHIP

Most women who visit physicians aren't aware of the lack of research into women's health, the difficulties in diagnosing women with cardiac disease, or the discrimination against women in medical school. What they *are* aware of is dissatisfaction with their physicians and with their health care in general. They base these opinions on what goes on in the doctor's office and the respect—or lack of it—they receive there. "The usual experience for a woman going to a gynecologist includes humiliation, depersonalization, even pain, and too seldom does she come away with her needs having been met," asserts gynecologist John M. Smith, M.D., author of *Women and Doctors*. And gynecologists are certainly not the only physicians guilty of this mistreatment.

Marianne J. Legato, M.D., associate director of the Center for Women's Health at Columbia–Presbyterian Medical Center, has toured the country talking with women about their experiences as patients. "The general mood is anger," she says. Women complained to her that their physicians were insensitive, uninterested, rushed, arrogant, and uncommunicative. Because women's health care is fragmented, with women seeing a gynecologist for reproductive health, an internist for a general physical, and other specialists for more specific problems, one woman told her she felt "like a salami, with a slice in every doctor's office in town."

None of this surprises Dr. Legato, who says that medicine is a mirror of the rest of society and its values. "Women, the old, the poor, children, and minority groups as a whole who haven't achieved economic power are taken less seriously and held in less regard... which kind of leaves the emphasis on white males."

Many physicians interact with their women patients based on a view of the female sex that was already archaic decades ago. "If she's premenopausal, she is dismissed as suffering from PMS; if she's postmenopausal, then she obviously needs hormone replacement therapy; if she's a homemaker, she has too much time on her hands; if she's a business executive, then the pressure of her job is too much for her. She just can't win," writes Isadore Rosenfeld, M.D.

Medical school textbooks from only two decades ago portray women not much differently from the "walking wombs" that physicians treated in the 1800s. In this century gynecologists embraced the idea that hormones were the long-suspected link between the uterus and the brain. This theory led them to believe that a pelvic exam could help diagnose mental problems. Conditions such as painful or irregular periods, excessive morning sickness or labor pain, and infertility became indications that a woman was battling her femininity. One 1947 obstetrics textbook, still on a practicing physician's shelf, introduces a chapter on such pregnancy problems as heartburn, nausea and vomiting, constipation, backache, varicose veins, and hemorrhoids with the sentence "Women with satisfactory self-control and more than average intelligence have fewer complaints than do other women."

Things still hadn't improved by the 1970s. A 1973 study of how women were portrayed in gynecology textbooks found that most textbooks were more concerned with the well-being of a woman's husband than with the woman herself. Wrote the authors, "Women are consistently described as anatomically destined to reproduce, nurture, and keep their husbands happy." A popular 1971 ob-gyn textbook portrayed women as helpless, childlike creatures who couldn't survive sex, pregnancy, delivery, or child raising without their doctors and added, "The traits that compose the core of the female personality are feminine narcissism, masochism, and passivity."

While current textbooks seem generally more sensitive and realistic, the physicians who trained on the older books are still in practice. When *JAMA*, a leading medical journal, ran an article in 1991 about gender disparities in medical care, they received a letter from a physician in Ohio who wrote that perhaps women's "overanxiousness" about their health and their greater use of health services "may be due to temperamental differences in gender-mediated clinical features of depression, which are manifested by women's less active, more ruminative responses that are linked to dysfunction of the right frontal cortex in which the metabolic rate is higher in females." In other words women are more anxious about their health because they are somehow brain-damaged. With doctors like this, no wonder women are unhappy.

### Women as Patients

Surveys show that women are more dissatisfied with their physicians than men are. And the dissatisfaction is not necessarily due to the quality of the medical care women receive, but to the lack of communication and respect they perceive in the encounter. In a 1993 Commonwealth Fund survey of twenty-five hundred women and a thousand men on the subject of women's health, women reported greater communication problems with their physicians, and were more likely to change doctors because of their dissatisfaction. One out of four women said she had been "talked down to" or treated like a child by a physician. Nearly one out of five women had been told that a reported medical condition was "all in your head."

The perception nationwide is that doctors and patients just don't understand each other. A study of one thousand complaints from dissatisfied patients at a large Michigan health maintenance organization found that more than 90 percent of the problems involved communication. "The most common complaints had to do with a lack of compassion on the physician's part," says Richard M. Frankel, Ph.D., associate professor of medicine at the University of Rochester School of Medicine and Dentistry. "Patients would complain their physician never looked at them during the entire encounter, made them feel humiliated or used medical jargon that left them confused."...

"Women are patronized and treated like little girls," says Ann R. Turkel, M.D., assistant clinical professor of psychiatry, Columbia University College of Physicians and Surgeons. "They're even referred to as girls. Male physicians will call female patients by their first names, but they are always called 'Doctor.' They don't do that with men. Women are patted on the head, called 'dear' or 'honey.' And doctors tell them things like, 'Don't you worry your pretty little head about it. That's not for you to worry about; that's for me to worry about.' Then they're surprised when women see these statements and reactions as degrading and insulting."...

There is also a perception among women that physicians don't take women's time seriously. How else to explain what happened to Roberta, a busy magazine editor who was on a tight deadline schedule the day of her doctor's appointment. "My office was just one city block from the doctor's office, so I called them five minutes before my appointment time to see if the doctor was running on schedule," she recalls. The receptionist assured her he was, so Roberta left her office and arrived at her appointment on time—only to be kept waiting for nearly an hour. "When I finally saw the doctor, I was practically shaking with rage, and my blood pressure was sky high," she says. Even though the doctor apologized and spent a lot of time talking with her after the checkup, Roberta decided to find another doctor.

"I think women are kept waiting longer for an appointment than men are," says Dr. Turkel. "I wouldn't go to a gynecologist who kept me waiting in the waiting room for an hour and a half, but I hear these stories all the time from women patients about their gynecologist's office."

Advice columnist Ann Landers even gave a rare interview to *JAMA* to let physicians know how dissatisfied women are with their doctors. "I can't say too often how angry women are about having to wait in the doctor's office," she said. "And, who do they complain to? The office manager, who is also a woman. Then, when the male doctor finally sees them—an hour later —the woman is so glad to see him that she soft-pedals the inconvenience. She wants to see the doctor as a 'knight in shining armor.' This should change. The doctor's time is no more important than the patient's and, while I can understand special circumstances, I can't understand why a doctor is *always* running late."

Doctors may treat women as if they are inferior patients, but studies show that they are anything but. Women tend to ask more questions—and receive more information because of their inquisitiveness. Women also show more emotion during office visits and are more likely to confide a personal problem that may have a bearing on their health to their physicians. Men, on the other hand, ask fewer questions of their physicians, give less information to the doctor, and display less emotion. During a typical fifteen-minute office visit, women ask an average of six questions. Men don't ask any....

Although physicians should be thrilled to have patients who are interested in their health, ask questions, and volunteer personal information, women's concerns are often dismissed as symptoms of anxiety, their questions brushed aside. In business, successful executives are often seen as having forceful, take-charge personalities, while women with similar attributes are described as aggressive or bitchy. In medicine, male patients seem to describe symptoms, while women complain. Instead of valuing women as active, informed patients, doctors are more likely to prefer patients who don't ask questions, don't interrupt, don't question their judgment, and—perhaps most important—get in and out of the office as quickly as possible. Researchers have actually found that physicians *like* male patients better than female ones, even when factors such as age, education, income, and occupation are controlled for.

Perhaps because of these attitudes, women often feel frustrated when they try to ask questions and receive explanations. One study reported that women received significantly more explanations than men—but not significantly more explaining *time*. Wrote the authors, "It is possible that many of the explanations they received were brief and perfunctory. Or, put differently, the men may have received fewer but fuller explanations than the women." The study also found that women were less likely than men to receive explanations that matched the level of technicality of the questions they asked. Doctors tended to talk down to women when answering their questions.…

## Miscommunication or Mistreatment?

Far more serious than patronizing attitudes and lack of consideration for women's time are the myths about women patients' complaints that jeopardize women's health care.

"Physician folklore says that women are more demanding patients," says Karen Carlson, M.D., an internist at Massachusetts General Hospital in Boston. "From my experience women are interested in health and prevention, desire to be listened to and treated with respect, want the opportunity to present and explain their agenda, and want their symptoms and concerns taken seriously."

But all too often women's symptoms are not taken seriously because physicians erroneously believe that these symptoms have no physical basis and that women's complaints are simply a sign of their demanding natures.

A 1979 study compared the medical records of fifty-two married couples to see how they had been treated for five common problems: back pain, headache, dizziness, chest pain, and fatigue. "The physicians' workups were significantly more extensive for the men than they were for women," reported the authors. "These data tend to support the argument that male physicians take medical illness more seriously in men than in women."

Another study found that women were shortchanged even in general checkups. Men's visits are more likely to include vision and hearing tests, chest X rays, ECGs, blood tests, rectal examinations, and urinalyses.

Dr. Carlson, speaking to a roomful of women physicians at an annual meeting of the American Medical Women's Association, cited evidence to show that women may actually complain *less* than men. "The myth is that women complain more, but studies show another truth," she says. Carlson cited studies showing that, compared with men, women with colon cancer are more likely to delay care and experience diagnostic delay. That women with chronic joint symptoms and arthritis are less likely to report pain. That women have more severe and frequent colds, but men are more likely to overrate their symptoms. That women delay seeking help for chest pain or symptoms of a heart attack. These studies point to women as being more stoic, yet when they finally do show up in the doctor's office, they are apt to be met with skepticism.

Betsy Murphy (not her real name) had been seeing the same doctor for years. "We had a perfectly fine relationship as long as I just went for my yearly checkups and didn't ask a lot of questions," she recalls. "But then I got my first yeast infection and had to go see him for a prescription—the medicine wasn't available over-the-counter then." Betsy told her doctor what she thought she had—she had talked to enough friends and read enough magazine articles to recognize the distinctive cottage-cheeselike discharge, yeasty odor, and intense itching. "But he ignored me when I told him what I thought was wrong. After he took a culture and examined it under the microscope, he sneeringly said, 'Well, Ms. Murphy, it seems as if your diagnosis is correct.'" Although he diagnosed the problem and prescribed the medication, Betsy left his office feeling insulted and patronized.

At a recent workshop on the patient-physician partnership, an auditorium full of physicians was asked how they would handle a "problem" patient. One of these "problems" was the patient who comes in and announces his or her own diagnosis. The physicians, almost unanimously, ridiculed the patient for daring to speculate what was wrong. They preferred that someone just present a description of symptoms, as specifically and articulately as possible. "It's no help for someone to come to me and say, "I have a cold and I just need some medicine,'" said a participating doctor to a journalist in the audience. "Instead the patient should describe how they feel as specifically as possible. And obviously some people are more articulate and some less; that's where the doctor's skill comes in." In other words, a patient should show up for an appointment and tell the doctor, "I have a stuffy nose and I keep sneezing," and then wait for the doctor, in his infinite wisdom, to pronounce, "You have a cold." For a patient, male or female, who is reasonably certain what is wrong, the suggestion seems ludicrous.

Women's dissatisfaction with their medical care can lead to serious health consequences. They may switch doctors so frequently that they receive no continuity of care. Or they may simply avoid seeing doctors altogether because they find the experience humiliating. When men without a regular source of health care are asked why they don't have one, they tend to reply that they don't need a doctor. But women are more apt to say that they cannot find the right doctor, or that they have recently moved, or that their previous doctor is no longer available. In the Commonwealth Fund poll, 41 percent of women (compared with 27 percent of men) said they had switched doctors in the past because they were dissatisfied. "If you brought your car in to be fixed and the person who fixed it did an okay but not great job, but was nasty, wouldn't you go to another mechanic? The same is true of physicians," says Frankel.

Physicians seem to realize there's a problem, but many of their efforts to remedy it are laughable. One 1993 article in the medical newspaper *American Medical News* advised doctors that if they wanted to make their practice "women-friendly," they should "create an atmosphere similar to that of a living room. This includes the seating, lighting and wall decorations." Yet it's difficult to imagine any woman listing "ugly wallpaper" as a reason for being dissatisfied with her health care. It's not the decor women are complaining about when they complain about doctors' offices.

Ob-gyn John Smith lists padded stirrups and speculum warmers as among the improvements women have gotten their doctors to make since the 1960s. But even those superficial improvements are not enough. What women really want are doctors who will listen to them, talk to them, and treat their medical questions and problems with respect and empathy....

## THE FUTURE OF WOMEN'S HEALTH

... Despite helter-skelter improvements in the care of women, the move toward special centers, nurse-run practices, and medical school curricula in women's health suggests a larger trend: the feminization of medicine. More women than ever are entering medical school. By the year 2010 the AMA estimates that one-third of all doctors will be women. ... Not surprisingly these women are bringing a feminine, and sometimes feminist, sensibility to the practice of medicine.

"Feminism is about empowering all our patients—men, women, and children —and treating them with respect," says Laura Helfman, M.D., an emergency room doctor in North Carolina. "We're doctors, we're not gods up on high." To Helfman this means taking the opportunity to do "a gentle and warm pelvic exam so I can reeducate the person receiving it that it doesn't have to be awful." To a gynecologist friend of hers it means making sure the patients never have to wait and that they always get to speak with the doctor. To a surgeon friend it means holding the patient's hand in the recovery room....

These practitioners are putting the rest of the health care system on notice. Women, both as physicians and as patients, are primed to transform the way medicine is practiced in this country. And so we celebrate the new female norm: the 60-kilogram woman. She has breasts and a uterus and a heart and lungs and kidneys. But she's much more than that. No longer a metaphor for disease, she's the model for health.... The time is right for a new woman-centered health care movement. It's the least women should demand.

# NO

Andrew G. Kadar

# THE SEX-BIAS MYTH IN MEDICINE

"When it comes to health-care research and delivery, women can no longer be treated as second-class citizens." So said the President of the United States on October 18, 1993.

He and the First Lady had just hosted a reception for the National Breast Cancer Coalition, an advocacy group, after receiving a petition containing 2.6 million signatures which demanded increased funding for breast-cancer prevention and treatment. While the Clintons met with leaders of the group in the East Room of the White House, a thousand demonstrators rallied across the street in support. The President echoed their call, decrying the neglect of medical care for women.

Two years earlier Bernadine Healy, then the director of the National In-stitutes of Health [NIH], charged that "women have all too often been treated less than equally in... health care." More recently Representative Pat Schroeder, a co-chair of the Congressional Caucus for Women's Issues, sponsored legislation to "ensure that biomedical research does not once again overlook women and their health." Newspaper articles expressed similar sen-timents.

The list of accusations is long and startling. Women's-health-care advocates indict "sex-biased" doctors for stereotyping women as hysterical hypochon-driacs, for taking women's complaints less seriously than men's, and for giving them less thorough diagnostic workups. A study conducted at the University of California at San Diego in 1979 concluded that men's com-plaints of back pain, chest pain, dizziness, fatigue, and headache more often resulted in extensive workups than did similar complaints from women. Hard scientific evidence therefore seemed to confirm women's anecdotal reports.

Men more often than women undergo angiographies and coronary-artery-bypass-graft operations. Even though heart disease is the No. 1 killer of women as well as men, this sophisticated, state-of-the-art technology, critics contend, is selectively denied to women.

The problem is said to be repeated in medical research: women, critics argue, are routinely ignored in favor of men. When the NIH inventoried all

From Andrew G. Kadar, "The Sex-Bias Myth in Medicine," *The Atlantic Monthly* (August 1994). Copyright © 1994 by Andrew G. Kadar. Reprinted by permission.

the research it had funded in 1987, the money spent on studying diseases unique to women amounted to only 13.5 percent of the total research budget.

Perhaps the most emotionally charged disease for women is breast cancer. If a tumor devastated men on a similar scale, critics say, we would declare a state of national emergency and launch a no-cost-barred Apollo Project–style program to cure it. In the words of Matilda Cuomo, the wife of the governor of New York, "If we can send a woman to the moon, we can surely find a cure for breast cancer." The neglect of breast-cancer research, we have been told, is both sexist and a national disgrace.

Nearly all heart-disease research is said to be conducted on men, with the conclusions blindly generalized to women. In July of 1989 researchers from the Harvard Medical School reported the results of a five-year study on the effects of aspirin in preventing cardiovascular disease in 22,071 male physicians. Thousands of men were studied, but not one woman: women's health, critics charge, was obviously not considered important enough to explore similarly. Here, they say, we have definite, smoking-gun evidence of the neglect of women in medical research —only one example of a widespread, dangerous phenomenon.

Still another difference: pharmaceutical companies make a policy of giving new drugs to men first, while women wait to benefit from the advances. And even then the medicines are often inadequately tested on women.

To remedy all this neglect, we need to devote preferential attention and funds, in the words of the *Journal of the American Medical Women's Association*, to "the greatest resource this country will ever have, namely, the health of its women."

Discrimination on such a large scale cries out for restitution—if the charges are true.

In fact one sex does appear to be favored in the amount of attention devoted to its medical needs. In the United States it is estimated that one sex spends twice as much money on health care as the other does. The NIH also spends twice as much money on research into the diseases specific to one sex as it does on research into those specific to the other, and only one sex has a section of the NIH devoted entirely to the study of disease afflicting it. That sex is not men, however. It is women.

\* \* \*

In the United States women seek out and consequently receive more medical care than men. This is true even if pregnancy-related care is excluded. Department of Health and Human Services surveys show that women visit doctors more often than men, are hospitalized more often, and undergo more operations. Women are more likely than men to visit a doctor for a general physical exam when they are feeling well, and complain of symptoms more often. Thus two out of every three health-care dollars are spent by women.

Quantity, of course, does not guarantee quality. Do women receive second-rate diagnostic workups?

The 1979 San Diego study, which concluded that men's complaints more often led to extensive workups than did women's, used the charts of 104 men and women (fifty-two married couples) as data. This small-scale regional survey prompted a more extensive national review of 46,868 office visits. The results, reported in 1981, were quite different from those of the San Diego study.

In this larger, more representative sample, the care received by men and women was similar about two thirds of the time. When the care was different, women overall received more diagnostic tests and treatment—more lab tests, blood-pressure checks, drug prescriptions, and return appointments.

Several other, small-scale studies have weighed in on both sides of this issue. The San Diego researchers looked at another 200 men and women in 1984, and this time found "no significant differences in the extent and content" of workups. Some women's-health-care advocates have chosen to ignore data from the second San Diego study and the national survey while touting the first study as evidence that doctors, to quote once again from the *Journal of the American Medical Women's Association*, do "not take complaints as seriously" when they come from women: "an example of a double standard influencing diagnostic workups."

When prescribing care for heart disease, doctors consider such factors as age, other medical problems, and the likelihood that the patient will benefit from testing and surgery. Coronary-artery disease afflicts men at a much younger age, killing them three times as often as women until age sixty-five. Younger patients have fewer additional medical problems that preclude aggressive, high-risk procedures. And smaller patients have smaller coronary arteries, which become obstructed more often after surgery. Whereas this is true for both sexes, obviously more women fit into the smaller-patient category. When these differences are factored in, sex divergence in cardiac care begins to fade away.

To the extent that divergence remains, women may be getting better treatment.

At least that was the conclusion of a University of North Carolina/Duke University study that looked at the records of 5,795 patients treated from 1969 to 1984. The most symptomatic and severely diseased men and women were equally likely to be referred for bypass surgery. Among the patients with less-severe disease—the ones to whom surgery offers little or no survival benefit over medical therapy—women were less likely to be scheduled for bypass surgery. This seems proper in light of the greater risk of surgical complications, owing to women's smaller coronary arteries. In fact, the researchers questioned the wisdom of surgery in the less symptomatic men and suggested that "the effect of gender on treatment selection may have led to more appropriate treatment of women."

As for sophisticated, pioneering technology selectively designed for the benefit of one sex, laparoscopic surgery was largely confined to gynecology for more than twenty years. Using viewing and manipulating instruments that can be inserted into the abdomen through keyhole-sized incisions, doctors are able to diagnose and repair, sparing the patient a larger incision and a longer, more painful recuperation. Laparoscopic tubal sterilization, first performed in 1936, became common practice in the late 1960s. Over time the development of more-versatile instruments and of fiber-optic video capability made possible the performance of more-complex operations. The laparoscopic removal of ectopic pregnancy was reported in 1973. Finally, in 1987, the same technology was applied in gallbladder surgery, and men began to enjoy its benefits too.

Years after ultrasound instruments were designed to look inside the uterus, the same technology was adapted to search for tumors in the prostate. Other pioneering developments conceived to improve the health care of women include mammography, bone-density testing for osteoporosis, surgery to alleviate bladder incontinence, hormone therapy to relieve the symptoms of menopause, and a host of procedures, including in vitro fertilization, developed to facilitate impregnation. Perhaps so many new developments occur in women's health care because one branch of medicine and a group of doctors, gynecologists, are explicitly concerned with the health of women. No corresponding group of doctors is dedicated to the care of men.

So women receive more care than men, sometimes receive better care than men, and benefit more than men do from some developing technologies. This hardly looks like proof that women's health is viewed as secondary in importance to men's health.

* * *

The 1987 NIH inventory did indeed find that only 13.5 percent of the NIH research budget was devoted to studying diseases unique to women. But 80 percent of the budget went into research for the benefit of both sexes, including basic research in fields such as genetics and immunology and also research into diseases such as lymphoma, arthritis, and sickle-cell anemia. Both men and women suffer from these ailments, and both sexes served as study subjects. The remaining 6.5 percent of NIH research funds were devoted to afflictions unique to men. Oddly, the women's 13.5 percent has been cited as evidence of neglect. The much smaller men's share of the budget is rarely mentioned in these references.

As for breast cancer, the second most lethal malignancy in females, investiga-tion in that field has long received more funding from the National Cancer Institute [NCI] than any other tumor research, though lung cancer heads the list of fatal tumors for both sexes. The second most lethal malignancy in males is also a sex-specific tumor: prostate cancer. Last year approximately 46,000 women succumbed to breast cancer and 35,000 men to prostate cancer; the NCI spent $213.7 million on breast-cancer research and $51.1 million on study of the prostate. Thus although about a third more women died of breast cancer than men of prostate cancer, breast-cancer research received more than four times the funding. More than three times as much money per fatality was spent on the women's disease. Breast cancer accounted for 8.8 percent of cancer fatalities in the United States and for 13 percent of the NCI research budget; the corresponding figures for prostate cancer were 6.7 percent of fatalities and three percent of the funding. The spending for breast-cancer research is projected to increase by 23 percent this year, to $262.9 million; prostate-research spending will increase by 7.6 percent, to $55 million.

The female cancers of the cervix and the uterus accounted for 10,100 deaths and $48.5 million in research last year, and ovarian cancer accounted for 13,300 deaths and $32.5 million in research. Thus the research funding for all female-specific cancers is substantially larger per fatality than the funding for prostate cancer.

Is this level of spending on women's health just a recent development, needed to make up for years of prior neglect? The NCI is divided into sections dealing with issues such as cancer biology and diagnosis, prevention and control, etiology, and treatment. Until funding allocations for sex-specific concerns became a political issue, in the mid-1980s, the NCI did not track organ-specific spending data. The earliest information now available was reconstructed retroactively to 1981. Nevertheless, these early data provide a window on spending patterns in the era before political pressure began to intensify for more research on women. Each year from 1981 to 1985 funding for breast-cancer research exceeded funding for prostate cancer by a ratio of roughly five to one. A rational, nonpolitical explanation for this is that breast cancer attacks a larger number of patients, at a younger age. In any event, the data failed to support claims that women were neglected in that era.

Again, most medical research is conducted on diseases that afflict both sexes. Women's-health advocates charge that we collect data from studies of men and then extrapolate to women. A look at the actual data reveals a different reality.

The best-known and most ambitious study of cardiovascular health over time began in the town of Framingham, Massachusetts, in 1948. Researchers started with 2,336 men and 2,873 women aged thirty to sixty-two, and have followed the survivors of this group with biennial physical exams and lab tests for more than forty-five years. In this and many other observational studies women have been well represented.

With respect to the aspirin study, the researchers at Harvard Medical School did not focus exclusively on men. Both sexes were studied nearly concurrently. The men's study was more rigorous, because it was placebo-controlled (that is, some subjects were randomly assigned to receive placebos instead of aspirin); the women's study was based on responses to questionnaires sent to nurses and a review of medical records. The women's study, however, followed nearly four times as many subjects as the men's study (87,678 versus 22,071), and it followed its subjects for a year longer (six versus five) than the men's study did. The results of the men's study were reported in the *New England Journal of Medicine* in July of 1989 and prompted charges of sexism in medical research. The women's-study results were printed in the *Journal of the American Medical Association* in July of 1991, and were generally ignored by the nonmedical press.

Most studies on the prevention of "premature" (occurring in people under age sixty-five) coronary-artery disease have, in fact, been conducted on men. Since middle-aged women have a much lower incidence of this illness than their male counterparts (they provide less than a third as many cases), documenting the preventive effect of a given treatment in these women is much more difficult. More experiments were conducted on men not because women were considered less important but because women suffer less from this disease. Older women do develop coronary disease (albeit at a lower rate than older men), but the experiments were not performed on older men either. At most the data suggest an emphasis on the prevention of disease in younger people.

Incidentally, all clinical breast-cancer research currently funded by the NCI is being conducted on women, even though 300 men a year die of this tumor. Do studies on the prevention of breast cancer with specifically exclude males signify a neglect of men's health? Or should a disease be studied in the group most at risk? Obviously, the coronary-disease research situation and the breast-cancer research situation are not equivalent, but together they do serve to illustrate a point: diseases are most often studied in the highest-risk group, regardless of sex.

What about all the new drug tests that exclude women? Don't they prove the pharmaceutical industry's insensitivity to and disregard for females?

The Food and Drug Administration [FDA] divides human testing of new medicines into three stages. Phase 1 studies are done on a small number of volunteers over a brief period of time, primarily to test safety. Phase 2 studies typically involve a few hundred patients and are designed to look more closely at safety and effectiveness. Phase 3 tests precede approval for commercial release and generally include several thousand patients.

In 1977 the FDA issued guidelines that specifically excluded women with "childbearing potential" from phase 1 and early phase 2 studies; they were to be included in late phase 2 and phase 3 trials in proportion to their expected use of the medication. FDA surveys conducted in 1983 and 1988 showed that the two sexes had been proportionally represented in clinical trials by the time drugs were approved for release.

The 1977 guidelines codified a policy already informally in effect since the thalidomide tragedy shocked the world in 1962. The births of armless or otherwise deformed babies in that era dramatically highlighted the special risks incurred when fertile women ingest drugs. So the policy of excluding such women from the early phases of drug testing arose out of concern, not out of disregard, for them. The policy was changed last year, as a consequence of political protest and recognition that early studies in both sexes might better direct testing.

\* \* \*

Throughout human history from antiquity until the beginning of this century men, on the average, lived slightly longer than women. By 1920 women's life expectancy in the United States was one year greater than men's (54.6 years versus 53.6). After that the gap increased steadily, to 3.5 years in 1930, 4.4 years in 1940, 5.5 in 1950, 6.5 in 1960, and 7.7 in 1970. For the past quarter of a century the gap has remained relatively steady: around seven years. In 1990 the figure was seven years (78.8 versus 71.8).

Thus in the latter part of the twentieth century women live about 10 percent longer than men. A significant part of the reason for this is medical care.

In past centuries complications during childbirth were a major cause of traumatic death in women. Medical advances have dramatically eliminated most of this risk. Infections such as smallpox, cholera, and tuberculosis killed large numbers of men and women at similar ages. The elimination of infection as the dominant cause of death has boosted the prominence of diseases that selectively afflict men earlier in life.

Age-adjusted mortality rates for men are higher for all twelve leading causes of death, including heart disease, stroke, cancer, lung disease (emphysema and pneumonia), liver disease (cirrhosis), suicide, and homicide. We have come to accept women's longer life span as natural, the consequence of their greater biological fitness. Yet this greater fitness never manifested itself in all the millennia of human history that preceded the present era and its medical-care system—the same system that women's-health advocates accuse of neglecting the female sex.

To remedy the alleged neglect, an Office of Research on Women's Health was established by the NIH in 1990. In 1991 the NIH launched its largest epidemiological project ever, the Women's Health Initiative. Costing more than $600 million, this fifteen-year program will study the effects of estrogen therapy, diet, dietary supplements, and exercise on heart disease, breast cancer, colon cancer, osteoporosis, and other diseases in 160,000 postmenopausal women. The study is ambitious in scope and may well result in many advances in the care of older women.

What it will not do is close the "medical gender gap," the difference in the quality of care given the two sexes. The reason is that the gap does not favor men. As we have seen, women receive more medical care and benefit more from medical research. The net result is the most important gap of all: seven years, 10 percent of life.

# POSTSCRIPT

## Does Health Care Delivery and Research Benefit Men at the Expense of Women?

"Nobody was paying attention to women's health," says Phyllis Greenberger, executive director of the Society for the Advancement of Women's Health Research in Washington, D.C. "For years, women's health issues were ignored because the men who were making the decisions didn't think they were important." This situation may be turning around. In 1987 only 14 percent of the $5.7 billion National Institutes of Health (NIH) budget was spent on women's health research. In 1994 the NIH spent over $1.4 billion dollars on health research related to women's diseases in hopes of finding treatments and cures for osteoporosis (bone thinning), heart disease, and breast cancer. In addition to increased funding, pressure from the Congressional Caucus for Women's Issues forced the NIH, the nation's largest research funder, to include women in all applicable clinical trials of medical treatments. The Food and Drug Administration (FDA) also issued guidelines in 1993 to include women in tests of new drugs.

These reforms, however, are not welcomed by all physicians and researchers. Professor Curtis Meinert of Johns Hopkins University doubts that the new approach will uncover significant differences between the genders either in treatment or in their responses to diseases. Meinert also feels that including women in all studies will require so many additional participants that research will become prohibitively expensive. Benjamin Wittes and Janet Wittes, employees of Statistics Collaborative, a company that designs clinical trials, echo Meinert's view in "Group Therapy," *The New Republic* (April 5, 1993). This viewpoint is also held by Marcia Angell, executive editor of *The New England Journal of Medicine*. Angell feels that claiming important biological differences between men and women as a rule is not plausible.

The effort to quadruple federal expenditures on breast cancer research has also been criticized. Some scientists have complained that designating so much money for one disease will be at the expense of research into cures and treatment for other illnesses. An article entitled "Equality Law Could Backfire on Researchers," *New Scientist* (August 7, 1993) argues that redressing past inequities by including women and minorities more often in research could backfire.

The claim that women with chest pains or other symptoms of heart disease are treated less aggressively than men has also been disputed. A study reported in "A Comparison of the Early Outcome of Acute Myocardial Infarction in Women and Men," *The New England Journal of Medicine* (January 1, 1998) found that women were treated as appropriately as men for their specific conditions and that gender was not a significant factor in doctors' deciding on a course of treatment. See also "The Sex Bias Myth in Medicine," *The Atlantic Monthly*(August 1994). In "Why Do Women Last Longer Than Men?" *New Scientist* (October 23, 1993), the reasons behind males' shorter life spans are discussed. Life span and longevity are also addressed in "Survey Shows Women May Live Longer, but Not Healthier Than Men," *Nation's Health* (August 1993).

Many articles, in both the popular press and the scientific literature, maintain that there is a gender bias in medicine. These include "Study Finds White Male Patients Get Better Heart Care Than Women, Minorities and Elderly," *Jet* (April 20, 1998); "Group Calls for Increased Funding for Women's Health," *Women's Health Weekly* (February 9, 1998);"What Doctors Don't Know About Women's Bodies," *Ladies Home Journal* (February 1997); "Men, Women, and Health Insurance," *The New England Journal of Medicine* (January 16, 1997); "Are Women the Weaker Sex?" *American Health* (July/August 1996); and "Did You Know That Women Continue to Get Shockingly Substandard Medical Care?" *Health Confidential* (January 1995).

For an overview on women's health, see "Women's Health Issues," *CQ Researcher* (May 13, 1994), which addresses such topics as hormone therapy debates, whether or not women's health should be a separate medical specialty, breast cancer, hysterectomies, and leading causes of death for men and women. See also "The Cost of Being a Woman," *The New England Journal of Medicine* (June 4, 1998) and "Women in the New World Order: Where Old Values Command New Respect," *Journal of the American Dietetics Association* (May 1997). Two books on gender bias in women's health are *Women and Health Research: Ethical and Legal Issue of Including Women in Clinical Studies* by Anna Mastroianni et al. (National Academy Press, 1994) and *Unequal Treatment: What You Don't Know About How Women Are Mistreated by the Medical Community* by Eileen Nechas and Denise Foley (Simon & Schuster, 1994).

# ISSUE 13

## Should Confidentiality Remain a Priority for People With AIDS?

**YES: Gabriel Rotello,** from "AIDS Is Still an Exceptional Disease," *The New York Times* (August 22, 1997)

**NO: William B. Kaliher,** from "How Federal and State Policies Spread AIDS," *The World & I* (May 1998)

### ISSUE SUMMARY

**YES:** Journalist Gabriel Rotello contends that there are good reasons to exempt AIDS from the traditional public health tracking of infectious diseases.

**NO:** Disease intervention specialist William B. Kaliher argues that treating the disease as a public health issue rather than as a political issue can help reduce the number of AIDS cases.

Acquired immunodeficiency syndrome (AIDS) can be called the world's most serious health concern since the bubonic plague, which killed one-third of the population of Europe in the fourteenth century. Although there are drugs to manage the progression of AIDS, currently there is no vaccine or cure.

It is not clear if AIDS is a "new" disease or one that has been around and only recently begun to spread. As early as 1977 medical journals printed articles about a pneumonia-like disease that affected mostly young homosexual males and intravenous drug users. In 1983 scientists isolated the virus responsible for AIDS and eventually called it the human immunodeficiency virus (HIV). HIV attacks white blood cells (T-lymphocytes) and weakens the immune system, damaging the body's ability to fight other diseases. Without a functioning immune system to ward off other germs, a person now becomes vulnerable to life-threatening diseases, such as pneumonia. AIDS initially appeared to affect mostly male homosexuals, but it became apparent that it also affected intravenous (IV) drug users and people receiving infected blood products. AIDS began to spread among the sexual partners of these individuals as well. The virus can also be transmitted to children during birth. People who are infected may not initially have symptoms but are capable of passing the virus on to others.

AIDS has become more prevalent each year in the United States, as reported instatistics from the Centers for Disease Control and Prevention (CDC). In the early 1980s approximately 150 cases of AIDS were reported. By early 1998 over 640,000 cases of HIV and AIDS were reported.

AIDS is currently the fifth leading cause of death among people 25–44 years old. Over 390,000 people in the United States have died from AIDS.

HIV and AIDS have also spread throughout the world. It is estimated that 33.4 million people are currently living with HIV worldwide. Deaths attributed to AIDS by the end of 1998 numbered 13.9 million.

To help reduce the spread of HIV in the United States, public health officials have proposed treating AIDS like many other sexually transmitted diseases. When someone is diagnosed as being HIV-positive their personal contacts, either needle-sharing or sexual, would be notified and tested. Since the beginning of the AIDS epidemic these traditional methods have not been used. Special interest groups argue that tracking contacts would cause discrimination in employment, housing, and other areas. They assert that a breach in confidentiality would deter people from seeking testing and treatment. Health officials who helped to develop the policy of "AIDS exceptionalism" continue to support it. HIV exposure notification raises difficult human rights questions. Most people would agree that a baby who is exposed to HIV at birth has the right to receive treatment. However, does this right overcome the privacy rights of the mother, whose HIV status is revealed through the infant's antibody test results? Similarly, an individual who shares a needle with an infected person or has sexual intercourse with an infected person has a right to know that he or she has been exposed to HIV. How can this be balanced against the privacy rights of the infected person?

The federal government has been criticized for not providing leadership on the issue of tracking. Each state is allowed to decide whether or not to track partners of HIV-positive people. In June 1998 New York State, which has the highest number of AIDS cases in the nation, passed a manditory partner notification law. California, which has the second-highest number of cases, continues to have voluntary notification. Currently the federal government's position is somewhat ambiguous. States that receive funding for HIV prevention and treatment are required to support some form of confidential partner notification program. These states are also mandated to make an attempt to notify the spouse of someone who tests positive for HIV. However, it is not clear exactly what partner notification entails. In many states it means that individuals are encouraged to notify their partners. As a result sometimes partners are contacted but not always. Although *requiring* partner notification may slow down the AIDS epidemic, many activists maintain that there is no good way to force people to disclose this sensitive information.

In the following selections, Gabriel Rotello contends that we cannot drop the confidentiality shield for AIDS because AIDS is still different from other communicable diseases. William B. Kaliher counters that we must separate AIDS from special interest agendas and begin infectious disease intervention.

# YES

**Gabriel Rotello**

## AIDS IS STILL AN EXCEPTIONAL DISEASE

In 1936, Thomas Parran, the director of the nation's anti-venereal-disease program, told a conference of medical professionals, "Every case must be located, reported, its source ascertained and all contacts then informed about the possibility of infection and if infected, treated."

And so it has been ever since for sexually transmitted diseases. Except for AIDS. And for good reason.

During epidemics of most sexually transmitted diseases, state public health authorities routinely test large numbers of people, sometimes without their knowledge, report names of the afflicted to health departments and try to trace and inform their sexual partners. The main goal is to identify people who do not know they are infected and get them into treatment as quickly as possible, before they can infect others.

AIDS has always been largely exempted from these traditional methods of managing public health. But now a major new debate is questioning "AIDS exceptionalism." And surprisingly, many of those questioning it are AIDS advocates themselves, the very folks who once drew a bright line between AIDS and other sexually transmitted diseases.

But there is reason to be cautious before we jettison laws or health policies that insure confidentiality for people infected with H.I.V.

For years, AIDS seemed to render traditional approaches to containing outbreaks of venereal disease not only useless, but also counterproductive. Useless because there were no effective treatments, so identifying victims was likely to produce despair rather than action. Counterproductive because society's stigmatization of gay men and intravenous drug users, the two populations most affected by AIDS, made these groups justifiably wary of anything that might expose them to further discrimination.

AIDS advocates feared that reporting the names of those with H.I.V. and contacting their sexual partners could easily lead to exposure and discrimination. Some even feared a slippery slope leading to eventual quarantine and criminalization of the H.I.V. positive.

It didn't help that many of those calling for traditional approaches in the 1980's were openly hostile to gay men and people with AIDS. As public health authorities quickly learned in dealing with the politically mobilized gay community, effective prevention is impossible if you drive the people most at risk away from the health care system.

Finally, it was argued that in populations with large numbers of sexual partners, contact tracing would be both very expensive and largely useless, since it requires individuals to remember everyone they had sex with.

It seemed far wiser to spend what little prevention money was available—and it has never been enough—on trying to get high-risk populations to alter behavior by emphasizing that everyone was at potential risk.

Now, however, new treatments are vastly improving and extending the lives of many people with H.I.V., although the rate of new infections remains high. Studies indicate that the earlier people enter therapy, the better the prognosis. If AIDS is no longer uniquely fatal and untreatable, advocates ask, should we keep treating it that way? Shouldn't we go back to the tried and true methods of the past?

Well, maybe, but not so fast. The new debate indicates a pragmatic desire to embrace whatever might work, and that's great. But it also holds potential dangers. The old methods were certainly tried, but were they necessarily true?

The fact is that practices like name reporting and contact tracing arose in the late 19th and early 20th centuries, before there was any scientific way of determining whether they worked. They may have satisfied a popular demand that health authorities do something, but the fact is, we don't really know how effective they were.

Contact tracing may have made a dent in rates of transmission, but epidemics of syphilis, gonorrhea, chlamydia and other sexually transmitted diseases raged on anyway.

Even some who advocate name reporting and contact tracing for people with H.I.V., like Marcia Angell, executive editor of The New England Journal of Medicine, acknowledge that evidence is lacking.

"Nobody can document or prove that traditional methods of control would work better at containing AIDS," Dr. Angell recently told The Atlantic Monthly, "because nobody has done what would be necessary to get such proof." Namely, studying two populations in which different methods were tried.

Even today, there is a long list of basic questions we do not have answers to— What makes some people practice safer sex? What encourages some people to enter the health care system? What drives others away? Does knowing whether you are infected affect your sexual behavior?

And there is still a lot of AIDS bashing out there. A new bill in Congress, sponsored by Representative Tom Coburn, Republican of Oklahoma, calls for a national registry of all H.I.V.-positive people (there is no such registry for any other disease), authorizes health professionals to refuse to perform invasive procedures until a patient has been tested for H.I.V., and allows funeral homes to refuse to perform procedures unless the deceased has been tested.

It ignores needle exchange, a technique that has now been scientifically proved to prevent H.I.V. transmission without increasing drug use. And shockingly, the bill provides not a penny in additional money, even though its provisions have been estimated to cost hundreds of millions of dollars per year.

Thankfully, most Congressional observers doubt that this punitive bill will pass. But it vividly illustrates the fact that authoritarian, anti-scientific attitudes about H.I.V. prevention are still powerful.

This is not to say that civil liberties are absolutes when it comes to dire threats to the public health. The rights of infected people must be balanced against the right of all people to protect themselves. If traditional methods can be shown to prevent new infections and bring treatment to the infected, they should be considered.

But the key is whether these methods can be shown to be effective.

\* \* \*

To do that, health authorities have an obligation to apply scientific rigor to their own methods and assumptions. And society has an obligation to insure that whatever methods are approved, they strive to balance civil liberties with public safety, encourage people to enter the health system rather than drive them away, and provide adequate financing and care to the afflicted.

The debate on AIDS exceptionalism is a healthy sign that AIDS advocates are open to new ideas. But it should proceed with caution, and with a healthy sense of what we still don't know, and what we need to find out.

# NO

William B. Kaliher

# HOW FEDERAL AND STATE POLICIES SPREAD AIDS

I am one of the few venereal disease investigators, if not the only one, who has been allowed to interview HIV-positive patients and trace HIV/AIDS contacts since 1985. I have observed many aspects of this disease not reported to the general public, and I have managed the case investigations of over nine hundred infected patients. We properly interviewed the majority of those individuals.

My twenty-five years' experience working with venereal diseases and my involvement in this aspect of AIDS has made me acutely aware of and concerned over the illogical public health decisions concerning AIDS. Scrutinizing the Centers for Disease Control and Prevention (CDC), one could conclude that this agency is concealing certain facts from the public, or one could think, as a respected doctor said after working at the CDC, "Every decision is being politically made." No matter your personal perspective, two observations are painfully clear: It is apparent decisions are not being made in the interest of public health, if that goal means retarding the spread of communicable diseases, and the decisions made are not maximizing the benefits from the public's tax dollars.

A venereal disease investigator appears to have the straightforward job of interviewing infected persons and bringing their contacts in for treatment. But the detective-like qualities of an experienced investigator allow intervention in more dramatic ways. In my area of South Carolina, with AIDS the above description is fairly accurate, except we bring the contacts in for counseling and testing by nurses instead of treatment. Unfortunately, for the American taxpayer and—more importantly—the people at risk, we are virtually the only area in the United States since 1985 that has dealt with AIDS as a communicable disease. Tabulation files of HIV/AIDS contacts are not being kept in any adequate way nationally.

A dramatic method of disease intervention and unpardonable problems with the national AIDS program are demonstrated by the case of a thirty-year-old non-IV-drug-using, HIV-positive heterosexual female. I describe her by her lack of risk factors because she was diagnosed when women without

From William B. Kaliher, "How Federal and State Policies Spread AIDS," *The World & I* (May 1998). Copyright © 1998 by *The World & I*, a publication of The Washington Times Corporation. Reprinted by permission.

risk factors were being ignored, avoided, or thought to be anomalies. She named four men as sexual contacts in the five years prior to her positive test. One contact, a one-night stand, was not located. A second was tested and found HIV-negative. Information concerning a third man, who had been fired from a bottling plant, was forwarded to another city. Because of our program structure, that was the end of his AIDS investigation. Had he been a syphilis contact, the investigators would have obtained his address from the company and traced him.

Her fourth contact, an alcoholic heterosexual, was located two months after being named. When tested, he was found to be EIA positive and western blot indeterminate, meaning another test was needed to determine if he was actually infected. While awaiting his initial test results, this man decided he did not want to be followed. With many less-dangerous STDs (sexually transmitted diseases), he could not legally refuse testing and possibly other follow-up, but with AIDS testing, that option was his right.

We tried to obtain a second and conclusive test, but he avoided us for over a year. On the occasions when we located him, he refused further testing. We eventually did what is called a cluster interview of the infected woman who named him. She identified two other women he was having sex with. We also learned of two additional women he was involved with during visits to his parents' home. In total, we discovered four other heterosexual contacts of this man's without interviewing him or having a positive test. Three of the four women tested positive. Two of those named over twenty contacts each, with one of them

having already spread the disease to two other men.

Three years after we located those four women, two other women were incidentally tested and found to be positive for HIV. They named this man, but we lack either the laws or more probably the leadership with the will to force this man to be tested and/or stop him from infecting others. The incidents concerning this case became known in 1989. In 1992 an additional four people who related directly to the original patients in this case has become infected, demonstrating the problems of controlling a communicable disease without having a program with "real objectives" and a clear, methodical method of tracing contacts.

## INEXPERIENCED LEADERSHIP AND HOMOSEXUAL LOBBYING

In many states, virtually anybody except physicians, nurses, venereal disease investigators, or epidemiologists was selected to manage AIDS programs. The selection of inexperienced leadership combined with homosexual lobbying resulted in many states lacking the essentials of a disease-control program. Name-reporting systems were often nonexistent. Anonymous reporting was encouraged. Accountability mechanisms to ensure patients were contacted and—even in the best-managed states —exceedingly poor interviewing and contact-tracking programs were put in place. Despite such poor quality, South Carolina has a program that is considered one of the nation's best. Its accomplishments in reducing the spread of AIDS have been achieved by local effects, not necessarily because of state leadership and definitely in spite of national leadership.

Nationally, proper interviews that could lead to disease intervention are not routinely obtained, and contacts are rarely followed. Nurses or counselors in most states were assigned the role of conducting intense interviews for sexual contacts without adequate training. In addition to their lack of training, these workers were not allowed to gain those skills by doing in-depth interviews on gonorrhea patients to determine what they could produce.

The results of such mindless experiments in disease control with perhaps the most dangerous disease of the century have been disastrous. A study by doctors at the University of North Carolina, published in the *New England Journal of Medicine*[1] and reported on by newspapers in January 1992, revealed the horrors and depth of the problem of having a national AIDS program in name only. They discovered that counselors located only half of all partners named, while infected people told only 7 percent of the people they exposed. Of the 534 people studied, almost half never returned to the clinic. Of the partners notified during the study, 94 percent were unaware they had been exposed to the virus.

Factors as basic as contact indexes, number of locatable contacts, and the number of cases relating to other infected individuals were not considered. Often those in charge of programs did not know the meaning of such basic terms or concepts. The ability to systematically transmit contact information from one county or state to another or to an accounting system to ensure every AIDS patient was either counseled or interviewed is still lacking.

It should have been obvious from the start, as poor results readily demonstrated, that a nurse could not properly conduct a quality sexual interview —pushing for hidden contacts—and still function as a nurse giving nurturing care to the same infected individual. Taking a gentle view, this was, and is, the philosophy of leadership guiding most programs in the nation, a leadership that has never wanted to examine facts and productivity or base decisions on such mundane reasoning. A leadership that in one small city allowed or caused hundreds of positive test results to be lost. Four years later, with no changes having been made, the same error recurred. Another hundred positive reports were discovered in a desk drawer. The positive HIV reports were simply set aside and ignored. The patients involved were never notified.

This is only one minor example of our country's AIDS programs. Should you think it couldn't be worse, then consider that during the past thirteen years most states have lacked programs that could even gather the hundred positive reports by name and address. The reason South Carolina's AIDS program is far superior to most is self-explanatory: There is little else adequate for comparison.

## INEFFECTIVE HEALTH EDUCATION

Exacerbating matters for the tax-paying public, the health educator contingent duplicates the media with their efforts. For thirteen years newspapers and TV have almost daily delivered facts concerning AIDS. One cannot imagine a normal human being in the United States being unaware of the three ways that the CDC claims AIDS is spread. Infected people with an IQ of sixty can explain how AIDS is spread. Despite this public awareness, health educators are still designing programs to reemphasize such basic knowledge during prime-time TV hours.

At some point the leaders in the war on AIDS should realize that people sitting home watching TV are not the most at-risk groups. Instead of working on their standard pamphlets and TV productions, health educators should travel to areas where crack users live and deal, where women perform oral sex on as many as fifteen men an evening. Perhaps then they could discover a more at-risk population and design more-effective messages. By ignoring these groups, educators find little to say beyond their standard messages. Such staid thinking abounds among our leadership.

In my small area of South Carolina, without bias and without a hidden agenda, our staff has for the most part been able to attack AIDS as a communicable disease. With data collection, the chips have fallen as they should. For thirteen years we have consistently found that nearly 35 percent of our HIV-positive people are heterosexual, non-IV drug users—a finding quite different from what has been nationally indicated. One woman has heterosexually infected nine men. This information has been known for ten years, and yet the CDC has never officially inquired how this happened or asked if we had similar cases. The case was discussed in the national news and still prompted no inquiry from either the CDC or the state AIDS program. Private physicians, such as Dr. J. D. Robinson, did inquire into these heterosexual cases, but these are not the people running the CDC. Those who inquired from the CDC have done so only unofficially.

Our basic data compiled in 1990 included the following information: of 203 infected individuals identified, 23 refused to name any contacts, but 180 named 836 contacts. (I am including cluster contacts with contacts to simplify this report, but the cluster numbers were not significant enough to alter the findings.) Of the 836 contacts, 116 tested positive and 404 were negative (in other words, about 20 percent of those tested were positive). The remainder either lived outside my area and were not checked or are pending. Some 92 of the 836 contacts lived in states that will not notify them—a good cause for virtually everyone to feel less secure.

## PROLONGING LIVES AND DETERRING AIDS

We who follow AIDS as a venereal disease make many observations that will be verified in time. If sexual contacts are notified and found to be positive in the early stage of the infection, they are able to immediately begin good nutritional habits as well as monitor their health before becoming sick. We estimate that with this process patients can prolong their lives in a healthy state for at least three years longer than people who find they are infected after becoming ill. Also, by discovering their infection earlier than they would have without a partner notification program, they can avoid unintentionally spreading the infection to others.

A realistic review of the ever-increasing number of babies being born to HIV-positive mothers should signal much greater concern than has been aroused. This increase in infected babies clearly demonstrates how inaccurate CDC assumptions and predictions have been. If you consider that most women who know they are infected do not get pregnant, then the constantly climbing figure for perinatal infection becomes more alarming. This indicates that the real heterosexual AIDS or HIV increase may be far larger than is imagined.

Many areas of AIDS infection seem paradoxical. One person may be exposed once or twice and become infected, while another with multiple exposures remains HIV-negative. This is not in the majority of cases, but it occurs enough to make one wonder. We see a healthy person deteriorate rapidly and a sickly person survive much longer than expected. Two people with T-cell counts of zero for over a year did well. We wonder why no one studies these apparent survivors. Do they have some unknown genetic makeup that allows them to remain healthy enough to work every day—and without medication?

Obviously, the AIDS program should have been put in the proper hands years ago. Many people have been needlessly infected because leadership shirked its responsibility to use trained interviewers and investigators to elicit and trace contacts and to require the testing of contacts. How can supposedly sane leaders have failed to push for laws to incarcerate the small percentage of infected individuals who have intentionally spread this infection? Many of the private AIDS organizations do no better in halting the disease. In June 1991, the International AIDS Society mailed an urgent letter asking people to write legislators and certain other individuals to protest the U.S. ban that kept infected individuals from entering our country. This group made itself into a political advocacy group and attempted to influence policy for political reasons, not medical ones. It also encouraged an international boycott against allowing any international AIDS conference to be held in the United States. Not a word in the letter mentioned doing anything to halt the spread of the disease. Could they possibly imagine that something as basic as reporting positively tested individuals by name might be important in slowing the spread of AIDS?

Too often, HIV-positive individuals return to the clinic with gonorrhea, signifying that they are not practicing safe sex but are spreading AIDS. A mind-boggling amount of AIDS or HIV virus can be spread in the pus from gonorrheal discharge during sex—a discharge loaded with white cells, the home of the virus.

How can the current leadership be allowed to stay in control of the AIDS program? Is there no one who can be held accountable when many infected people are not notified? Can anyone be held responsible for the AIDS program being totally ineffective in slowing the disease's spread? The sad reality is that when AIDS programs falsely give the appearance of working toward controlling the disease, they protect themselves from being properly monitored and thereby actually help spread the disease.

## SECRECY MUST GO

The other side of the AIDS disease control question must be brought out. Secrecy should never be allowed in nonmilitary, tax-supported organizations. More public health employees would gladly speak out to condemn the national AIDS effort, but they fear losing their jobs. Two health officers in New York City paid the price for trying to build a real AIDS program. Recently we saw a national uproar over Darnell McGee, who was reported to have infected at least eighteen women in Missouri, and over Nessbawn Williams, who allegedly infected at least nine women in Mayville, New York. Several years ago there was a similar uproar over Edward Savitz exposing children to AIDS in Philadelphia. But unknown to the public, some workers have questioned the AIDS leadership and even accused them of knowingly making decisions that would ensure the continued destructive behavior of the McGees and the Savitzes of this world.

Last but not least, it is time to separate AIDS control from the homosexual agenda. It is past time we add disease intervention to the title of the AIDS program. The current omission of these words tells the story.

## REFERENCES

1. S. E. Landis, V. J. Schoenbach, et al., "Results of a Randomized Trail of Partner Notification in Cases of HIV Infection in North Carolina," *New England Journal of Medicine* 336:2 (9 Jan. 1992): 101–107.

# POSTSCRIPT

## Should Confidentiality Remain a Priority for People With AIDS?

Traditional means of disease tracking and partner notification for HIV have been implemented by only a few state and local health departments. The CDC maintains that since many of those infected with HIV have multiple sexual partners, tracking would be extremely difficult. The CDC has concluded that the risk of discrimination due to breaches of confidentiality outweigh any potential benefit of tracking those who test positive for HIV.

Nevertheless, public health authorities are moving closer to requiring mandatory name-based reporting and partner notification, practices that have long been in place for tuberculosis and sexually transmitted diseases. The HIV policy that places confidentiality over disease prevention is often referred to as the "AIDS exceptionalism." Because of the stigma against AIDS, health officials believe that name reporting and partner notification would cause people to refrain from HIV testing and treatment. See "No One Left to Track," *Advocate* (April 14, 1998) and "Gay Doctors Warn Against HIV Name Reporting," *AIDS Weekly Plus* (December 8, 1997). Current treatments are extending the lives of people with HIV, but only if they receive treatment early. As a result, there is now a major push in many states to end AIDS exceptionalism and to establish a system of mandatory name reporting and partner notification. In 1997 Representative Tom Coburn (R-Oklahoma) introduced a bill that would establish confidential HIV reporting nationwide. See "Dr. Tom Coburn's Bill Would Bring Back Public Health Measures," *Saturday Evening Post* (January/February 1998). The American Medical Association backs this bill, but AIDS activists have denounced it as a means of stigmatizing people with AIDS. They also argue that there is no evidence that traditional public health measures would have an impact on reducing the number of AIDS cases. Coburn counters that there is no evidence that traditional measures would *not* be effective since they have not been tried.

For a comprehensive overview of the AIDS confidentiality issue see "The Secret Weapon Against AIDS?" *Self* (August 1998) and "The AIDS Exception: Privacy vs. Public Health," *The Atlantic Monthly* (June 1997). Other articles concerning tracking and partner notification include "Proposal Would Allow Better Tracking of HIV Patients," *AIDS Weekly Plus* (March 23, 1998); "Public Health and Human Rights" *The Lancet* (March 7, 1998); "Progress on AIDS Brings Movement for Less Secrecy," *The New York Times* (August 21, 1997); and *Human Rights and Public Health in the AIDS Pandemic* (Oxford University Press, 1997).

# ISSUE 14

## Should Partial-Birth Abortion Be Banned?

**YES: Robert J. White,** from "Partial-Birth Abortion: A Neurosurgeon Speaks," *America* (October 18, 1997)

**NO: John M. Swomley,** from "The 'Partial-Birth' Debate in 1998," *The Humanist* (March/April 1998)

### ISSUE SUMMARY

**YES:** Professor and neurosurgeon Robert J. White states that Congress should completely ban late-term, partial-birth abortion.

**NO:** John M. Swomley, a professor emeritus of social ethics, maintains that the increased medical risk caused by banning late-term, partial-birth abortion is reason enough for Congress to allow the practice.

Few issues have created as much controversy and resulted in as much opposition as abortion, particularly late-term, or partial-birth, abortion. Those involved in the abortion debate not only have firm beliefs, but each side has a self-designated label—pro-life and pro-choice—that clearly reflects what they believe to be the basic issues. The supporters of a woman's right to choose an abortion view individual choice as central to the debate. They maintain that if a woman cannot choose to end an unwanted pregnancy she has lost one of her most basic human rights. The pro-choice supporters assert that although the fetus is a potential human being, its life cannot be placed on the same level with that of a woman. On the other side, the supporters of the pro-life movement argue that the fetus *is* a human being and that it has the same right to life as the mother. They contend that abortion is not only immoral; it is murder.

Although abortion appears to be a modern issue, it has a very long history. In the past women in both urbanized and tribal societies used a variety of dangerous methods to end unwanted pregnancies. Women consumed toxic chemicals, or various objects were inserted into the uterus in hopes of expelling its contents. Modern technology has simplified the abortion procedure and has made it considerably safer. Before abortion was legalized in the United States, approximately 20 percent of all deaths from childbirth or pregnancy were caused by botched illegal abortions.

In 1973 the U.S. Supreme Court's decision of *Roe v. Wade* determined that an abortion in the first three months (trimester) of pregnancy is a decision between a woman and her physician and is protected by a right to privacy. The Court ruled that during the second trimester an abortion can be performed on the basis of health risks. During the final trimester an abortion can be performed only to preserve the mother's life.

Since 1973 abortion has become one of the most controversial issues in America. The National Right to Life Committee, one of the major abortion foes, currently has over 11 million members, who have become increasingly militant. Demonstrators have also become more aggressive and violent. In 1993 David Gunn, a physician who performed abortions in Pensacola, Florida, was gunned down by a pro-life fanatic. Gunn's replacement, Dr. John Britton, was killed along with his bodyguard in August 1994 by a regular protester at an abortion clinic. In Massachusetts later ttat year, several people, including a receptionist, were gunned down in two women's health clinics that performed abortions. In spring 1997 abortion protestors targeted high schools across the United States that taught students about pregnancy termination.

In 1995 the Partial Birth Abortion Act was passed by both houses of Congress but was vetoed by President Bill Clinton in 1996. It passed again in the House of Representatives in 1997. This bill permits late-term abortions only if the mother's life is threatened. Although it is expected that the president will again veto the bill, over 25 states have passed laws banning partial-birth abortions. In Wisconsin, possibly the state with the most extreme abortion laws, violators are subject to life in prison for providing late-term abortion services. Many legislators that are considered pro-choice have voted in favor of banning late-term abortions.

In the following selections, Robert J. White maintains that partial-birth abortions should be banned. John M. Swomley argues that there are medically valid reasons to continue providing women with late-term abortions.

# YES

Robert J. White

## PARTIAL-BIRTH ABORTION: A NEUROSURGEON SPEAKS

I do not come before you as an obstetrician or a gynecologist. I come before you as a brain surgeon and as a neuroscientist. When I was undergoing my training at Harvard Medical School and was working at Children's Hospital in Boston, I saw the efforts that the pediatricians and the neonatologists were putting forward to save the lives of children, infants, yes, even extremely small preemies, even in those days. It has left a mark on my consciousness and on my future medical practice. I have been trained through all of my years, including many years at the Mayo Clinic, to save lives—not to take life.

I come from a time in American medicine when abortion was abhorred by the medical profession. One of the things we have to consider here is the fact that we are dealing with a human being, for a fetus is a human person. By the 20th week of gestation, the fetus has in place the neurocircuitry to appreciate noxious stimuli. Scientific studies are available demonstrating that fetuses of these ages can perceive and respond to painful sensations. As a matter of fact, there are studies suggesting that even at earlier ages (8 through 13 weeks' gestation) there is sufficient neuroanatomical development that noxious stimuli could be recognized.

It is well to remember that, at this particular time, the 20th week of fetal maturation and later, the neurofiber systems, in the form of small nerves, are in place providing sensory information from the surface of the skin to the spinal cord, from which sensation can be conducted to special areas of the brain. This includes pain, where it can be localized to subcortical and even cortical regions of the brain. But the neurosystems that are equally important in the modulation and suppression of pain are not yet as mature as those that conduct pain. Consequently some authorities feel that fetuses at these early ages (20 weeks or more) perceive pain to a greater degree than the adult. So I would like to emphasize that, within the framework of fetal nervous maturation, pain can be recognized and appreciated.

* * *

Now, as I have testified, I am not an obstetrician. But as I view and understand this particular abortive procedure, the partial-birth abortion—with its tissue compression, its pulling of limbs and body, its anatomical distortion—must be an extremely painful experience for the fetus as it is advanced into and through the birth canal. But what is most disturbing for me is the surgical procedure itself. Here we are talking about a brain operation on a living human fetus who has reached an age at which, if it were outside the womb, it would be a candidate for neurosurgery.

We operate on preemies within this age range, conducting brain surgery to save their lives. We would never consider any procedure giving us surgical access to a preemie's central nervous system without sophisticated neuroanesthesia to eliminate pain.

I have read, as you have, that this procedure to terminate the fetus's life requires the opening of the scalp or neck to enter the upper spinal canal. Now I am wondering if the people who perform this procedure really know what they are doing, in a technical sense. When we operate in this same anatomical region on the infant brain beyond the 24th week of gestation, optical magnification is required. Some of the most sophisticated surgical instrumentation employed in medicine today is used to allow us to enter these same neuroanatomical areas that are apparently crucial to this late-term abortion procedure.

I can imagine that these untrained people would actually "suck out" the brain without eliminating the pain of the procedure. The anatomical area where they plan to divide the upper cervical spinal cord, using a large scissors, is a region that has come to public attention because it is the part of the spinal cord where Mr. Christopher Reeve (aka Superman) has been injured. While medical science is bringing to bear the best technology to improve Mr. Reeve's body functioning and he is being treated by some of the finest neurosurgeons in this country, we are justifying abortion surgery in the same area to kill infants!

* * *

The obstetrician who conducts this type of partial late-term abortion is attempting brain surgery. There is no description in any of the doctors' articles or responses from those who do these procedures to indicate whether they are grossly severing the upper cervical spine (spinal cord) or acting on the brain stem (the anatomical structure that connects the cord to the upper brain). The truth is, they really do not know where they are.

It is true that once you sever or damage central nervous tissue in that area, the capability for breathing and other essential physiological functions has been eliminated, as has happened to Mr. Reeve. The physicians conducting this abortion procedure are not trained neurosurgeons. Even though they are attempting to terminate the child's life by removing its brain, the poor infant's pain neurocircuitry could remain intact, allowing the fetus to experience severe discomfort for some time.

Nowadays, as I spend hours at the operating table using sophisticated instrumentation, concentrating intensely to remove blood from the brain, to direct specially developed miniaturized hydraulic tubing into the fluid passages of the brain of infants of this age or perhaps a little older, all of these maneuvers directed to save their lives, it disgusts me to think that other medical professionals are undertaking destructive operations in the same brain and spinal cord areas to terminate human life!

I would also remind you that powerful groups in this country have displayed great concern over animal research, particularly as it relates to alleged pain in medical experimentation when animal models are employed. It seems to me that we have already reached a point where far greater care would have to be exercised by the veterinarian or the medical scientist experimenting on animals to reduce or eliminate pain than is employed by these doctors doing surgery on the central nervous system to destroy a living being. I am sure that the animal rights groups in this country would be able to bring sufficient political pressure on Congress and within the media to have painful, late partial-abortion in animals totally eliminated.

* * *

To sum up: The fetus in a late-term partial-abortion is at an age of gestation where pain can be perceived, possibly more exquisitely than by an adult. The procedure itself is a brain operation. But the details of it are so gross and so ghastly that it seems to me impossible to believe that medical colleagues of another specialty would carry it out.

# NO

**John M. Swomley**

# THE "PARTIAL-BIRTH" DEBATE IN 1998

As the 1998 elections draw near, the Republican-controlled Congress is expected to attempt another override of President Clinton's veto of the so-called Partial-Birth Abortion Act of 1997. After consulting with their religious allies, congressional Republican leaders will no doubt organize such an override attempt to take place on a date determined to have maximum impact on the elections. Legislation prohibiting this particular type of late-term abortion first passed in the 1996 session of Congress and was vetoed by the president on the grounds that the bill permitted such abortions only if the mother's life were threatened, not if her health were in danger. It then became an issue in the presidential campaign of 1996, leading to new legislation by congress and another presidential veto in 1997.

Given this continuing threat to reproductive freedom, it is compelling to review a few public cases of women whose lives would have been endangered had this legislation been law at the time of their pregnancies.

\* \* \*

**VIKKI STELLA** from Naperville, Illinois. Parents of two daughters, Vikki and her husband Archer discovered at thirty-two weeks of pregnancy that the fetus had only fluid filling the cranium where its brain should have been, as well as other major problems. The Stellas made "the most loving decision we could have made" to terminate the pregnancy. Because the procedure preserved her fertility, Vikki was able to conceive again. In December 1995, she gave birth to a healthy boy, Nicholas.

\* \* \*

**MARY-DOROTHY LINE** from Los Angeles, California. In the summer of 1995, Mary-Dorothy was told at twenty-one weeks of pregnancy that her fetus had an advanced, textbook case of hydrocephalus—an excess of fluid on the brain. It was so acute and so advanced that it was untreatable. Practicing Catholics, she and her husband Bill sought a medical miracle but were told that no surgery or therapy could save their baby. Indeed, the medical experts who reviewed the case told her that her own health was at risk, and so the Lines decided to end the pregnancy. Mary-Dorothy was able to become pregnant again and gave birth to a healthy baby girl in September 1996.

* * *

COREEN COSTELLO from Agoura, California. In April 1995, seven months pregnant with her third child, Coreen and her husband Jim found out that a lethal neuromuscular disease had left their much-wanted daughter unable to survive. Its body had stiffened and was frozen, wedged in a transverse position. In addition, amniotic fluid had puddled and built up to dangerous levels in Coreen's uterus. Devout Christians and opposed to abortion, the Costellos agonized for over two weeks about their decision and baptized the fetus in utero. Finally, Coreen's increasing health problems forced them to accept the advice of numerous medical experts that the intact dilation and extraction (D&X) was, indeed, the best option for Coreen's own health, and the abortion was performed. Later, in June 1996, Coreen gave birth to a healthy son.

* * *

MAUREEN MARY BRITELL from Sandwich, Massachusetts. Maureen and her husband Andrew, practicing Catholics, were expecting their second child in early 1994 when, at six months' gestation, a sonogram revealed that the fetus had anencephaly. No brain was developing, only a brain stem. Experts at the New England Medical Center in Boston confirmed that the fetus the Britells had named Dahlia would not survive. The Britells' parish priest supported their decision to induce labor and terminate the pregnancy. During the delivery, a complication arose and the placenta would not drop. The umbilical cord had to be cut, aborting the fetus while still in delivery in order to prevent serious health risks for Maureen. Dahlia had a Catholic funeral.

* * *

CLAUDIA CROWN ADES from Los Angeles, California. In 1992, in the twenty-sixth week of a desperately wanted pregnancy, Claudia and her husband Richard were told after an ultrasound that the male fetus she carried had a genetic condition called trisomy-13. Its anomalies included extensive brain damage, serious heart complications, and liver, kidney, and intestinal malformations. Its condition was incompatible with life. After consulting with many physicians, Claudia and Richard chose the D&X as the medically appropriate procedure for Claudia and the most compassionate procedure for their would-be son.

* * *

There are, of course, other cases wherein severely handicapped children would have been born had Congress succeeded in enacting the "partial-birth" legislation. The crucial question is whether medical decisions should be made by qualified physicians or by politicians.

The major medical associations oppose government intervention. The American College of Obstetricians and Gynecologists said, "The physician, in consultation with the patient, must choose the most appropriate method based upon the patient's individual circumstances." A legislative ban would force doctors in many cases to select what they consider a second-best method in order to avoid criminal prosecution.

Dr. Allan Rosenfield, an obstetrician and dean of New York's Columbia School of Public Health, says, "I am also concerned that the medical community is being used—and abused—to further the political agenda of individuals who do not support access to safe, legal abortion. To many this legislation appears to be simply the first step in a 'procedure by procedure' attempt to make the constitutional right to choose meaningless." The American Nurses Association concurred, stating, "It is inappropriate for the law to mandate a clinical course of action for a woman who is already faced with an intensely personal and difficult decision."

New Jersey lawyer John Tomasin has proposed that any such ban should include the following language:

PROVIDED:

(a) If the potential parents and best medical evidence clearly show that the potential child will probably be severely handicapped and unable to take care of itself for the rest of its life, and

(b) The federal government forces the parents to have said child anyway, and

(c) If said child is in fact born severely handicapped and unable to take care of itself for the rest of its life,

(d) Then the federal government shall pay 51 percent of the costs of taking care of said child for the rest of its life, and, if the child is institutionalized, the federal government shall pay 100 percent of said costs, and

(e) If legal action is necessary to enforce such obligations, interested parties shall recover proper judgment, plus reasonable legal fees and costs.

Such a proposal, which would almost certainly be rejected, sheds light on the fact that the religious anti-abortion movement and its congressional allies are concerned only with religious doctrine and not with the consequences of the legislation they advocate and adopt.

This same motive is also responsible for perpetuating false information about the subject. For example, the term *partial-birth abortion*, which was used in the House and Senate bills, is not found in any medical dictionary or textbook. It is a term that originates in the anti-abortion movement, organized by the Catholic bishops and by the authors of the legislation in response to that movement. The Catholic bishops' "Plan for Pro-Life Activities" specifically demands "passage of federal and state laws and adoption of administrative policies that will restrict the practice of abortion as much as is possible."

It is also important to note that the anti-abortion movement always refers to embryos and fetuses as "babies." This is a propaganda device known as *prolepsis*, which *Webster's Dictionary* defines as "describing an event as if it has already happened" when, in fact, it may be months away or may never happen. For example, a normal person who eats a fertilized egg does not say, "I have just eaten a chicken," nor is the crushing of an acorn the destruction of an oak tree.

In order to understand the meaning of *partial-birth abortion* it is essential to note that there are two types of abortion: elective and emergency. An elective abortion, which is chosen by the woman, must take place either in the first trimester (within twelve weeks of pregnancy) or in the second trimester (twenty-four weeks). The Supreme Court has held that a woman is constitutionally entitled to have an abortion of a nonviable fetus for whatever reasons she finds compelling. Therefore, physicians performing second-trimester abortions must first determine that the fetus is too underdeveloped to survive outside the womb.

After twenty-four weeks of pregnancy, which is the approximate date of viability and the beginning of the third trimester, the abortion procedure is not elective but emergency, in that the fetus is gravely or fatally impaired, or the woman's life or health is at risk, or both.

According to the most recent data, 90 percent of all abortions are performed in the first trimester and 99 percent within twenty weeks, or near the midpoint of the second trimester. No national data are available on abortions past twenty weeks, but the Allan Guttmacher Institute has estimated, based on limited data collected by the Centers for Disease Control and Prevention, that approximately 320 to 600 abortions annually are performed after the twenty-sixth week, hence, in the third trimester of pregnancy.

The term *partial-birth abortion* was defined in the 1996 legislation as one wherein "the person performing the abortion partially vaginally delivers a living fetus before killing the infant and completing the delivery." The nearest medical term that to some degree meets that definition is an *intact dilation and extraction*, which involves the deliberate dilation of the cervix, usually over a sequence of days. The fetal body, excepting the head, can then be readily extracted; the fetal head cannot until the doctor reduces the size so it can pass through the fragile and narrow cervical opening. That reduction requires partial evacuation of the intracranial contents.

This raises certain questions. Why is this procedure sometimes necessary? Why not induce labor with drugs? The cervix, which holds the uterus closed during pregnancy, is very resistant to dilation until about thirty-six weeks.

Inductions done before this time take two to four days and are physically painful. Because of the danger of uterine rupture, the woman requires constant nursing supervision.

Another question: Isn't there another option, such as a cesarean section? A cesarean delivery usually involves twice as much blood loss and, before thirty-four weeks of pregnancy, the lower segment of the uterus is usually too thick to use a standard horizontal incision, so a vertical incision is necessary. Any uterine incision complicates future pregnancy, but a vertical incision jeopardizes both the mother's health and future pregnancies, which would also require a cesarean.

The safest and, hence, better option in some situations is the D&X procedure. Using intravenous anesthesia, the physician can insert small dry cylinders into the cervix that expand gradually as they absorb fluid from the woman. She can usually return home except for twice-daily visits to the clinic or office to be sure that she is dilating and to replace the dilators if required. This, plus a spinal needle to remove some fluid from the fetal head, reduces the chance of lacerating the cervix.

There are still other questions, such as why not let the woman wait until the thirty-sixth week and go into labor? Fetuses with severe defects have a high chance of dying in utero well before labor begins and therefore create a serious threat to the mother. When a fetus dies, its tissues begin to break down and enter the mother's bloodstream. This can cause clotting problems, making it more difficult for her to stop bleeding. This may then require a surgical delivery or an emergency hysterectomy.

These and other problems are the reason the physician—not the politician

—must be able to exercise judgment as to which method to pursue. The "partial-birth" legislation, however, makes the physician liable to criminal penalties if he or she chooses the D&X method, thus deterring doctors from using such procedures.

Dr. Rosenfield says, "The reasons these abortions are performed late [in the third trimester] is because these women were pursuing wanted pregnancies and then something went terribly wrong," such as "severe fetal abnormality" or serious health threats to the women that developed late in pregnancy.

All abortions require the termination of a fetus, but the government should not require a woman to bear an increased medical risk because one method of abortion may seem more brutal than another. Many medical decisions—ranging from invasive surgery to amputation—seem harsh but may be necessary to save a patient's life.

The focus of the original legislation, which President Clinton vetoed in 1996, was on catastrophic third-trimester pregnancies. It should be noted that the ban proposed in 1997 was not limited to the last few weeks of pregnancy, when one might expect a viable birth. Rather, it would ban D&X abortion in the second, as well as the third, trimester. Thus it is intended to ban abortions *before* viability as well as *after* viability.

It should be obvious that the abortion of a fetus well before viability cannot be a partial birth, because the fetus could not survive after the procedure. It is also true that some women during the second trimester need an abortion for medical, and not just elective, reasons. They therefore may need the same emergency care as if they were in the third trimester. However, the anti-abortion movement opposes all abortions—no matter what happens to the woman.

There is at least one other important argument against this legislation: one or a few religious organizations ought not to be able to legislate their religious dogma about abortion into law. If they are unable to persuade their own members not to have an abortion, they ought not use the police power of the state to send physicians to jail to prevent these women from having one. Nor should religious zealots be allowed to coerce women of other religions or no religion to accept *their* church's dogma. Separation of church and state is always better than theocracy.

# POSTSCRIPT

## Should Partial-Birth Abortion Be Banned?

The abortion issue continues to be complex and polarizing. In 1983 and 1986 the Supreme Court reaffirmed its support of abortion rights. However, the Court has become more conservative and pro-life in recent years. With pressure and support from pro-life groups throughout the country, *Roe v. Wade* may continue to come before the Supreme Court for reconsideration. Pro-life groups have been successful in keeping the abortion issue in the media and in the political arena, particularly the issue of partial-birth abortion.

The literature on abortion is often passionate and judgmental. Many recent articles decry the outbreaks of violence directed toward doctors who perform abortions and clinics where abortions are performed. Pro-life supporters often assert, however, that in some cases the end justifies the means. In "The Right-to-Life Rampage" *The Progressive* (August 1993), Operation Rescue founder Randall Terry is quoted as saying, "If there are no doctors to do abortions, it doesn't matter whether abortion is legal." Articles addressing the violence at clinics include "Abortion Case Verdict," *The New York Times* (March 6, 1994); "Antiabortion Violence: Cause and Effects," *Women's Health Issues* (Fall 1993); "One Doctor Down, How Many More?" *Time* (March 22, 1993); and "Bomb Squad," *The Village Voice* (February 4, 1997).

Despite the increased violence at abortion clinics, the morality of abortion continues to be a central theme in many articles and books. In "On Abortion," *Commentary* (January 1994), James Q. Wilson writes, "What kind of people are we that we cannot say, legislatively, that human life is precious, that an infant's life is perhaps the most precious of all?" "Abortion and the Politics of Morality in the USA," *Parliamentary Affairs* (April 1994) discusses the role of abortion and the politics of morality in American life.

In "Abortion Is Morally Wrong," *The World & I* (1989), Nancy Meyers, media director of the National Right to Life Committee, states that abortion is never justified and that it is a violation of human rights. William F. Buckley, in "Abortion: The Debate," *The National Review* (December 1989) concurs. However "Killing Babies Isn't Always Wrong," *Spectator* (September 16, 1995), argues that in some circumstances abortion is justified.

Many people believe that if abortion becomes illegal again, the number of self-induced and back-alley abortions would increase. Whether or not legalized abortion has improved women's health is still the subject of controversy. In *The Choices We Made* (Random House, 1991), Angela Bonavoglia asserts that legalizing abortion saves women's lives. She notes that of the 1.6 million legal abortions performed each year in the United States, only 6 women die annually from the procedure. However, in Mexico, where abortion is not legal, 140,000 women die annually from the procedure.

David C. Reardon, in *Aborted Women: Silent No More* (Loyola University Press, 1987), counters that the legalization of abortion has not improved the health of women. Although the number of deaths from legal abortions is low, Reardon maintains that infection and bleeding rates are high. He argues that since abortion rates have climbed since 1973, the health risks associated with abortion have increased due to the number of women having abortions.

There are thousands of articles and books addressing this issue. The following selections discuss the particular concerns surrounding late-term abortion: "Partial-Birth Abortion, Congress, and the Constitution," *The New England Journal of Medicine* (July 23, 1998); "Partial Truth," *National Review* (June 22, 1998); "Out of This Nettle, Danger . . . ," *Crisis* (June 1998); "A Heinous Procedure," *American Spectator* (April 1998); "Dead Reckoning," *National Review* (January 26, 1998); and "They Lied Through Their Teeth," *Human Events* (March 14, 1997).

Although many decry late-term abortions, some believe that they remain a medical necessity. See "Lights Out on Abortion," *The Progressive* (July 1998); "Fetal Distraction," *The Village Voice* (January 27, 1998); "The Dead-Baby Boom," *George* (January 1998); and "Separating Fact from Fiction," *Ms.* (May/June 1997).

# ISSUE 15

## Will Most Postmenopausal Women Benefit from Estrogen Replacement Therapy?

**YES: Michael Castleman,** from "Hormonious Heart," *Mother Jones* (July/August 1997)

**NO: Julie Felner,** from "Dr. Susan Love Cuts Through the Hype on Women's Health," *Ms.* (July/August 1997)

### ISSUE SUMMARY

**YES:** Health columnist Michael Castleman asserts that unless a woman has a history of breast cancer, the benefits of postmenopausal hormone replacement therapy far outweigh the risks.

**NO:** Writer Julie Felner interviews physician Dr. Susan Love, who states that she is alarmed that many physicians prescribe hormone replacement therapy for all menopausal patients indefinitely.

Women of the baby boom generation are now approaching middle age. Millions of these women will go through menopause, a normal part of the aging process caused by a gradual decline in the production of the female sex hormone estrogen. Menopause increases the risk of age-related diseases, such as osteoporosis, heart disease, and Alzheimer's disease. Menopause can also produce uncomfortable symptoms, including skin flushing, urinary tract infections, and uterine cramps. In the past fewer women lived long enough to reach the age of menopause and those who did tended to suffer silently. Baby boomers have generally rejected many of the stereotypes of middle and old age and have sought to redefine these later years. Given their large numbers, baby boomers represent a huge consumer market in items such as anti-wrinkle creams, cosmetic surgery, nutritional supplements, and hormone replacement therapy (HRT). HRT drugs are generally prescribed to women at or approaching menopause to relieve menopausal symptoms and to help prevent heart disease and osteoporosis.

Although the medical industry in general heavily promotes HRT, it is a controversial treatament. Many studies indicate that HRT lessens or eliminates menopausal symptoms and also significantly reduces heart disease, the leading cause of death among women. HRT can also help prevent bone loss leading to osteoporosis, a major cause of death and disability among older women. Newer evidence has also shown that HRT may help reduce the risk of Alzheimer's. However, HRT has been found to it significantly increase the risk of breast and uterine cancer, especially among long-term users. When HRT was first introduced, women were urged to consider it for short-term use only to relieve menopausal symptoms. In recent years, women have been encouraged to receive HRT on a long-term basis, sometimes for the rest of their lives, to help prevent heart disease and osteoporosis. Women's health advocates and feminists argue that the normal aging process has been medicalized by placing women on HRT permanently. They also state that the pharmaceutical and medical industries are biased toward HRT due to the financial benefits they receive from drug sales. Premarin, the major brand of estrogen, is the largest selling prescription drug in the United States. Some maintain that there are nonhormonal alternatives to prevent heart disease and osteoporosis, including exercise, healthy diet, and quitting smoking.

Medical and pharmaceutical companies have generally promoted HRT, but there is disagreement among physicians and health providers about the risks versus the benefits. Some physicians believe that estrogen should be prescribed to all women unless there is a specific reason not to do so. Other physicians believe that estrogen should not be routinely prescribed to all women. Complicating the issue are the frequent contradictions in the scientific literature. The benefits and drawbacks of HRT can be difficult to weigh against each other. A National Institute on Aging study entitled "Estrogen Replacement Therapy and Longitudinal Decline in Visual Memory: A Possible Protective Effect?" *Neurology* (December 1997), found that women who took estrogen for up to 16 years after menopause reduced their risk of developing Alzheimer's by slightly over 50 percent. Shortly after that study was published, an article entitled "Postmenopausal Hormone Therapy and Mortality," *The New England Journal of Medicine* (November 22, 1997), suggested that for women that have a low risk of heart disease, the benefits of long-term estrogen treatment may be offset by an increased risk of breast cancer. The article reported on the 43 percent increase in breast cancer rates among women who used HRT for over 10 years. Another article, entitled "Effect of Postmenopausal Hormone Therapy on Lipoprotein (a) Concentration," *Circulation* (March 17, 1998), stated that HRT may reduce the risk of heart attack and strokes.

In the following selections, Michael Castleman states that HRT significantly reduces a women's risk of heart disease, osteoporosis, Alzheimer's disease, and colon cancer. Although women may reduce their risk factors through lifestyle changes, Castleman argues that many American women are not willing to make these changes. Julie Felner interviews Susan Love, who claims that she is against the routine prescribing of HRT for all women.

# YES

Michael Castleman

# HORMONIOUS HEART

I never thought I'd write the following sentence, but the evidence has become pretty overwhelming: Unless a woman has a history of breast cancer or has some other condition aggravated by estrogen, the benefits of postmenopausal hormone replacement therapy (HRT) far outweigh the risks.

For the past 15 years, I've been very skeptical about the safety of estrogen in both HRT (estrogen plus the hormone progestin), which women use to ease the passage into menopause, and in birth control pills (see box). Many studies have shown that HRT increases the risk of breast cancer in postmenopausal women; others have shown no association. On balance, I felt that estrogen was a bad idea.

However, studies have also shown that estrogen helps prevent heart disease, osteoporosis (postmenopausal bone-thinning), and colon cancer, and can even reduce the risk of Alzheimer's. Women faced a stark decision: What are you more afraid of? Breast cancer? Heart disease? Osteoporosis? But the terms of the debate have changed—and as a result, I've changed my tune.

*  *  *

It's been a long road for yours truly. For years, I've been astonished at the number of scientists who gamely argued that HRT poses no breast cancer risk. That seemed ridiculous. For decades, estrogen has been widely recognized as a stimulator of breast tumors in both animals and humans. It stood to reason that as growing numbers of women took estrogen, over time, we would see a steady increase in breast cancer—and we have, at a rate of about 1 percent per year. Contrary to what some experts have claimed, the increase cannot be fully explained by earlier detection (i.e., mammography).

In addition, it has become increasingly clear that compounds which mimic estrogen—chemicals unrelated to the hormone but that bind to cellular estrogen receptors—have been disrupting mammalian wildlife reproduction and, quite possibly, contributing to the higher incidence of human breast cancer....

Meanwhile, arguments in favor of estrogen to ward off heart disease and osteoporosis rubbed me the wrong way. It made no sense to throw a cancer-promoting hormone at women to prevent diseases that could be checked as effectively and more safely by quitting smoking, a low-fat diet, regular exercise, stress management, and supplemental calcium.

But now the equation has changed. Here's why: During the past few years, a scientific consensus has emerged that HRT does indeed, when used for 10 to 15 years, increase the lifetime risk of developing breast cancer (by 20 to 30 percent). Ironically, however, the latest research shows that, in addition to other health benefits, women taking HRT actually enjoy a decreased lifetime risk of breast cancer death.

\* \* \*

Menopause marks not only the end of a woman's reproductive years, it also signals the beginning of her major-risk years for heart disease. Heart disease is by far the No. 1 killer of both older men and women, but while heart disease takes a considerable toll on men in their 40s, estrogen protects women until after menopause. Then, as their natural levels of estrogen decline, their risk of heart disease soars.

Unfortunately, few women appreciate this. Not long ago, the Gallup Organization asked women to name the leading cause of female death. Forty percent said breast cancer, while 19 percent said heart disease. In fact, 35 percent of women die from heart disease, while only 4 percent succumb to breast cancer. And among postmenopausal white women, the lifetime probability of death from heart disease is even higher—46 percent.

The survey respondents' mistaken assumption was to some extent understandable. Breast cancer begins claiming a significant number of lives while women are in their 40s. Heart disease doesn't surpass it until women are well into their 50s. As a result, fear of breast cancer hits hard premenopausally, and lingers long after the risk from heart disease has dwarfed it.

Recently, Dawn B. Willis, scientific program director for the American Cancer Society, provided some welcome perspective on the risks and benefits of HRT. On the risk side, a decade or so of HRT increases the risk of breast cancer by as much as 30 percent. However, HRT also significantly reduces a woman's risk of heart disease.

Some simple math shows what these figures mean: At age 50, a white woman has a 9 percent risk of developing breast cancer over the next 30 years. HRT increases that risk by approximately a third, or 3 percentage points, to about 12 percent. However, the same woman faces a 46 percent risk of developing heart disease. HRT cuts it 12 percentage points to 34 percent. Even if breast cancer and heart disease killed the same number of postmenopausal women, these numbers would argue in favor of HRT—a 12-point reduction in heart disease risk outweighs a 3-point increase in breast cancer risk. But heart disease is much more lethal than breast cancer, which argues even more strongly in favor of HRT.

As for osteoporosis, one-quarter of white women over 45 have detectable bone-thinning, and by age 75, the figure is 90 percent. In a study of women over age 50, HRT reduced hip fracture risk from 15 to 12 percent.

As I mentioned, both heart disease and osteoporosis can be prevented without

---

### PILLING TIME

Most birth control pills contain estrogen, which raises the red flag of breast cancer risk. Some studies have shown increased risk in current and former Pill users. Recently, Pill users got good news from Dr. Valerie Beral, chief of cancer epidemiology at Oxford University, who has performed the most comprehensive review ever of the research investigating the link between the Pill and breast cancer: 54 studies in 25 countries involving more than 150,000 women. Beral found that birth control pills raise a woman's breast cancer risk 24 percent while she is taking them. But as soon as she stops, that risk begins to decline. After 10 years post-Pill, a woman will again have only an average breast cancer risk.

The Pill is generally a young woman's contraceptive. Women take it during their teens and 20s, and then usually switch to another method during their 30s. Breast cancer becomes a health concern for most women during their 40s. According to Beral, if women stop using the Pill by their mid-30s, their years on it won't increase their risk of breast cancer when the disease becomes a health concern.

—M.C.

---

estrogen. But doing so requires lifestyle changes many American women seem unwilling to make. I'm all for encouraging a healthier lifestyle, but from a public health perspective, it's callous to insist on lifestyle transformations when HRT provides significant benefits quickly and easily without them.

What's more, two recent studies show that estrogen may help prevent Alzheimer's (which is currently destroying the minds of some 2 million American women) because it helps preserve the neurotransmitters in the brain that become impaired by the disease. Researchers from the National Institute on Aging who followed 472 postmenopausal women for 16 years found that, compared with those who had used estrogen, those who had never taken it were more than twice as likely to develop Alzheimer's. A similar study in New York showed that women taking estrogen had a 2.7 percent risk of being diagnosed with Alzheimer's; among those not taking the hormone, the risk was 8.4 percent.

In addition, HRT helps prevent colon cancer. After 50, 6 percent of white women develop colon cancer; new research shows that HRT cuts this risk to just 3 percent.

Still, breast cancer is the disease women fear most, and despite the evidence of HRT's benefits, women have rejected it in droves because of breast cancer-phobia. Fewer than 25 percent of postmenopausal women who could take HRT do so.

Which brings me to the research showing that while HRT increases risk of developing breast cancer, it also reduces risk of dying from it by a whopping 22 percent. These findings come from American Cancer Society researchers who followed 422,000 postmenopausal women for nine years. This study's enormous number of participants and its long duration give its findings considerable scientific weight.

How could a hormone that increases risk of developing breast cancer simultaneously reduce the risk of dying from it? No one knows for sure, but most studies have shown that HRT use decreases women's risk of death from breast cancer.

Don't get me wrong: I'm not urging every postmenopausal woman to take HRT. The current consensus is that those with a history of breast cancer should not take it. HRT also increases risk of gallstones, asthma, and, more rarely, blood clots in veins.

But for women who have a low risk for these conditions, and especially for those with family histories of heart disease, colon cancer, osteoporosis, or Alzheimer's, HRT is definitely something to consider.

# NO                    Julie Felner

## DR. SUSAN LOVE CUTS THROUGH THE HYPE ON WOMEN'S HEALTH

Dr. Susan Love's modus operandi can best be summed up by one of the bumper stickers adorning her car: "Subvert the Dominant Paradigm." One of the country's leading experts on breast cancer and the author (with Karen Lindsey) of "Dr. Susan Love's Breast Book," she has spent much of her professional and personal life challenging the status quo—from her outspoken critique of conventional breast cancer treatments to the landmark lesbian adoption case that she and her partner, Helen Cooksey, won in 1994.

Love's fierce devotion to her patients—and to the truth—is eloquently captured in "To Dance with the Devil," Karen Stabiner's harrowing account of a year at the UCLA Breast Center, where Love served as director until last May. A faculty member at the UCLA School of Medicine, where she does breast cancer research, Love has now brought her honesty, compassion, and critical eye to the subject of women and hormones with "Dr. Susan Love's Hormone Book: Making Informed Choices About Menopause" (Random House).

Former "Ms." health editor Julie Felner talked with Love about hormone therapy, the controversy surrounding mammography for women under 50, and the latest in breast cancer research.

JULIE FELNER: In most of the reviews of your new book, the general tenor seemed to be, "Susan Love has seen the enemy and it's hormone therapy," "Susan Love thinks estrogen is poison," and so on. There's no doubt that the book decries the medicalization of menopause and the rush to put all women on hormones. But a lot of the concerns you raise reflect what feminists have been saying for years. While the mainstream press is focusing on how you're bucking the orthodoxy of the medical establishment, you're also knocking some feminist orthodoxies, in saying that, actually, short-term hormone therapy to relieve perimenopausal symptoms doesn't appear to do any harm and may in fact be a good idea for some women. You say that hormones are "neither the fountain of youth nor an evil empire." For all the talk about the radical Susan Love, the book seems to me to have a very moderate, reasoned, thoughtful approach.

SUSAN LOVE: I think the press likes to polarize, so they would like to have you be on one extreme. And really the reason I wrote the book is that I didn't see any moderate voice in there. People were either saying hormones are wonderful, the fountain of youth, or they're the devil and you should never take them. And it's usually somewhere in between. It reminds me of arguments about childbirth—where we went from being drugged and not knowing you'd given birth to "you have to do it naturally, or else," and there were some people who were suffering a whole lot and could benefit from an epidural.

But what alarms me is this rush toward "every woman should be on hormones forever." I think there are a lot of things that haven't been very well explained. One of the problems is that we have very little research on menopause, and what we do have is based on women who've had hysterectomies. So, the assumption has been that the ovaries shut down, dry up, and become useless. But it turns out that the ovaries continue to produce hormones well into your 80s —estrogen, testosterone, androsterone —and that natural menopause is a very different process from surgical menopause, and you can't extrapolate. And because of using the hysterectomy model, the notion is that menopausal symptoms come from low estrogen, and that since your estrogen levels are going to stay low, your symptoms are going to last forever—when in fact there are growing data that say it's not that at all, that the majority of symptoms happen before you have your last period.

Menopause is sort of puberty in reverse, and, as with puberty, it's transient.

So, if you are suffering a lot—and it's not everyone, it's about a third who suffer enough to need something—take hormones for four or five years and then slowly taper off, because if you stop abruptly you get your symptoms back. The average time for symptoms is two years, so if you say four or five years you should be over the hump. The reason I use five years as a limit is that the breast cancer risk seems to start around five years. So short-term use is, as far as we can tell, pretty safe, but it's the forever use that I'm much more concerned about.

J.F.: Which is one of the things you go into great detail about in the book—the risks of taking hormones long-term to prevent heart disease and osteoporosis.

S.L.: I think the problem is that it's not being very well framed. We have the most data on osteoporosis. The initial data looked like every woman lost bone at menopause, but then when they started doing studies that followed the same woman over time, they found that some of the women had a big loss at menopause and some of them didn't. And then there's a second time of bone loss, in your 70s, which may in fact be more significant, because the average hip fracture is at 80. Maybe it's that second loss that really tips you over, rather than the first one.

Estrogen will help prevent that loss, and as long as you're taking it, you will maintain your bone—you won't build it, but you'll maintain it—and it does ultimately decrease fractures. The problem is that we've oversold osteoporosis. And we've redefined osteoporosis. It used to be defined as having fractures in your 80s, and now it's defined as having an abnormal test [i.e., an increased risk of fracture].

It's like saying that high cholesterol is the same thing as heart disease.

When they redefined it, they made the parameters so broad that every woman who gets a fracture will fit the definition. So, it means that a lot of women are being told "You have osteoporosis," and they're afraid they're going to crumble tomorrow. And it leads you to the idea that you have to take something.

The drug companies are now marketing diseases instead of drugs—if we can scare people that they're going to get a disease, then they're much more likely to take drugs. What's fascinating is that I have a newspaper clip about how in England, they're trying to figure out which women are fast [bone] losers... so they can save the other women from taking hormones. And here we do the opposite. We say if there's any risk at all we should put every woman on them. God forbid we should pick the right people, because drug companies make more money on prevention. If you're only treating a disease, you treat one person. If you're treating prevention, you can treat the three other people who are at risk but who are never going to get it.

There was a very interesting study recently that found that the women who started on hormone therapy in their late 60s had the same bone density in their 70s as the women who had taken it from 50 on, so it may be that if there's any role for hormone therapy, it's in secondary prevention, later on.

J.F.: Secondary prevention, meaning you've already had a fracture and then go on it?

S.L.: Yeah, or starting later. Maybe look at bone density in your late 60s, see who's at risk then, and put those women on it.

The other interesting thing about osteoporosis is what I call the "no-free-lunch" data—that if you have high bone density, you have four times the risk of breast cancer. And if you have low bone density, you have 60 percent less breast cancer. So if you have a lot of natural estrogen, you'll have good bones/bad breasts, and if you have low natural estrogen, you'll have bad bones/good breasts. But you can't have both.

J.F.: And one of the points you make is that we're talking about taking hormones to avoid a wrist or hip fracture in your 80s. Meanwhile, you may die of breast cancer in your 60s as a result.

S.L.: Exactly. The breast cancer risk is 64; the heart disease is 76 or 77; and the hip fractures are in the 80s. So, we're not measuring things at the same time.

J.F.: What about the data that suggest hormones will protect against heart disease?

S.L.: The claim about heart disease is trickier because it hasn't been proven at all. It's being based on these observational studies of women who are already on hormones, and there's a big selection bias there—the women who are on hormones are at a high socioeconomic level, are more likely to go to a doctor, are more likely to exercise, eat well, all that stuff. So just those factors alone would explain a 50 percent reduction in [heart disease] risk—without the hormones.

I think we're vastly overemphasizing the benefit in terms of heart disease. Elizabeth Barrett-Connor [a researcher at the University of California at San Diego], who in fact was the first person to show that there was any benefit, thinks the same thing. [Estrogen] does lower your cholesterol, but that's probably not [why it seems to reduce heart disease], because you have to be on estrogen to get the benefit. [If you go off estrogen, your risk returns to what it was before], and if it were just about lowering your cholesterol, if you had ten more years of lowering cholesterol, it should put off heart disease for ten more years, but it doesn't.

Now, if you drip estrogen directly on blood vessels, it seems to do good things. So, it may have some value for women who already have heart disease. But that's very different from putting every 50-year-old on it.

J.F.: But don't you say in the book that women shouldn't take estrogen right after a heart attack?

S.L.: Well, it's not clear. There's always been this worry about clots... and some of the heart data come from that study on high doses [of estrogen] and men, so it's not clear. But there's a study going on right now, the HERS study [which is investigating estrogen and progesterone for women with preexisting artery disease], so we'll have data pretty soon for women who already have heart disease. And I'm sure that what's going to happen is the media will then say, "Aha! Well, if it's good for women who have heart disease then it must be even better for prevention," which is not necessarily true.

Now, they say that over a lifetime, one out of two women will die of heart disease, and only one out of eight gets breast cancer, but under age 75, there are three times more deaths from breast cancer than heart disease, and if you take the smokers out, six times more deaths from breast cancer than heart disease, so it's not an even match. And the breast cancer risk does go up the longer you're on hormones. If you are on hormone therapy, and if you've been on it for over five years, particularly over ten years, you see an increased risk of breast cancer.

J.F.: And you would have to stay on it that long to see any benefit in terms of heart disease.

S.L.: Yes—unless, you say, "Let's start in the late 60s." If the average age for a heart attack is 76, then that will ensure you're going to be on it in time. And then you're talking about the risk of getting breast cancer in your 80s instead of your 60s. If there's any case for hormones for prevention, at least at this moment, it looks like it's at a much later time.

J.F.: You say repeatedly throughout the book that there are no definite answers and that we won't really have any reliable information until 2007, when we'll have the results of the Women's Health Initiative [which is examining the effects of Premarin, medroxy progesterone, calcium, vitamin D, and low-fat diet on heart disease, breast cancer, colorectal cancer, and osteoporosis].

S.L.: Right, and even that will be limited, but at least then we have a randomized controlled trial. One of the things this brings us to, which also ties in with the issue of mammograms, is what's really been absent in medical reporting—and it's the fault of the medical profession as much as the media—is that we don't always tell the truth. We get caught in wishful thinking and sound bites, and then we say those enough times that we start believing them. And so we say, "It may prevent heart disease," and then after we've said that for a couple of years, we start saying it does—even without having to prove that it does.

One of the things we lose sight of is that menopause is not a disease. We're talking about a normal process, and we're talking about prevention. You may be willing to take some risks if you have a life-threatening disease that you're treating. But if you're healthy, then do you want to risk a life-threatening disease in order to potentially prevent something which you don't even know you're going to get?

J.F.: Do you think that this whole shift in medicine toward pharmacological prevention has done more harm than good?

S.L.: Absolutely. What you never hear in the discussion are the lifestyle changes that will do the same thing. In *JAMA [Journal of the American Medical Association]*, they had an article talking about the benefits of hormone replacement therapy, and they used the example of a woman who smokes, has high blood pressure, high cholesterol, and one first-degree relative with breast cancer. They used a mathematical model to add up all the risks and benefits and found that if she takes hormones for the rest of her life, she'll add six months to her life. What they don't say is that if she quit smoking, cleaned up her diet, and exercised, she'd add a couple of years to her life, probably more! So it's either drugs or nothing. But the first step should be look at your lifestyle. If you've maximized that and it doesn't work, then you might want to consider drugs.

J.F.: Why are doctors so reluctant to talk about lifestyle changes? Is it because no one stands to make money off diet and exercise or because they just don't think that women will be disciplined about it?

S.L.: I think it's a combination. They automatically say, "Well, they're not going to do it anyway—all they want is a pill." And they don't try. I think we give lip service to it. We say, "Well, of course you should exercise and do a good diet, and here's a prescription and this is how you take it." But if I sat down and said, "O.K., I think exercise is key to your survival, so let's look at your schedule and see when you could do it and what

you could do, and let's set a plan, and come back in two weeks and let me check up on how you're doing," you'd be much more likely to start. And we don't do that. I think part of it is, it takes longer—it's quicker to give somebody a pill. And another thing is that we just assume that nobody's going to want to do it and then it becomes a self-fulfilling prophecy. And I think the drug companies are marketing very, very strongly.

J.F.: It just seems that doctors are severely underestimating women. I mean, look at the example of Susan Love, who used to be a chain-smoker and crash dieter, who used to take the Pill continuously so as not to have periods at all. Now you're a tofu lover who exercises for 45 minutes every day, and you've sworn off hormones during your own menopause. So, if you can do it . . .

S.L.: Yeah, people can do it. It just has to be a high enough priority.

There are a number of things that feed into it, but we certainly don't emphasize healthy behavior. Take quitting smoking: smoking brings on menopause two years earlier, it causes more heart disease, more osteoporosis, more breast cancer, more wrinkles, the whole bit, and still, as a country, we subsidize tobacco growing.

J.F.: Let's talk specifically about hormones and African American women.

S.L.: Zero data on African American women, and the little bit of data that we have is so selected. Take, for example, the Alzheimer's study that came out a little while ago—they said this is a good study because it has African American women and Hispanic women in it. But it's still an observational study, which means that you don't know why they were put on hormones to start with. And if you think it's a select population of white women who get on hormones, it's an even more select population of African American and Hispanic women. So we have no data. We do know that African American women have much less osteoporosis.

J.F.: And a higher risk of stroke and lupus, not to mention a higher breast cancer mortality rate...

S.L.: Right. But also a much higher hysterectomy rate. If anything goes wrong reproductively in the slightest, they are hysterectomized. It's much higher. In this country one out of three women will have a hysterectomy by age 60 overall—and it's only 10 percent in Europe, and that's not because our uteruses are more damaged, either—and I think it may be one out of two for African American women. Because there's no attempt to do anything else. And I think in some subtle way, or maybe not so subtle way, it's birth control. If you have the slightest problem, a fibroid or bleeding or whatever, and the provider thinks you've had enough kids, then you know, you get everything taken out. I don't know that it's a conscious bias, but I think it's true.

J.F.: But given that set of risk factors—the lower osteoporosis but the higher lupus, stroke, breast cancer—it seems to me that African American women should avoid hormone therapy.

S.L.: Yeah, the same thing is true for Hispanic women. So obviously, these things are not universal. You know, in Japan, they don't even have a word for hot flashes. They have less osteoporosis, less heart disease, less breast cancer, and a longer life expectancy with no hormones. I hate it when people say osteoporosis and heart disease are the consequences of menopause. No! Osteoporosis and heart disease are diseases that are more common as you get older. And, you know, there may be a reason to take drugs

to prevent them, but they are not the consequences. Men get osteoporosis, men get heart disease—without menopause!

J.F.: You have been one of the most vocal critics of mammography for women under 50. And up until recently you had the National Cancer Institute [NCI] agreeing with you. Now, the NCI, which has flip-flopped back and forth, has changed its mind again, saying, "O.K., we recommend mammography every one to two years starting at 40." We have the American Cancer Society [ACS] actually recommending annual mammograms after 40. We've got the American Medical Association, the American College of Obstetrics and Gynecology, we've got all these other groups all endorsing mammography for high-risk women in their 40s. And then we have Susan Love on the other side—

S.L.: —and the American College of Physicians. I mean there are other groups —the National Breast Cancer Coalition—

J.F.: Yeah, the NBCC, which you co-founded. My point is that we have all these cancer organizations recommending it, and you saying it's a bunch of hooey. What's going on?

S.L.: O.K., well, let me tell you the mammogram story. Because it's a very telling saga of what happens in this country when we don't tell the truth.

When the ACS came out with their first guidelines, all they had was the HIP [Health Insurance Plan] study in New York, which showed a benefit over 50. They also had the BCDDP [Breast Cancer Detection Demonstration Project], which was a demonstration project with a very select population, so there might have been a benefit under 50, but it wasn't clear. So, the ACS made up the guidelines. They said baseline at 35—with no basis for that. They said every other year from 40 to 50—again with no particular basis.

And they said every year after 50. Now, it's O.K. to make it up, because basically, at some point, you have to come up with some kind of recommendation, but what you should say at that point is, "We're making this up. This is our best guess. Stay tuned. Things may change as the information comes in." But no, they didn't say that. They said this is the truth.

And after a while, they dropped the baseline-at-35 part, because they realized that it was ridiculous—your breast at 35 has nothing to do with your breast at 50, so it's silly to compare them. But they were still saying every other year from 40 to 50, and the NCI was going along with that. And then several years ago, the data started coming in. There were several randomized controlled studies in Europe and the big one in Canada, and none of them had shown any real benefit in women under 50. So it's not like we didn't have the studies anymore—we had the studies and they didn't show a benefit. And there probably are a number of reasons why. One, because cancer is less common under 50. Number two, the breast tissue is less dense and so the chance of seeing something is less—it's like looking for a polar bear in the snow. And it may be that the radiation is more [damaging] for women in their 40s. So the number of women that you would have to mammogram to find some with cancer in order to find a percentage [for whom there's a decrease in mortality because of the mammogram] is so enormous that we haven't been able to demonstrate any benefit.

So in 1993 the NCI came out and said, we've looked at the science and it really doesn't support this, so we're going to change our guidelines—which was correct from the scientific standpoint. The American Cancer Society said, we can't do that, we've been saying this was the truth all these years. Women will get confused if we change our guidelines, we're going to stick to our guns. And you've got to know that there are a lot of radiologists in the ACS, and the ACS has staked its institution on early detection working, and has sort of oversold early detection, and so it really meant changing everything. So now you've got these two different opinions and a lot of flak, because we've spent so much time and energy convincing women that everybody should be getting it and that early detection worked, that women don't understand why we're depriving them of their God-given right to get radiated.

And so Richard Klausner, the new head of the National Cancer Institute, comes along and says, we'll hold another consensus conference. So he sets it all up, they look at all the data very carefully, and in January they come out saying, you know what, the data does not show a benefit; basically there may be some women whom it would benefit, but we cannot make a global recommendation that every woman from 40 to 50 should be getting mammography because there's not the data to support it. Klausner says, "Wrong answer!"

And so then he throws it to the National Cancer Advisory Board to decide, and in March, the NCI changed the recommendation. There was enormous political pressure to change it. And there are enormous vested interests, one of the biggest being the American College of Radiology, but also the ACS and all kinds of groups who said women need a clear message.

And I think that should enrage women. Because what they're saying is, even if it's not true, they need a clear message.

Sometimes the clear message is "Hey, guess what, there's no clear message," and women are perfectly capable of making decisions based on inadequate information—we do it all day, every day.

There were two editorials in the *New England Journal of Medicine* talking about how it's important to tell people when it's a toss-up and let them decide based on their own values. But the way it was presented to the media, or the way the media picked it up, was, "We can't decide, so it's really up to the woman." And what they were really saying is there's not enough of a benefit to make a global recommendation; there may be people for whom it's beneficial; we don't want to say never do it; so each woman's going to have to sit down and look at her own situation. And I think that's perfectly reasonable.

J.F.: What about the Swedish study that did find a benefit?

S.L.: Well, the Swedish study found that if they followed women long enough there was a benefit, but by then the women were well into their 50s, so you don't know if the benefit was because they started at 40 or if the benefit was because they started at 50. And that's the problem. So, if you follow women for 17 years from their first mammogram at 40, you will see a benefit. But by then they've gone through menopause. I mean, what's the magic of 50? It's menopause.

J.F.: Right, let's clarify the terms we're using here. It's not that at age 50 mammography suddenly makes sense. We're talking about the benefits for premenopausal versus postmenopausal women.

S.L.: Yes. The reason we say 50 is because the average age of menopause is 50, but basically, unless you take HRT [hormone replacement therapy]—and actually if they take HRT, a third of women will have their breasts get more dense, which may actually make this whole debate a moot point—but basically, as your hormones go away, your breast tissue becomes less dense and also cancer becomes more common, so now you see a benefit. But it's only a 30 percent benefit for women over 50. It's not 100 percent.

We say things like: "Mammography will see something like 85 percent of cancers." True. Some of them are the size of a grapefruit, but it'll see them. And then we say: "Mammography can find cancer early." It's absolutely true. It doesn't always, but in some women it can. And then we say: "Cancer that's diagnosed early has a 95 percent five-year survival rate." It's true. And when you say those three sentences together quickly, you get the impression that mammography can find 85 percent of cancers when they're 95 percent curable, which is not true at all! So we've oversold this notion that early detection always works, which it doesn't, and now we've got all these people who feel like we're depriving them, when in fact it was because we were overselling them the stuff in the first place.

J.F.: What about the argument that the studies don't show a benefit because they're based on older equipment and less effective imaging techniques?

S.L.: You know, the problem is that imaging is not the answer. By the time you see cancer on a mammogram, it could have been there eight to ten years. And improving the imaging has improved the numbers by 1 percent, 2 percent, but it's not going to do it by 30 or 40 percent.

What we need is a blood test or something that will find cancer very early on—in the first year or two—or really, what we need is prevention. What

## JUDY MAHLE LUTTER: INFO-SOURCE ON WOMEN'S HEALTH

As president of the St. Paul, Minnesota-based Melpomene Institute for Women's Health Research, Judy Mahle Lutter documents and celebrates the importance of physical acitvty and play for women and girls of all ages, sizes, and backgrounds. "Healthy does not mean skinny," says Lutter. "It does mean active, engaged, and informed."

Lutter founded the institute (named after the Greek woman who defied officials to run in the 1896 Olympic marathon) 15 years ago along with Susan Cushman, a Twin Cities OB/GYN. "At the time, there was very little research on how much exercise is reasonable for pregnant women," says Lutter. And we also wanted to know more about the link between amenorrhea [missed periods] and women runners and other athletes." Within a few years, Lutter secured a $15,000 grant from Tambrands, Inc., which was used in part to fund the institute's first major study on amenorrhea.

Today, the budget is near $300,000, and the institute employs seven part-timers as well as a staff of interns and fellows who manage research projects; run a resource center; maintain the institute's Web site, at http://www.melpomene.org; and produce a newsletter, books, pamphlets, videos, and self-help guides. One of the institute's recent studies found that girls who participated in physical activity or sports reported higher levels of self-satisfaction and feelings of confidence and competence than girls who didn't. Lutter, a mother of three and former project director at the University of Minnesota, has strong opinions about the link between exercise and empowerment. "Almost 20 years ago," she says, "I started jogging as a way to claim time for myself. It changed my life completely."

—Jill Petty

bothers me the most about this is that we spend all this money and energy arguing. You know that if there's this much disagreement, it can't have a big effect. Even if it's positive, it can't be big! Because if it were big, we'd agree. And so it obviously is a very small effect. So let's take that money and put it into prevention. Let's put it into finding something that does work in younger women. Let's not kid ourselves that we have something that's working when we don't. That's what happens: we get lulled into this sense—and this is the breast self-exam story, too—into this wishful thinking. And it's particularly feminists who wish it would work. And guess what —it doesn't.

J.F.: Let's talk about breast self-exam. You basically caused quite a stir when you came out against BSE—

S.L.: Not against BSE—

J.F.: But basically you're saying, it's not an effective tool, it doesn't decrease mortality, it makes women scared, and it alienates them from their bodies, sending them on a kind of search-and-destroy mission every month.

S.L.: Right, and it wastes money on shower cards.

J.F.: And while I find your argument very convincing, I have to say that every time I've gone to see an OB-GYN, they ask me in that guilt-tripping way, "Do you do BSE?" and I reply, "No, because Dr. Susan Love says..." and they always respond in the same exact way. They say, "Well, I totally respect Susan Love and her work and I think she's got a point, but BSE is the only thing we've got and I urge my patients to do it." Why are doctors so reluctant to give up BSE?

S.L.: Well, it's been drummed into their brains forever, and they want to be able to give patients something. We don't want to admit that we don't have anything good for early detection in younger women, because that makes us feel impotent. We want to act like we can do something, and we figure it won't hurt. What's the harm? But there is a harm in terms of alienating women from their bodies, and there's a harm in terms of masking the fact that we haven't gotten further along than we have. And so we spend all this money on shower cards, by having all these campaigns—Hanes spends all this money to put BSE info in their stocking packages, and Tampax in their tampon boxes and whatever—when we should take that money and spend it on prevention or finding something that works.

So we get lulled into thinking early detection works. And it backfires in a number of ways. I'll talk to someone and she'll say, "I had this friend and she had this big cancer and I'm so mad at her because I know that if she had done BSE she would have found it early and wouldn't be dead." And in fact, it's probably that her friend just wasn't very lucky.

J.F.: But also another point you make is that for younger women, their cancers are more aggressive and by the time you actually feel a lump—

S.L.: —it could have been there eight to ten years. Whether you find it this month or next month is not the critical factor. Now, people have misunderstood me, and they think I'm saying: you should never touch your breasts again in your life. And I'm not saying that. I think we should touch our whole bodies, we should get to know them. You should touch your breasts not just after your period, but before your period—all kinds of times. Most women find their own lumps. It's not doing BSE. It's rolling over in bed, in the shower, a lover finds it, something hurts and you poke around and find it. In your own body you can feel from the inside out and the outside in, so you're much more likely to feel something. So I'm not saying don't touch yourself. I'm saying you don't have to go through this formal song and dance every month. We need to get beyond that, get beyond imaging, and let's find something that really works, that's really early detection.

J.F.: The whole corporate BSE campaign reminds me a bit of Keep America Beautiful, which is basically this so-called environmental group that's bankrolled by aluminum can manufacturers and corporate polluters, and puts out all those ads about how you can make a difference cleaning up the side of the road, meanwhile—

S.L.: They're the ones making the garbage! Right. Well, it allows companies to say, "Look what we're doing for women."

J.F.: There's this really poignant and funny moment in Yvonne Rainer's new film, MURDER and murder, where she talks about the fact that the company that makes the tamoxifen she's taking to treat her breast cancer also produces pesticides and paints—

S.L.: And funds National Breast Cancer Awareness Month.

J.F.: Right. So on the one hand, this company cosponsors National Breast Cancer Awareness Month, and on the other hand, it was sued for allegedly dumping millions of pounds of DDT and PCBs in the Pacific Ocean.

S.L.: I don't think these people are evil. I don't think they sit down and say, "Let's cause breast cancer so we can cure it." I think it's two divisions of the company and they never put two and two together. It's just like I don't think gynecologists are evil because they're pushing hormones. I think they're busy, they don't read the articles, they don't look at the statistics, and they're being marketed to very strongly. But we have to be the conscience and we have to be aware these things are going on, because women, feminists, are very critical in a lot of fields, but when it gets to medicine, they tend not to be. And part of it is that we get scared when we get sick. Where we'll reinvent history everywhere else, we'll just accept medicine.

J.F.: But, on the other hand, you supported the tamoxifen trial while there were women's health activists who demanded that the trial be stopped. I mean, there is a long history of feminist health activism—and there were many women's health activists who said, "We do not trust this drug. We think this trial should be stopped." And you said it should continue.

S.L.: Because it's a study. The only way we're going to have an answer is if we do a randomized controlled study, if we do a good study. It's the same thing with

the Women's Health Initiative. I think it's a great thing. I don't think hormones are probably good, but I would very much like to know the answer and so if they are good, that's fine. I'll be a believer. I always will support studies, because that's the way we're going to get the answers. But when you put women on hormones with no study, not collecting the data, then it's a big experiment, not well designed, and you're never going to get an answer. That's what I object to.

I think the tamoxifen study had been started—it was halfway through. If you stop in the middle you're going to end up with nothing, no data, and women who were willing to do it—we're not coercing women to be on the study, they were volunteers. And so I think you ought to do the full study and see what answers you get out of it.

J.F.: I just read *To Dance with the Devil*, which I thought was quite an incredible book. And one of the things I found so sobering about it is that it exposes just how primitive breast cancer treatments are and how little we know about the disease.

S.L.: This is again what we've masked. When you look at how much improvement in survival you get from chemotherapy, overall it's 8 to 10 percent. Tamoxifen is 4 to 5 percent. We have taken chemotherapy, radiation, and surgery as far as we can take them—just like we've taken imaging as far. And I really feel very strongly that if we're going to get anywhere, we've got to go down a whole new path, we've got to change the paradigm. We have to have better treatments. And I think it's on the horizon.

J.F.: In the fight against AIDS, we've seen a remarkable transformation this past year. I don't want to overstate the case, but protease inhibitors have made a huge difference in terms of treatment options and quality and length of life. Is there anything in the research pipeline that's going to make the same kind of difference for breast cancer patients?

S.L.: There are a couple of things. I think that people are really changing the paradigm. We used to think of breast cancer as an evil invader. We thought of it the way we thought of infection. We had to kill every last cancer cell and it was a war to the end. Thus we radiated, we slashed, burned, and poisoned. And what we're starting to recognize is that it's really a regulatory problem, that these are our own cells and that the regulation of their growth has gone a little off. And that potentially we could reverse that. There's evidence that you could either make the cells dormant or reverse them, and so maybe we don't have to kill them at all.

Look at people who get treated, are fine, and then 10 years later, the cancer comes back again. What were those cells doing for 10 years? They were asleep. Well, what put them to sleep? What woke them up? And if we can keep them asleep for 10 years, why not 50 years? Likewise, in the old days, prior to chemotherapy, we used to treat premenopausal women with breast cancer by taking their ovaries out. And guess what? It worked as well as chemo. Now, that doesn't kill cancer cells. What does it do? It changes the environment that the cells find themselves in, which may in fact put them to sleep, or reverse them or whatever. Tamoxifen doesn't kill cells, but it changes the environment. So, what we're looking at now is ways of doing that, and it will be much more subtle.

I think we'll look back on this era and think we were totally crazy that we did these barbaric things to people for breast cancer. You know, it's sort of like the iron lung and polio. So I really do think we're on the verge, there's a lot of stuff going on in laboratories right now, research that I think is close to being clinical. I think that certainly within my lifetime, probably within the next five to 10 years, we're going to see a revolution in the way we look at this disease.

J.F.: Tell me a little about your own research on duct endoscopy.

S.L.: Well, the idea is that breast cancer starts in the lining of the milk duct, and we have no access to that. With cervical cancer, you can do a Pap smear. With colon cancer, you do colonoscopy. But we have no way to do that [with breast cancer]. So when we're imaging or feeling, it's beyond something in the milk duct, which is microscopic. In fact, nobody's actually even figured out the anatomy of the milk ducts or even figured out how many holes there are, which is something that we're working on. But it occurred to me that if milk comes out, we ought to be able to go in the other direction. So I have this tiny, little half-a-millimeter scope and a tiny little catheter, and I can thread it in through a hole—there are six to nine milk ducts, I think—and I can actually look around and I can get cells back. If we can get into the ducts on a reliable basis, we can find what the early changes are, what comes before DCIS [ductal carcinoma in situ, a noninvasive cancer]. And then you could also do prevention research. You could sample the lining of the duct, give someone soy for a year, go back and sample the same spot and see if you've made any difference. Right now, if I want to do prevention, I have to put you on soy, wait ten years, and see if you get breast cancer or not. Now, there are still a few hurdles. The question is, can I do this whenever I want to whichever duct I want? When you look at your nipple, you don't actually see six to nine holes looking back at you. . . . So, we're working on a technique to make that happen, and if we can get that to happen then it will be great because you could also treat DCIS by just squirting something down the duct, Drāno or something, just clean it out, drain the duct once a year, instead of cutting it off.

J.F.: Is there any new information about lesbians and breast cancer? There was a real scare a few years ago when a study suggested lesbians were at greater risk.

S.L.: What happened was that a researcher at the NCI looked at the risk factors in some data on lesbians and looked at the risk factors for breast cancer. She did a mathematical model and said that if all this is true, then lesbians are two or three times more likely than heterosexual women to develop breast cancer. She did it not so much to scare the lesbian community but to let people realize that there was a reason why we should specifically do research on lesbians. And it worked —it did convince the larger studies on women that there was a value in identifying this subgroup and not just assuming that lesbian health problems were going to be the same as those of the rest of the population. Now the Women's Health Initiative is asking a question on sexual orientation. We've got a question on sexual orientation in the Nurses' Health Study questionnaire. So we will get data. But the problem with doing research on lesbians is you're really only doing it on those women who are out. So that limits your denominator significantly.

J.F.: You told the Boston *Globe* that you think you're probably the only doctor you

know who thinks that managed care is good.

S.L.: [Laughs] One of the few.

J.F.: I mean, you hear horror stories every day about decreasing quality of health care. Do you really believe that managed care is in fact good for us?

S.L.: Yes. I think it's going to be much better for patients. See, what's happening now is really a very strong media campaign—helped along by the AMA. But what we're losing sight of is that health care was not very good in the old way—all the economic incentives were to overtreat. And we did. There was no accountability. A third of what we do has never been proven to work, but that's never stopped us. There was nothing spent on prevention, no reimbursement. Through most of my career, they didn't cover mammograms unless you wrote down fibrocystic disease, they didn't cover well-baby care, they didn't cover immunizations. All of our education as doctors and all of the insurance was based on diseases.

So we had no prevention and it was not a very good system. And it seems disingenuous for doctors to complain, "They're only letting me spend 15 minutes per patient," when most of them never spent more than 15 minutes before!

J.F.: But what about managed care companies not paying for necessary procedures?

S.L.: The problem is we oversell. . . . I'll give you an example. The CDC says the recommendation for Pap smears is every one to three years, if you're monogamous and have had a normal one.

J.F.: Three years?

S.L.: Three years—and that has been the recommendation for a long time. And that's perfectly adequate for [detecting] cervical cancer. In most parts of the country it's done every year. In L.A., it seems to be six months.

J.F.: Well, if someone started telling me I could only have a Pap smear every three years, I'd think they were crazy.

S.L.: Right. But I'll tell you, I haven't had one in three years. I certainly wouldn't have it every year. I know that you don't need it that often.

You know, people say, "Oh, it's terrible, the economic incentive is to undertreat," and they never talk about the enormous incentive we had to overtreat and how we've done it for years. Again, one out of three women have hysterectomies in this country, and it's not because we have abnormal uteruses! So, I think managed care is going to be good for women in the long run.

J.F.: But how do you ensure that the pendulum doesn't swing the other way?

S.L.: Well, we'll have accountability. It's actually to the advantage of the managed care companies to have evidence-based medicine, because they don't want to pay for things that don't work. And you don't have an incentive to overtreat. What I think is going to happen—if you look at what happens in a free market—is that once the prices are down, everybody will be about the same price, and then they have to compete on quality. And I think that then you're going to see much more emphasis on prevention.

And you're going to see more alternatives. Because it was the AMA, the doctors, that blocked alternative medicine. But if a managed care company is paying for it, acupuncture's a lot cheaper than disc surgery. The doctors were not going to change it. We were in fat city. We could do whatever we wanted to whomever we wanted, charge whatever we wanted, and get paid for it. Why would we change a system like that? And now you hear

them saying things like "I don't want an insurance company telling me what to do," and the translation is "I never had to justify what I did to anybody before. The nerve—that I actually have to prove that what I do works!"

Now, I think it's critical that people get involved who really care about the quality stuff, and I think you have to be bilingual to do that. That's why I'm going to business school. Because I think you have to speak business and medicine. I think that the reforms had to come from business because they were paying the bill. But they have more trouble with the quality piece, mostly because they don't know what they can throw out and what they can't. And they don't realize that it's not so simple.

The drive-through mastectomy story is a good example. I did same-day mastectomies for years. There's no medical problem with it. But if you're going to do it, you have to set it up right. You have to spend some time with the patient ahead of time. You have to teach them how to do the drains, you have to make sure they have the people at home, that it's going to work. You can't just suddenly say, "O.K., we're going to do them the same day." So I think that that's where the business people lack the finesse to do some of what they have to do, and they need to have people who are bilingual, who can help with that.

J.F.: Why did you decide to retire from surgery? The only analogy that I can think of is that it's like Michael Jordan giving up basketball.

S.L.: Well, I've been taking primary care of women with breast cancer for 20 years. And there's a high burnout rate. If you really pay attention, empathize, try to be there for your patients, it takes a lot out of you over the years. Also, it gets harder and harder to do as you get older, because the difference between you and the patient vanishes. You know, when you're young and the patient's old, you can say, oh well, [they have breast cancer] because they're old. But when the difference between you and them is luck, that becomes harder. And also it's harder and harder for me to sell the standard treatments, and yet I don't have any alternative to sell. It's hard for me to enthusiastically promote things that I'm not sure are going to make a big difference and yet at the same time not take people's hope away.

It was a combination of things—the burnout, and probably menopause, too. You know, the other thing that didn't occur to me at the time but came up later, is that women at this time of life do step back. It is a time when you say, I've been taking care of everybody and maybe I need to stop for a minute and take care of myself. I have a nine-year-old. I don't want to miss the next 10 years. And I also want to do research and I want to do the political stuff, and I can't do it all. Whether it's forever or not I don't know. But it feels right for now. I haven't said I will never come out of it.

I think that one of the important things —and this goes full circle to HRT—is the message that you're not making a forever, life-and-death decision. Things change. You're going to make the best decision you can make based on your values and what you know today, and next year we may have something entirely different. I'm not taking hormones, but you know what? Next year if I have such bad hot flashes that I can't stand it, I'll take them.

J.F.: What do you think about all the controversy surrounding the 63-year-old woman in Los Angeles who gave birth?

S.L.: Well, I had my daughter when I was 40, and I tried to get pregnant again for a year or two after that. But I think that once you're getting up into your 60s, it does seem to me that we can't have it all. Particularly in southern California, we think that death is optional. And we think we can control everything. And to me one of the real lessons that I couldn't control everything was not being able to get pregnant a second time.

You know, your fertility does end. I think that menopause is programmed in because we're not supposed to have high hormones our whole lives, that we are not fertile our whole lives because it probably isn't good for us. So I do believe in some degree of biological fatalism. Not entirely. But I think it's hard. I love being a mother and I'm very glad I got it in.

You know, the one other thing that I didn't get to say before is that this whole notion of menopause being estrogen deficiency and a disease and implying that premenopausal is normal —it's all in the framing. The other way to frame it is Margaret Mead and postmenopausal zest: We have all these powerful postmenopausal women —Margaret Thatcher, Indira Gandhi, Madeleine Albright—as well as eight- and nine-year-old girls who are full of beans, and then they hit puberty and they lose it. So maybe the answer is that we have too much estrogen. Maybe we need estrogen enough to reproduce the race, and then we can get liberated from it with menopause!

# POSTSCRIPT

## Will Most Postmenopausal Women Benefit from Estrogen Replacement Therapy?

In "Relationship Between Estrogen Levels, Use of Hormone Replacement Therapy, and Breast Cancer," *Journal of the National Cancer Institute* (June 3, 1998), Graham Colditz summarizes nearly 100 related studies and concludes that, based on his review of the literature, it is evident that HRT causes breast cancer. Colditz questions how this should be viewed from a public health perspective since HRT also reduces the risk of heart disease and osteoporosis. From a population perspective, women who used HRT for 10 or more years had a 20 percent reduction in overall deaths. This benefit, however, was more pronounced for women who were at high risk for heart disease.

In *Dr. Susan Love's Hormone Book: Making Informed Choices About Menopause* (Random House, 1997), Love argues that most of the studies linking HRT to a reduced risk of cardiovascular disease were not valid, since the majority of women taking the drugs were at the lowest risk for heart disease to start. These women ate a healthy diet, exercised, and were less likely to smoke. Love believes that the lifestyles of these women skewed the results. See "Prior Use of Estrogen Replacement Therapy: Are Users Healthier Than Nonusers?" *American Journal of Epidemiology* (May 15, 1996). Love also questions studies linking HRT to reduced incidences of osteoporosis. She believes that lifestyle changes, including a high-calcium diet and more exercise, may improve bone density and reduce fractures better than HRT. There are also nonhormone drugs available to increase bone density. For further reading about Dr. Love, see "The Estrogen Question: How Wrong Is Dr. Susan Love?" *The New Yorker* (June 9, 1997); "Sometimes Mother Nature Knows Best: Efficacy of Hormone Therapy for Menopause," *The New York Times* (March 20, 1997); and "Estrogen Therapy: Should You or Shouldn't You?" *Good Housekeeping* (February 1997). The relationship between alcohol consumption and HRT is reported in "Alcohol May Pose Problems for Women on Estrogen," *Tufts University Health & Nutrition Letter* (February 1997).

Numerous studies have indicated that HRT is beneficial in reducing disease among postmenopausal women. For further reading on the benefits of HRT, see "HRT Therapy May Reduce Risk of Heart Attack and Stroke," *Geriatrics* (June 1998); "Look Who's Taking Estrogen," *Health* (April, 1998); "Estrogen Helps to Protect Memory into Old Age," *The Lancet* (January 3, 1998); and "Postmenopausal Hormone Therapy and Mortality," *The New England Journal of Medicine* (June 19, 1997).

# On the Internet . . .

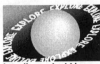

## Calypte Biomedical's Chronicillnet

The Chronicillnet features a directory of online resources pertaining to chronic illnesses, sponsored by Viaticus, Inc., and Calypte Biomedical of Berkeley, California. There are lists and links to the latest news and information sources on illnesses such as Gulf War syndrome and chronic fatigue syndrome.
*http://www.chronicillnet.org*

## The U.S. Environmental Protection Agency

The U.S. Environmental Protection Agency's Global Warming site focuses on the science and impacts of global warming and on actions by governments, corporations, and individuals.
*http://www.epa.gov/globalwarming/*

## Agency for Toxic Substances and Disease Registry Science Corner

The Agency for Toxic Substances and Disease Registry (ATSDR) Science Corner is a gateway to environmental health information and resources. New resources are cited, searched, and documented as they come online.
*http://atsdr1.atsdr.cdc.gov:8080/cx.html*

# PART 5

## Environmental Issues

*Many of today's environmental concerns are related to modern technology. Since World War II, thousands of new chemicals have been developed for the manufacturing and agricultural industries and for the military. But technological growth often has negative effects. Persian Gulf War veterans, for example, returned from the conflict claiming that environmental exposure to chemicals in the Persian Gulf have caused both minor and severe health problems in the soldiers. Energy needs have increased, resulting in the release of environmental pollutants, including greenhouse gases. Also, as the world population continues to grow, how can food production keep pace without increased environmental degradation and exposure to toxic pesticides? This section discusses controversies related to environmental health issues.*

■ Is the Gulf War Syndrome Real?

■ Is Pesticide Exposure Harmful to Human Health?

■ Public Policy and Health: Is Global Warming a Real Threat?

# ISSUE 16

## Is the Gulf War Syndrome Real?

**YES: Dennis Bernstein and Thea Kelley,** from "The Gulf War Comes Home: Sickness Spreads, But the Pentagon Denies All," *The Progressive* (March 1995)

**NO: Michael Fumento,** from "Gulf Lore Syndrome," *Reason* (March 1997)

### ISSUE SUMMARY

**YES:** Journalists Dennis Bernstein and Thea Kelley maintain that there are some four dozen disabling, sometimes life-threatening medical problems related to environmental and chemical exposure affecting thousands of soldiers who fought in the Persian Gulf War.

**NO:** Author Michael Fumento argues that Gulf War veterans are not suffering from illnesses at an extraordinary rate. They do not show evidence of more cancers, birth defects, and miscarriages than those who did not serve in the Persian Gulf.

Since Operation Desert Storm—the 1991 international effort to drive invading Iraqi forces out of Kuwait—more than 45,000 veterans out of the approximately 650,000 troops who served in the Persian Gulf War have complained of symptoms that have collectively become known as the Gulf War Syndrome. These symptoms include rashes, fatigue, headaches, vision problems, infections, joint and bone pain, birth defects in babies conceived after the war, and cancer.

The syndrome has been compared to the afflictions suffered by veterans of the Vietnam War. Unlike the health problems of the Vietnam veterans, however, the causes of the Gulf War veterans' varied symptoms are less clear. A number of entities are currently searching for an explanation. The American Legion claims that toxins from a long list of possible environmental origins —including fumes from burning oil wells and landfills, contact with hydrocarbons, pesticides sprayed over military vehicles, poor sanitary conditions, local parasites, inoculations, and insect bites—may be to blame. The U.S. government is exploring other causes, such as exposure to depleted uranium and the drug *pyridostigmine bromide*, an experimental pharmaceutical issued to soldiers to protect them against a possible nerve gas attack. The drug (as yet not approved for general use) was administered under a special waiver from the Food and Drug Administration, to be distributed with the informed consent of soldiers after the Department of Defense conducted its own research. Troops ordered to take the drug were reportedly never warned about its possible side effects. In addition, research on the drug was conducted only on men, so the drug's effects on women were unknown.

Another explanation being proposed is that veterans' health problems are the result of exposure to depleted uranium. Uranium was used to coat some artillery shells and tanks to protect them from enemy fire. On impact, however, depleted uranium releases radioactive particles of a related compound. The government claims that a relatively small number of personnel were exposed to this material and that none of them have shown any adverse symptoms. In Britain, allegations that the defence ministry is covering up evidence of Gulf War syndrome has created a political row. The Armed Forces minister in that country has admitted that troops were not properly advised of the dangers of radioactive contamination from depleted uranium shells. He has insisted, however, that there is no evidence of a link between serving in the Gulf War and veterans' subsequent health problems, even though over 20 British war veterans have been hospitalized with kidney and lung ailments typical of depleted uranium exposure.

There have been documented cases of illnesses among soldiers who served in the Gulf War, but less is known about the health of their families. One study conducted by outgoing senator Donald Riegle found that of 1,200 ill male veterans, 78 percent of their wives, 25 percent of children born to them before the war, and 65 percent born after suffered various illnesses and birth defects. Wives have reported bizarre symptoms concerning their husband's semen, which burns on contact. These women also complain of vaginal infections, cysts, bleeding sores, and blisters.

Despite widespread reports of health problems among Gulf War veterans, the Department of Veterans Affairs and the Pentagon insist that the symptoms are either psychological or due to chance. Major-General Ronald Blanck, commander of the Walter Reed Army Medical Center in Washington, D.C., in addressing Congress, said, "Extensive evaluation and thorough epidemiological investigations have failed to show any commonality of exposure or unifying diagnosis to explain these symptoms." Many politicians, however, are fighting back and have vowed not to allow the Gulf War Syndrome to become another Vietnam-style denial by the government.

In the following selections, Dennis Bernstein and Thea Kelley argue that, although the Pentagon denies it, exposure to environmental and toxic substances in the Persian Gulf is responsible for illnesses experienced by thousands of veterans and their families. Michael Fumento counters that many illnesses suffered by Gulf War veterans have been attributed to the syndrome without sufficient evidence. He also asserts that there is no proof that any specific agent has caused physical sickness to soldiers or their families.

# YES

**Dennis Bernstein and
Thea Kelley**

## THE GULF WAR COMES HOME: SICKNESS SPREADS, BUT THE PENTAGON DENIES ALL

The Persian Gulf War is not over. It drags on in the lives of tens of thousands of Gulf War veterans. Gulf War Syndrome, or Desert Fever as it is often called in Britain, is a set of some four dozen disabling, sometimes life-threatening medical conditions that afflict thousands of soldiers who fought in the war, as well as their offspring, their spouses, and medical professionals who treated them.

The symptoms suggest exposure to medical, chemical, or biological warfare agents, but the Pentagon denies such exposure occurred and claims it can't identify any common link among those who suffer from Gulf War Syndrome. Don Riegle, the recently retired Senator from Michigan who held hearings on the subject beginning in the fall of 1992, doesn't buy it. He believes the Pentagon may be engaged in a massive cover-up of this serious health problem.

The scale of the problem is enormous. More than 29,000 veterans in the United States with symptoms of Gulf War Syndrome have signed onto the Veterans Administration's Persian Gulf War Registry, 9,000 more have registered separately with the Pentagon, and the Pentagon's list is growing by 1,000 veterans a month.

"These are horrendous statistics that show the true scale of this problem," said Riegle last October when he released his final report on Gulf War Syndrome. Riegle condemned "the heartlessness and irresponsibility of a military bureaucracy that gives every sign of wanting to protect itself more than the health and well-being of our servicemen and women who actually go and fight our wars. To my mind, there is no more serious crime than an official military cover-up of facts that could prevent more effective diagnosis and treatment of sick U.S. veterans."

Birth defects are one of the most alarming problems associated with Gulf War Syndrome. One National Guard unit from Waynesboro, Mississippi, reported that of fifteen children conceived by veterans after the war, thirteen had birth defects. An informal survey of 600 afflicted veterans conducted by Senator Don Riegle's Banking, Housing, and Urban Affairs Committee last fall found that 65 percent of their babies were afflicted with dozens of medical problems, including severe birth defects.

Another disturbing phenomenon is the apparent transmission of the syndrome from soldiers to their family members. Riegle's study found that 77 percent of the wives of these veterans were also ill, as well as 25 percent of the children conceived before the war.

Riegle believes the Pentagon knows that U.S. veterans were exposed to chemical or biological weapons in the Gulf War. "The evidence available continues to mount that exposure to biological and chemical weapons is one cause of these illnesses," Riegle said. "I have evidence that despite repeated automatic denials by the Department of Defense, chemical weapons [were] found in the war." Riegle added that "laboratory findings from gas masks" showed the presence of biological warfare materials "that cause illnesses similar to Gulf War Syndrome."

The cover-up is not limited to the U.S. Government, however. Britain's Ministry of Defense is also being less than forthcoming. It has "a policy of denying Desert Fever for fear of big compensation claims," the British newspaper *Today* reported on October 10. A British Defense spokesperson told the paper, "We have no evidence that this illness exists." More than 1,000 out of the 43,000 British troops who served in the Persian Gulf have cited symptoms of Gulf War Syndrome.

* * *

At 3 A.M. on January 19, 1991, Petty Officer Sterling Symms of the Naval Reserve Construction Battalion in Saudi Arabia awakened to a "real bad explosion" over head. Alarms went off and everybody started running toward their bunkers, Symms said. A strong smell of ammonia pervaded the air. Symms said his eyes burned and his skin was stinging before he could don protective gear. Since that time, he has experienced fatigue, sore joints, running nose, a chronic severe rash, open sores, and strep infections. Symms and other soldiers described several such chemical attacks to Riegle's committee in May 1994.

One of the men interviewed by the committee who requested anonymity wrote home to his mother about the attack: "I can deal with getting shot at, because even if I got hit, I can be put back together—a missile, I can even accept that. But gas scares the hell out of me.... I know they detected a cloud of dusty mustard gas because I was there with them, but today everyone denies it. I was there when they radioed the other camps north of us and warned them of the cloud."

Front-line officers assured their troops that it was not a chemical attack, that what they heard was a sonic boom. "Members of Symms's unit were given orders not to discuss the incident," says Senator Riegle's report dated May 25, 1994.

Former U.S. Army Sergeant Randall L. Vallee served in the Persian Gulf as an advance scout. Vallee told Congress back in 1992 that he was convinced Iraqi Scud missiles were armed with chemical or biological warfare agents. "I was in numerous Scud missile attacks when I was in Dhahran," says Vallee. "It seemed like every time I was back there we'd come under fire."

Vallee has been afflicted by at least a half dozen serious medical conditions that started shortly after the Scud attacks. He had been in "perfect health" before his Gulf War service. Vallee supported what scores of veterans have already told Congress: that after every Scud attack, hundreds of alarms signaling chemical and biological attacks would sound, to the point where they were routinely shut off and reset as a matter of course.

Vallee and other members of his detail questioned their superiors about the alarms and about the presence of chemical-warfare agents in the Gulf. "After the whole ordeal was over, we asked about it and they said, 'No, the alarms are just acting that way because they're sensitive.' They gave us stories like, 'Oh, it's because of supersonic aircraft' or 'sand in the alarms.' There was always a story as to why the alarms sounded."

Last August, Vallee received a phone call from the Pentagon's Lieutenant Colonel Vicki Merriman, an aide to the Deputy Assistant Secretary of Defense for Chemical and Biological Matters.

"She asked me about my health and my family," says Vallee. But after some small talk, "the colonel's attitude turned from one of being concerned about my well-being to an interrogator trying to talk me out of my own experiences. She started using tactics of doubt regarding my statements. She said in regard to chemical and biological agents that there was absolutely no way that any soldiers in the Gulf were exposed to anything. Her exact words were, 'The only ones whining about problems are American

troops, why aren't any of our allies?' And that was her exact word, 'whining.'"

* * *

British Gulf war vet Richard Turnball was surprised to hear Lieutenant Colonel Merriman's suggestion that only U.S. vets complained of Gulf War Syndrome. Turnball, who lives just outside Liverpool, served eighteen years in the British Royal Air Force. During the war against Iraq, Turnball built nuclear, biological, and chemical shelters, and instructed British troops in use of chemical monitoring and protective clothing. Turnball was based in Dhahran, Saudi Arabia.

Turnball is convinced there was widespread use of chemical-warfare agents. "People got sick in the chest and eyes, they got infections and skin rashes," he says. "One lad had his whole body covered with spots from head to toe" soon after a Scud attack that Turnball is convinced was chemical in nature.

"Within seconds of the warhead landing on January 20, every chemical-agent monitoring device in the area was blasting the alarm. We were put into the highest alert for twenty minutes," says Turnball, "and then we were told it was a false alarm caused by the fuel from aircraft taking off."

Corporal Turnball carried out two residual-vapor-detection tests for chemical and biological agents on January 20, shortly after the Scud hit "and both were positive," he says. Field supervisors dismissed the test results, claiming that jet fuel set off the indicators. Turnball was skeptical. "We tried on umpteen occasions, when aircraft were taking off in mass numbers," he says. "We stood on the side of the runway closer to the area where the aircraft were taking off, we carried out tests, and we got no readings."

At one point, Turnball says, he was warned to drop the case, and that if he kept it up he might be subject to secrecy laws under which he could be imprisoned. "I've had a very, very senior officer friend of mine ring me up and say, 'Richie, back off, you're kicking over a can of worms.'"

Before he went to war, Turnball said, he was in top condition, worked out every day, and was an avid scuba diver. Since his return, he has had twenty-four separate chest infections, and he has been forced to give up scuba diving because he "can't take the pressure below a few feet." Turnball can no longer run or swim or even take long walks. He said he has been put on steroids and uses two inhalers to help ease serious respiratory complications.

Turnball says the allies "used us as guinea pigs for new drugs" and chemical-weapons testing. He believes "probably both" chemical warfare agents and experimental drugs are responsible for his illness. "I feel we were subject to a chemical attack that affected us," he says. "As a serviceman, I can accept that, it's my job. But I believe more damage was done due to experimentation by our government. Many people got sick after taking some of the drugs. I came down with a high fever, I was sweating excessively. I actually stopped breathing a couple of times."

After three years of illness and fighting with the defense ministry, Turnball is still amazed by the denials that come out of the various bureaucracies. "We were always told that there was a 99.999 percent possibility of a chemical attack. We were expecting it. That was in our intelligence briefings. 'Inevitable' was the word used. And now they deny it."

* * *

Dr. Vivian Lane has never been to the Persian Gulf and is not a wife or mother of a Gulf War vet. The forty-three-year-old former squadron leader and former chief medical officer at the Royal Air Force base in Stafford, England, said she became seriously ill after treating a half dozen "very sick" British soldiers upon their return from the Persian Gulf. Dr. Lane says she was forced to move in with her elderly parents after she could no longer care for herself. Her parents, now in their eighties, are sick and suffering from lesions "very similar" to the ones she is suffering from, she says. "Nobody in this country can tell us why or what they are."

From December 1990 through June 1991 Dr. Lane treated at least six veterans who had the syndrome. Since that time, the aviation medical specialist, a former athlete, has been in great pain. She remembers waking up at four o'clock in the morning "with a terrific, excruciating, crushing type of chest pain and abdominal pain. When I got to the toilet, I didn't know whether to sit on it or stand over it. It just got worse from there. I managed somehow to get myself down to the medical center on base. All I remember was the excruciating chest pains. Next thing I know, I'm in intensive care. My parents had been brought to my bedside because everyone thought I was going to die. They didn't know what was wrong with me."

Dr. Lane offers a different angle on the hundreds of inoculations the soldiers were given before they left for the Persian Gulf. The protective shots were issued by the fistful, says Lane, and it's a wonder more people didn't have serious reactions. "With the amount we were banging into them, I'm surprised we didn't have more people falling over. We were attacking both arms, both buttocks, and their legs to get it all into them all at once. I think anybody with that amount of injections being shoved into them all within a couple of minutes of each other, would not feel terribly well."

Dr. Lane is one of several hundred former British soldiers suing the Ministry of Defense for medical redress. She says she is not holding her breath for results, though. "Frankly, I don't mean to be nasty, but I think they've bitten off more than they can chew."

Corporal Terry Walker was in the Persian Gulf from January to April 1991. Walker was a driver for the British Army's Fourth Armoured Brigade, First Armoured Division in Saudi Arabia. He has been sick ever since. He says his whole family suffers from Gulf War Syndrome.

In a recent interview, Walker described what he, too, believes was the Iraqi chemical Scud attack on January 20. "I was at the docks at Al-Jubayl about 2:30 in the morning," he said. "There was a couple of mighty bangs above our heads and suddenly all the chemical alarms went off and there were soldiers just running around in sheer panic, running around trying to get on their chemical suits." He says an "ammonia-like smell" filled the air after the sirens went off.

Walker, who had trouble getting his gas mask on, became ill soon after the Scuds hit. "I was feeling the burning sensation under the chin, around the back of the head as well. And ever since I've come back from the Gulf I've been ill." Walker suffers from chest infections, rashes, and headaches. Many of the people he served with were also sick after the attack, he says.

"As soon as the bangs happened, all these alarms went off and it was obvious that there was a chemical attack," says Walker, "but our superiors told us it was the jet fighters flying over with the sonic booms, and that it was also the fumes from the jets that set the alarms off."

"The thing is," says Walker, "they never went off before. The planes were flying day in and day out, and the alarms never went off at all, and on January 20, for about a ten-mile, fifteen-mile radius, these alarms went off."

Walker, who has since left the military, is furious with the military establishment in his country for "covering up what happened and the real risks" that would be faced by allied forces. "When they sent us out to fight the war, we expected them to look after us. Instead, when we came back they just tried to cover it up. They said there was nothing wrong at all because the general public would go against them if they found out about the exposures to chemical and biological warfare and how it gets into your whole family."

It is his family's illnesses that he objects to the most. "We knew there was a risk of being killed," he says, "but we didn't know that we would come back from the war so ill, and that our families would be getting sick, too. The wife has been ill since I've come back."

Walker's wife has had chronic abdominal pain and has been hospitalized at least seven times in the last three years. "She's been cut open twice but they couldn't find what was wrong," says Walker. The Walkers are extremely troubled about the health of their six-week-old child who has been plagued with a cold and respiratory problems "from day one."

* * *

Canadian legislator John O'Reilly recently raised the issue of Gulf War Syndrome in the House of Commons. O'Reilly asked the Defense Minister's Parliamentary Secretary, Fred Mifflin, what the government was doing to assist "deserving Canadians" who have been ill after serving in the Persian Gulf. Mifflin responded that the veterans had been cared for by Defense Department doctors and were experiencing "no difficulty whatsoever."

If Mifflin had spoken to Canadian Navy Lieutenant Louise Richard, he might have thought twice before painting such a rosy picture. Lieutenant Richard is an active-duty medical officer stationed at the National Defense Medical Center in Ottawa, the largest military hospital in Canada. Lieutenant Richard volunteered for service in the Persian Gulf as an operating-room nurse. She treated Americans, Britons, and Iraqi prisoners of war.

After eight years of commended service, Richard will be discharged from the Canadian Navy in September because of severe illness. She suffers from many of the same medical conditions afflicting some two dozen veterans interviewed for this article: severe respiratory problems, short-term memory loss, bronchitis, asthma, and pneumonia.

When Richard began to make a ruckus over her war-related illness and threatened to take it to the media, she ran into a stone wall of official denials and intimidation. "They've basically threatened me and said, 'It's all in your head, it's bullshit, don't go forward with it in the media.'" Richard says the threat from her medical superiors, whom she refuses to name for fear of further retribution, ran the gamut of intimidations. "It was the whole thing," says Richard, "your career, your pension—you know, the package."

She's frustrated at the lack of attention to the problem in Canada. "There doesn't seem to be anything happening since we're back," she says. "There's no research, no follow-up, there's nothing going on to help us." She said that she knows of many people in her position who have chosen to remain silent. "People fear to disclose anything because they don't want to ruin their pension or their career or whatever," she says. "I'm angry, because we were valued individuals when we were sent there, and now we're back, and we're not valued individuals at all. We're basically treated like mushrooms in a dark room."

* * *

Dr. Saleh Al-Harbi is an immunologist in Kuwait's Ministry of Public Health, and director of the immunogenetics unit of Kuwait University Medical Center. He says many people in Kuwait and Iran are suffering from what appear to be illnesses involving exposure to chemical and biological warfare agents.

"After the war we were getting diseases, respiratory diseases and unknown blood diseases such as leukemia, but not the typical kind, and for unknown reasons," he says. He is currently investigating with U.S. researchers the underlying causes of the medical conditions that have been plaguing Kuwaitis since the war. "Birth-related problems increased dramatically after liberation," he says, "and those kinds of cases have been reported to me."

He, too, is under pressure to keep a lid on his findings and concerns. "The authorities here are also standing with the Europeans' and Americans' point of view, but we believe that this is something political. I'm independent in mentioning this, and hopefully I will not get any threats from the superiors regarding this matter. They don't want the bad news and rumors to go around."

Dr. Al-Harbi characterizes the syndrome as a form of multiple chemical sensitivity, an explanation that is gaining favor in the United States as well.

Senator Riegle's report says that British and U.S. Army specialists, using sophisticated detection devices, made at least twenty tests that were positive for the presence of chemical-warfare agents. According to his report, "The Kuwaiti, U.S., and British governments all received reports on the discovery and recovery of bulk chemical agents."

Riegle's report also confirms that the alarms used in the war to warn troops of the presence of chemical warfare agents sounded thousands of times. In some cases, the report says, the alarms were sounding so frequently that they were simply turned off.

"The Defense Department told us at a hearing that they were all false alarms," says a former Riegle aide. "There were 14,000 of those chemical-alarm-monitoring units used during the war, and they're telling us that every time they went off, on all 14,000, they were false alarms. That's a little hard to believe."

According to a letter from Riegle to Veterans Affairs Secretary Jesse Brown, eighteen chemical, twelve biological, and four nuclear facilities in Iraq were bombed by the U.S.-led allied forces. Debris from the bombings was dispersed upwards into upper atmospheric currents, as shown by a U.S. satellite videotape obtained by Congress.

The Veterans Administration has only recently admitted that there is a problem with some "mystery illness" afflicting vets and their families. But the Pentagon denies there is any connection to chemical or biological warfare exposures.

In a May 25, 1994, "Memorandum for Persian Gulf Veterans," Defense Secretary William Perry and Joint Chiefs Chairman John Shalikashvili wrote:

"There have been reports in the press of the possibility that some of you were exposed to chemical or biological weapons agents. There is no information, classified or unclassified, that indicated that chemical or biological weapons were used in the Persian Gulf."

On June 23, 1994, the Defense Department's science board reported the results of an investigation into chemical and biological exposures in the Persian Gulf War. According to the report, "there is no evidence that either chemical or biological warfare was deployed at any level, or that there was any exposure of U.S. service members to chemical or biological warfare agents."

*   *   *

On December 13, 1994, the Pentagon released a report that says there was no single cause for Gulf War Syndrome. Veterans' groups were highly critical of this report. "It is more lies by the Pentagon to confuse and cover up the real causes of Gulf War Syndrome," says Major Richard Haines, president of Gulf Veterans International. In January, the Institute of Medicine of the National Academy of Sciences released a report critical of the Pentagon's research on Gulf War Syndrome.

Pentagon spokesman Dennis Boxx still maintains "we do not have any indication at this point that these things are transmittable to children or spouses."

Such declarations are consistent with the official British Ministry of Defense line. According to a July 14, 1994, letter from the Chemical and Biological Defense Establishment to the Pentagon's Lleutenant Colonel Vicki Merriman, "there was no evidence of any chemical warfare agent being present" in the Persian Gulf.

Ironically, when Senator Riegle first approached officials at the Department of Defense about veterans' possible exposures to chemical and biological warfare agents in the Persian Gulf, he was told by Walter Reed Army Medical Center commander Major General Ronald Blank that the issue was not even explored because "military intelligence maintained that such exposures never occurred."

While the Pentagon has refused to admit that chemical and biological warfare agents were present during the Gulf War, Senator Riegle stated on October 8, 1994, that "these Department of Defense explanations are inconsistent with the facts as related by the soldiers who were present, and with official government documents prepared by those who were present, and with experts who have examined the facts."

According to official Pentagon documents, at least eight members of the U.S. military who served in the Persian Gulf, in fact, received letters of commendation for locating and identifying chemical-warfare agents during the war. Army Captain Michael Johnson was awarded the Meritorious Service medal for overseeing the "positive identification of a suspected chemical agent." The certificate that accompanied Private First Class Allen Fisher's bronze star medal stated that his discoveries were the "first confirmed detection of chemical-agent contamination in the theater of operation."

In a memorandum dated January 4, 1994, to "Director, CATD," Captain Johnson of the Nuclear Biological and Chemical Branch of the Army wrote to his superiors: "Recent headlines have aroused considerable interest in the possible exposure of coalition forces to Iraqi chemical agents. Much of this interest is the result of health problems by Gulf War veterans that indicated exposure to chemical agents. Although no government officials have confirmed use, there is a high likelihood that some coalition forces experienced exposure to chemical agents."

Captain Johnson stated that he believed "coalition soldiers did experience exposure to Iraqi chemical agents." Johnson, who was commander of the 54th Chemical Troop, had cited in his report an example of a British soldier who was exposed. According to Johnson, "the soldier had an immediate reaction to the liquid contact. The soldier was in extreme pain and was going into shock." Captain Johnson first notified his superiors of his concerns in August 1991.

"This official dissembling and effort to obscure the facts are a continuation of Defense Department tactics," said Riegle in a written statement accompanying his October report. "The serious question remains as to why we were not provided with an official report dating from the time of the incident by the Department of Defense."

"If you look at the symptoms associated with biological and chemical contamination," says a former aide to Senator Riegle, "you'll see the same symptoms that are present in these veterans to varying degrees. The common denominator in all their illnesses is the breaking down of their immune system just as AIDS [acquired immunodeficiency syndrome] does, making them sicker and sicker as the days and years go by, and eventually incapacitating and killing some of them. And it's somehow being passed along to other people. We were getting hundreds of calls from people saying, 'He brought home this duffel bag, and we opened it up, and my eyes and hands started burning, and now I'm sick. What's wrong? What's happened?'"

# NO

Michael Fumento

# GULF LORE SYNDROME

"For Some, a Day of Betrayal," ran a headline in Denver's *Rocky Mountain News* the day before Veterans Day. A Persian Gulf vet said to be suffering the effects of the mysterious Gulf War Syndrome (GWS) was profiled, and the story by reporter Dick Foster contained a startling figure: "Cancers have developed in Gulf veterans at three to six times the rate among the general population." That news must have shot around Colorado faster than a Scud missile. Many vets probably spent their Veterans Day searching for lumps, bumps, sores, or anything else that might be a sign of cancer.

Three days later, a study appeared in *The New England Journal of Medicine*. Using the latest data available, it reported the cancer rate of Persian Gulf vets was slightly *below* that of comparable vets who didn't deploy to the Gulf, and far lower than that of the comparable civilian population.

Welcome to the world of Gulf Lore Syndrome. It is a world in which science is replaced by rumor, in which vets are presented as medical experts while real medical experts are ignored. It is a dimension in which authoritative review studies by eminent scientists are scorned and disdainfully labeled "Pentagon studies" because they reach the "wrong" conclusions—even if done by civilian organizations. Yet incredible accounts of such symptoms as skin-blistering semen and glowing vomit are taken as gospel. It is a "reality" constructed by crusading reporters, activists, demagogic congressmen, and, sadly, by Persian Gulf vets who have become convinced they are the victims of a conspiracy deeper and broader than anything on *The X-Files*. The sick vets live in this world of Gulf Lore Syndrome. Until reality is allowed to reach them, they will remain trapped in it.

I have been writing on GWS since 1993, and to the best of my knowledge I was the first writer to say that there is no Gulf War Syndrome in the accepted sense of the term. Since then, studies by some of the most prestigious scientists in the country have backed up that position. The early studies included two by the Department of Defense, one by the National Institutes of Health, and a preliminary report by the Institute of Medicine, an arm of the National Academy of Sciences. All said that the term *Gulf War Syndrome* was a misnomer. All said that the various theories of what might be making Persian

From Michael Fumento, "Gulf Lore Syndrome," *Reason* (March 1997). Copyright © 1997 by The Reason Foundation. Reprinted by permission.

Gulf vets sick lacked any scientific basis. And every one of these studies' conclusions bounced off the reporters, the activists, and the sick vets like bullets off an M1 tank.

Some things *have* changed: When I began writing on the topic there were perhaps a hundred news reports about GWS; there are now over 4,000. Back then there were a few thousand Persian Gulf vets who claimed to have the illness; now, depending on who's counting, there are anywhere from 40,000 to more than 100,000. GWS studies continue to appear. The most recent include:

- The final report from the Institute of Medicine, which said in October that there is no "scientific evidence to date demonstrating adverse health consequences linked with [Gulf War] service other than [about 30] documented incidents of leishmaniasis [a parasitical disease caused, in this case, by sand fly bites], combat-related or injury-related mortality or morbidity, and increased risk of psychiatric [problems from] deployment."
- A draft copy of the final report of the Presidential Advisory Committee on Gulf War Veterans' Illnesses (commonly called the PAC), leaked in November to *The New York Times* and *The Washington Post*, which found "no support for the myriad theories proposed as causes of illnesses among Persian Gulf war veterans, or even evidence there is a 'Gulf War Syndrome,'" according to the *Post*.
- The article in the November 14 *New England Journal of Medicine*, which found that Persian Gulf vets had the same death rate from disease as non–Persian Gulf vets, and a much lower rate than the comparable civil-ian population. An accompanying article looked at hospitalizations, finding Persian Gulf vets and non-Persian Gulf vets hospitalized at the same rate.

Will these findings make any difference? Within days of the PAC draft report's release, President Clinton announced a doubling of the budget to investigate GWS. A few weeks later, he announced that the PAC final report would not be a final one after all, that he was going to keep the committee going albeit perhaps dumping some old members and assigning new ones. Rep. Chris Shays (R-Conn.) called two days of highly publicized hearings to denounce the government and parade one sick soldier after another to testify before his congressional panel, each claiming that his symptoms were beyond doubt the result of GWS. Apparently, science is still reaching the wrong conclusion.

## MYTHS FIT TO PRINT

What pulled me back into the fray was the recent series of revelations concerning the demolition of bunkers at Khamisiyah, Iraq. The unit that blew up those bunkers was the 37th Engineer Battalion (Combat) (Airborne). In May, the Pentagon said U.N. inspectors had found that one of those bunkers and a nearby open pit contained Iraqi rockets marked to indicate a nerve gas called sarin. Thus, while the Pentagon could (and did) continue to say that there had been no offensive use of chemical weapons against U.S. troops, it was now clear that American soldiers had been close enough to exploding chemical weapons to be exposed to them. The 37th was my sister unit when I was in the 27th Engineers at Ft. Bragg, a decade earlier. I had lived in the same barracks and worn those same silver wings that mark the Army's proud elite, the paratrooper. I knew these soldiers in ways other reporters did not. What they would tell me in weeks of interviews taught me a great deal about GWS.

I interviewed eight of these men, beginning with former Pfc. Brian Martin. Martin is by far the most prominent 37th Engineer vet, having appeared on *60 Minutes* twice, on *Nightline, Geraldo, Montel Williams,* and *Tom Snyder,* and having been quoted by news wires, newspapers, and magazines, including the Associated Press, Gannett, *The Detroit News, Newsday, Playboy,* and one of a series of articles by *The New York Times*'s Philip Shenon. Martin, 33, is also co-president (with his wife) of International Advocacy for Gulf War Syndrome. Being a disabled vet is his life; indeed, his Web page lists his occupation as "disabled veteran," while his e-mail address is "dsveteran."

Martin is quick with a sound bite, such as, "I used to jump out of airplanes and now I can't even jump up and down." Sometimes he walks with a cane; other times he uses a wheelchair. We talked about our old brigade a bit. He explained to me the process of destroying the bunkers at Khamisiyah, and then I asked him to tell me about his symptoms. That was the first hint that something was seriously amiss about Pfc. Martin.

His long list of symptoms included such things as lupus—an autoimmune disease rarely found in men—and "early Alzheimer's." Sensationalist reporters just eat up things like this, but to a medical writer such symptoms were like flapping red flags.

Then *the* red flag unfurled. Martin told me what he would later tell a congressional panel headed by Shays on September 19, 1996. After returning from the Gulf, he told the panel, "during PT [physical training] I would vomit Chemlite-looking fluids every time I ran; an ambulance would pick me up, putting IVs in both arms, rushing me to Womack Community Hospital. This happened *every* morning after my return from the war." (Emphasis as noted in the official transcript.)

Chemlites are tubes that, when snapped, glow. In two conversations with me, Martin repeatedly referred to his vomit as being "fluorescent" and said these daily vomits lasted from "March 11 to December 31," 1991. Thus, we are dealing with a man who insists both that his vomit glows and that his NCOs and officers heartlessly insisted that he do physical training for 10 months, knowing that "every morning" he would end up in the hospital with IV tubes in his arms.

If Martin volunteered the vomiting story during both of my interviews with him, it's very likely he told it to every other reporter who interviewed him. Yet they all used Martin as a credible witness, omitting this peculiarity from their accounts.

There are two reporters that we know with certainty did this, because they attended the September 19 hearings and wrote about Martin's testimony. One was AP reporter Donna Abu-Nasr. I called her and asked why she didn't mention the glowing vomit remark. "I didn't notice it," she said. Did she think it impugned Martin's credibility? No, she said. "You have to remember he's been on talk shows, and they've written a lot about him." She then said, "Are you going to quote me?" I told her that was my job as a reporter, but I wouldn't if she insisted.

Not good enough. "I think that's very dishonest of you," she said, and hung up.

The other reporter who covered the hearing was John Hanchette at Gannett News Service, the chain that owns *USA Today*. Hanchette, a 1980 Pulitzer Prize winner, has probably written more articles on GWS—over 80—than any other single reporter, sometimes alone and sometimes with Norm Brewer. Given his reputation and sheer volume, he's certainly had a big impact on the perception of GWS. The titles of his stories show his slant: "Active-Duty Soldiers Tear into Pentagon Over Gulf Syndrome"; "Are Gulf Veterans Getting Needed Treatment?"; "Several Gulf Units Plagued by Unusually High Illness Rate"; "White House Panel: Pentagon Can't Be Trusted in Persian Gulf War Syndrome Probe"; "Persian Gulf Illnesses-the Lingering War"; "Gulf War Parents with Birth Defect Children: All They Want Are Answers."

In his coverage of Martin's testimony, Hanchette chopped Martin's symptom list down to nine, omitting the glowing vomit. Nor is that all he did.

Rather than merely attributing the laundry list of symptoms to Martin, Hanchette wrote that these symptoms were supported by "federal medical exams," making Martin's symptom list sound far more credible. But I had called Martin's doctors (with numbers Martin provided), and while Department of Veterans Affairs rules prohibit them from talking about any specific patient, I got around this by asking them if *any* of their patients had the various symptoms Martin claimed. Often, the answer was no. Some of the illnesses the doctors said they had not observed in any of their patients—such as lupus—were among those Hanchette listed as confirmed by

Martin's "federal medical exams." What exams could Hanchette possibly have been referring to?

I politely called Hanchette four times just to say I wanted to talk about his story. He didn't call back. I called twice more to say that I had reason to believe he had engaged in unethical conduct and that I wanted to give him a chance to respond. He still hasn't called back.

So I called Hanchette's editor, Jeffrey Stinson. In defending his reporter, Stinson noted twice that Hanchette was a Pulitzer winner, called my questions "a crock," and said he really couldn't comment further without seeing the relevant material. I faxed over Martin's testimony, Hanchette's write-up, and a list of questions. Stinson's response: "Our stuff is good; it's accurate. You're full of it, pal. Bye." Then he hung up. . . .

## SYNDROME OVER SCIENCE

To doctors, bizarre symptom claims like glowing vomit are a ready indicator that they are dealing with a patient suffering hysteria. "It's an old joke around ER; we ask if people's stools glow in the dark or if their hair hurts," Dr. Scott Kurtzman, assistant professor of surgery at the University of Connecticut School of Medicine, told me. But to the media, such symptoms are the makings of a great story. Kate McKenna's article, "The Curse of Desert Storm," in the March 1996 *Playboy*, didn't mention Brian Martin's vomit but said that he is "often confined to a wheelchair" because of "a *diarrhetic* condition that has damaged his spine." (Emphasis mine.) Perhaps the makers of Kaopectate should advertise that it may be effective in preventing spinal injury. . . .

A key component of Gulf Lore Syndrome entails suspending the laws of science whenever necessary. Consider the first death widely attributed to GWS, that of Army Reservist Michael Adcock. Adcock died in 1992 at the age of 22 from what began as a lymphoma (cancer of the lymph glands) and then spread to the rest of his body. Without doubt he believed—as his mother Hester testified before Congress—that he had contracted the lymphoma from exposure to something in the Gulf. His last words, she said, were, "Mama, fight for me. Don't let this happen to another soldier." The congressmen listened solemnly, and the media faithfully reported the story. But Army Surgeon General spokeswoman Virginia Stephanakis told me that Adcock "had rectal bleeding [the first symptom of his lymphoma] six days after arriving, and the family blamed it on the Gulf." It is universally accepted by the medical community that lymphomas take years to develop, perhaps 10 or more years on average. Not months, not weeks, and certainly not days.

Likewise, former Navy Seabee (combat engineer) Reservist Nick Roberts claims to have contracted his lymphoma within weeks of what he claims was a nerve gas attack. Roberts is almost as popular with reporters as Brian Martin. The AP, USA Today, States News Service, The Atlanta Journal and Constitution, and Esquire in its cover story on GWS have all portrayed Roberts as a prototypical GWS victim, using such headlines as "Walking Wounded" and "Trail of Symptoms Suggests Chem-Arms." I've talked to Roberts, and I'm sure he's convinced of what he says. But his claim is a medical impossibility, and none of the stories about him bothered to make that clear.

Roberts appeared before Shays's committee on the same day as Martin, so I called Robert Newman, the Shays staffer who invited them both to testify. I asked Newman first about Martin's daily spewing of glowing vomit. "In the overall scheme of things," Newman told me, "that's got to be a minor point." Well, OK. What about Roberts's lymphoma? "Do you know how long it takes a lymphoma to develop?" I asked Newman. "It takes a long time to develop," Newman said. "So you're willing to concede that Roberts's lymphoma couldn't have had anything to do with exposure from something in the Gulf?" I asked. "I'm not going to concede anything," he said.

No, he certainly wasn't. It is part of the strategy of the lore spreaders that you never, ever admit that any vet's claims are incredible, or that even a single veteran anywhere might be suffering psychosomatic illness. Newman ended our conversation by saying, "You caught me at a bad time because I'm in another crisis. Call me tomorrow." I did, and several times after that. We never talked again.

It is bad enough that the media and Congress always treat Persian Gulf vets as experts in self-diagnosis, but they're even considered experts in diagnosing others. Roberts told a congressional panel in November 1993 that of the 33 members in his military reserve unit, 10 in addition to him have been diagnosed with lymphomas. Were that true it would probably be the most amazing cancer cluster in history. He also held up a list of what he said were 173 cancer-stricken Gulf veterans, and the media duly reported his comments. Yet five months later, an update of the Persian Gulf Registry showed only eight lymphomas out of all the Gulf vets in the country, with 38 cancers of all types.

There have been reports of mysterious illness clusters throughout the GWS scare. Vets or their spouses will call other vets, essentially doing their own epidemiological study. Often they conclude that they are suffering an abnormal amount of illness. They then contact the media, who publicize these "findings," gingerly referring to them as "unofficial investigations.

The Institute of Medicine looked at three such reports, including one involving Nick Roberts's reserve Seabee unit. In all three cases, the IOM found that, while the symptoms tended to be the same among the three groups, these were classic psychosomatic manifestations. The outbreak studies, said the IOM, "were not successful in demonstrating that these symptoms occurred at a higher rate among PGW [Persian Gulf War] veterans than among [other] PGW-era veterans, or that these symptoms could be linked to specific medical diagnoses or exposures."

The most famous of the self-diagnosed clusters occurred in Mississippi, involving alleged defects in the babies of vets. These reports added a whole new dimension to the disease. Among the heart-wrenching stories built around the "cluster" were "Gulf Syndrome Kills Babies," "A Town in Torment," and *Ladies Home Journal*'s "What's Wrong with Our Children?"

The basic story, as *Nightline*'s reporter told it, was, "In Waynesville, Mississippi, 13 of 15 babies born to returning members of a National Guard Unit were reported to have severe and often rare health problems." It didn't say the report was "prepared," as it were, by the parents themselves. The Mississippi Department of Health investigated the alleged cluster and found that of 54 births to returning Guardsmen in that state, both major and minor defects were well within the expected range. There were also no more premature or low-birth-weight children than would be expected.

Since then, several birth-defect and miscarriage studies have looked for exceptional rates among the offspring of Persian Gulf vets. They have found none. In addition, all live births to Persian Gulf vets are being tracked, with birth defect compared to those in the offspring of non-deployed soldiers. When last analyzed, the children of the Gulf War vets had the same percentage of birth defects as the children of the comparison soldiers.

But of all the media outlets that originally reported on the alleged Mississippi cluster, only CNN later told its audience of the state's report. So the "Town in Torment" remains a staple of Gulf Lore. Dr. Russell Tarver, who headed up the study, told me, "It's unconscionable to frighten people out of reproducing unless you have some good data to support that contention." He called it "a crime against those veterans." ...

## POST GULF, ERGO PROPTER GULF

Much of what drives the GWS myth is the simplest of fallacies: that if something happens after a given event, it must have been caused by that event. The GWS fallacy works like this: The vets were obviously healthy when they went to the Gulf, or they wouldn't have been sent. Now they're sick. Therefore it must have been something in the Gulf that made them ill.

Appearing on *Nightline*, Sen. John D. (Jay) Rockefeller IV (D-W.Va.) invoked the fallacy repeatedly with such statements as: "They were totally healthy when they went over to the Persian Gulf. No problems whatsoever. They come back and all of the sudden their children are [born] defective, they can't have children, or they [the children] die."

So what happened to these vets? It depends not just on whom you ask, but what day you happened to ask them. Consider just the headlines from some of the stories authored or co-authored by Hanchette:

"Experimental Drugs on Gulf Troops Rapped by Panel"

"Key to Gulf War Syndrome May Be Flies"

"Doctor Says Gulf Illnesses Stem from Vaccines"

"CIA Document: Scud Fuel May Be Involved in Gulf War Illnesses"

"U.N. Intelligence Representatives Show Iraq Could Have Spread Deadly Aflatoxin"

Just can't make up our minds, can we? It's not uncommon for a vet or activist or reporter to insist that one thing is absolutely, definitely the cause of GWS, and later to insist that something else is absolutely, definitely the cause. Sometimes the media or activists will even use a sort of shotgun approach.

Nightline's GWS show in October, which left no doubt that GWS was both real and spreading, first indicated the cause was nerve gas. That nerve gas symptoms couldn't possibly spread from person to person was apparently considered inconsequential. The Nightline reporter then proceeded to blame pyrodistigmine bromide (PB) pills the vets had taken. Then it was exposure to fumes from oil wells. Again, neither of these could possibly cause symptoms that are communicable, but that too seemed not to matter.

Vets and their families will often be influenced by these shifting fads, as in the case of Michael Adcock, the Persian Gulf vet who died of cancer. In May 1993, the fad cause of GWS was multiple chemical sensitivity, and that month Adcock's mother, Hester, told The Washington Times, "Beyond a shadow of a doubt, I believe Michael died of multiple chemical exposure" in the Gulf. She cited oil well fires, fresh paint on vehicles, and lead in the diesel fuel used in lanterns and heaters. Six months later the fad cause of GWS was nerve gas, and Mrs. Adcock testified before Congress, doubtless sincerely, that her son's disease was from nerve gas released by a Scud missile the day before his first symptom of lymphoma appeared.

Though the fads come and go, the main two so far have been PB and Iraqi chemical weapons. PB was given to many of the troops because of evidence from animal experimentation that it could provide some protection if they were hit by one type of nerve gas. A Nexis search shows no fewer than 175 stories implicating PB as a possible cause of GWS.

But the focus on PB has more to do with confusion over terms than with science. Time and again, the media have described PB using the fear-triggering word *experimental*. Hanchette and Brewer at Gannett did so in two different articles, calling it "unlicensed" in a third. The soldiers "had no idea they were taking an investigational drug," Ed Bradley told 60 Minutes viewers, with a follow-up quote from a vet in combat fatigues saying, "We've been used as guinea pigs."

What virtually no one out there in media- and activist-land says is that PB was "experimental" or "investigational" only insofar as its ability to prevent illness from nerve agents went. The drug itself comes from a class of pharmaceuticals that has been in use since 1864. Far from being "unlicensed," it was licensed by the FDA in 1955 to treat a neuromuscular disease called myasthenia gravis. Moreover, the dose given to myasthenia gravis patients ranges from 360 to 6,000 milligrams daily. In contrast, U.S. soldiers in the Gulf were given a one-week supply of PB, with three 30-milligram pills to be taken daily.

This is why both the NIH and IOM panels rejected out of hand the notion that PB could be causing illness among Persian Gulf vets, with the NIH saying that even at the massive doses taken by the myasthenia gravis sufferers, PB has shown "no significant long-term effects." Yet one newspaper, in attributing the ills of Persian Gulf vet Carol Picou to the PB pills, went so far as to tell its readers that PB has never even been tested on women and was only the subject of a single test on men.

The second main culprit, nerve gas, has become a popular GWS suspect for reasons more psychological than scientific. "Chemical weapons are not useful as tactical weapons," FDA specialist Peter Procter told a wire service reporter during the 1990 Gulf buildup. Only 3 percent of Iranians gassed during the Iran-Iraq war died. It was hardly because Hitler was a humanitarian that he refrained from using sarin, the new nerve gas his scientists had invented, but rather because his experts convinced him that the old-fashioned high explosive shells and rockets were far more effective. But the received wisdom among American civilians, soldiers, reporters, and even government officials is that chemical weapons are incredibly efficient killing machines, so much so that they

are regularly lumped into the category "weapons of mass destruction," alongside hydrogen bombs.

Such weapons are mostly effective "as weapons of terrorism," the FDA's Proctor said six years ago. "The greatest fear among the soldiers on the line," wrote one reporter shortly before the Persian Gulf ground war began, "is the likelihood that the enemy artillery will be firing rounds of mustard gas and nerve gas. Thus, it's only natural that Gulf War vets seeking a cause for their symptoms would convince themselves that they must have been gassed.

But there are many problems with the gassing scenario. One is that, as the October IOM report stated, "there are no confirmed reports of clinical manifestations of acute nerve agent exposure." True, some vets are *now* claiming they remember being gassed, but not one of them reported to clinics then.

Chemical alarms went off constantly during the war, supposed evidence of gas attacks. But chemical alarms are made to be hypersensitive, for obvious reasons. Even a "confirmed" gas detection doesn't necessarily indicate the presence of gas; it's just a more specific test than the initial one....

That's it. Readers could conclude that GWS resulted from multiple chemical attacks, or a combination of such attacks and drugs. In fact, a [New York] Times reader could conclude anything or nothing about what the IOM had really said.

## MEDICINE AND 'MIRACLES'

Journalists aren't the only ones feeding the vets good stories that don't quite add up. Dr. Howard Urnovitz is one doctor beloved by vets who believe they have

GWS. Last year he said his discovery of a mystery virus in Persian Gulf vets explains how, "Like rubella, it is being passed on as a virus and can, we believe, explain the birth defects in children of the veterans."

Urnovitz is not, however, a disinterested scientist. Although he may believe what he's saying, he also appears to be appealing to the vets' fears to raise money for his biotech company, Calypte Biomedical of Berkeley, California. After all, as Calypte's Web page (ChronicIllnet) informs readers, "ChronicIllnet feels that much of the current breakthroughs in understanding IMMUNE SYSTEM IMBALANCE SYNDROMES, such as cancer, will come from the MIRACLES occurring with the new treatments being explored in Persian Gulf War related illnesses." (Emphasis theirs.)

No responsible physician would use the term *miracle* to describe his treatments; that's huckster terminology. As it happens, *miracle* is a hypertext link. If you click on it, the link takes you to a story about a Gulf vet who claims that his GWS symptoms were cured by doxycycline. Somehow a general-purpose antibiotic developed in 1966 doesn't seem like the sort of thing that will lead to a cure for cancer.

But it's not just cancer that these "miracle" cures will finish off. "If we can find a cure for Gulf War Syndrome," Urnovitz said at a 1996 symposium in Denver, "we'll be able to cure cancer and AIDS and chronic fatigue syndrome and other immune system disorders. They're all linked together." Maybe that cure will start your car on a cold winter morning, too.

Another doctor who is revered by sick Persian Gulf vets and has testified before the Presidential Advisory Committee is

Garth Nicolson. Nicolson is a highly regarded cancer researcher who says he and his wife Nancy, a molecular biophysicist, left the M. D. Anderson Cancer Center in Houston to pursue a cure for GWS after his stepdaughter, a Gulf War vet, fell ill.

Like Urnovitz, the Nicolsons claim great success with doxycycline. Unlike Urnovitz, the Nicolsons blame not a virus but a bacterium, specifically mycoplasma fermentans (MF). They claim that using a special form of the polymerase chain-reaction (PCR) test, they have detected MF in about half of the vets with GWS symptoms. With PCR you take some blood from a person and use a chemical procedure to enlarge parts of the DNA of an organism (such as MF) that you think might be in the blood. If you use the chemical that would enlarge the DNA of MF and it works, then you know the MF is there. If the chemical doesn't enlarge it, you don't have MF. So far, so good.

But the same sensitivity that makes PCR a useful tool in finding what's in blood also makes it liable to find what's not there. Improperly cleaned and sterilized equipment will have all sorts of DNA strands on it that didn't come from the blood of the specified patient. In the most famous case of PCR contamination, Dr. David Ho—recently named *Time*'s "Man of the Year" for his promising work on AIDS—published a study in the mid-'80s which, using PCR, detected the AIDS virus in numerous people who had tested negative in the standard blood test. It was a frightening result, but no one could duplicate his findings and Ho was forced to admit that his testing must have suffered contamination.

As with Ho's results, other doctors are finding they cannot duplicate Nicolson's PCR work on MF. This includes the man universally acknowledged as the leading expert on MF, Dr. Shyh-Ching Lo of the Armed Forces Institute of Pathology. "We've never found one" Persian Gulf vet with the bacterium, says Lo. "The Nicolsons claim their technique is different," allegedly using "a special form of PCR that's more sensitive," says Lo. Specifically, they claim their test can better find MF when it's hiding in the nucleus of the cell only. Lo says that's possible, "but we never truly get the detail of how [the Nicolsons] process PCR. They just give us the statements of their results." In late December [1996], Garth Nicolson announced that he will divulge his testing technique, but he had not done so at this writing.

I asked Nicolson if there were any scientists who had duplicated his work. He named only one, Aristo Vojdani, himself a GWS advocate and doctor who specializes in multiple chemical sensitivity. MCS is an alleged ailment that mainstream organizations, such as the American Medical Association, find questionable, if not outright nonsense. Vojdani is also now among the shrinking number of researchers claiming that silicone breast implants are harmful.

The other way of judging the merit of the Nicolsons' PCR work would be to see where it has been published. One National Institutes of Health MF expert, who asked not to be identified, conceded that Nicolson had indeed published in this area, but only in "garbage journals." Indeed, of the seven pieces Nicolson sent me, six were in journals that specialize in MCS or related fields. The seventh was in *The Journal of the American Medical Association*—but it was only an unrefereed letter to the editor.

None of which conclusively proves that the Nicolsons' research is invalid. But even if their unique test does detect MF, it may have no connection to Gulf War Syndrome. For one, nobody knows how many perfectly healthy people carry around MF in their bodies, just as we carry around myriad types of benign and even helpful bacteria. More important, medical science so far has identified MF as a probable cause of just one health problem, rheumatoid arthritis. There is also some evidence it may be involved in acute respiratory problems. Sure, some Gulf vets have complained of aching joints and others of breathing troubles. But what of the 100-plus other problems they claim?

Further, the very idea of MF as a biological weapon, as the Nicolsons claim it was, is ludicrous. The purpose of biological weapons is to cripple, kill, and terrorize on the battlefield—not to cause aching joints in vets years later.

Nor does it help the Nicolsons' credibility that they suggest they are targets of a conspiracy because their work threatens the GWS coverup. Garth told the *Houston Press*, an alternative weekly, that while he and his wife were at M. D. Anderson, their faxes and letters were repeatedly intercepted, and their phone had been tapped so many times that "it was a record." Nancy also claims there have been six attempts on her life, but "assassins told her they saw her face and just couldn't pull the trigger." ...

## THE MYSTERY SOLVED

Of the many reasons the media perpetuate Gulf Lore Syndrome, one is that reporters—and readers—love a mystery. Indeed, a Nexis search in November found 630 stories referring to the "mystery" of GWS. The allure of a mystery is often such that it refuses to die no matter how much light is shone on it. So it is with GWS. But there is no mystery.

Why are there so many sick Persian Gulf vets? First, because there are so many Persian Gulf vets, period. Take 697,000 vets, add their spouses and children, and you have a pool of well over a million people. In such a pool you're going to have every illness in the book. Because modern medicine is not an exact science, you're also going to have a certain number of illnesses for which no firm cause is identified.

"Among approximately 697,000 people over a period of several years, there will be poorly understood ailments and a number of obscure diseases," as the October IOM report put it. The question is, Are Gulf War vets having these illnesses at an extraordinary rate? The flat answer is: no—no more deaths (except vehicle accidents), no more cancers, no more birth defects, no more miscarriages. Persian Gulf vets have these problems because everybody has these problems. The difference is the media have convinced them that a neighbor's miscarriage is just a miscarriage, but *their* miscarriage is GWS.

Indeed, for all the talk of the "commonality" of symptoms of GWS, I have compiled a list of over 100, including hair loss, graying hair, weight gain, weight loss, irritability, heartburn, rashes, sore throat, kidney stones, sore gums, constipation, sneezing, leg cramps, insomnia, herpes, and "a foot fungus that will not go away." It is no exaggeration to say that every ailment any Persian Gulf vet has ever gotten —or that anybody has ever gotten—has been labeled a symptom of GWS.

According to Dr. Edward Young, former chief of staff at the Houston VA Medical Center, one of the three centers set up to investigate ailments among Gulf War vets, "We're talking about people who have multiple complaints. And if you go out on the street in any city in this country, you'll find people who have exactly the same things, and they've never been to the Gulf." In an interview with the *Birmingham Daily News,* he said, "It really rankles me when people stand up and call it 'Persian Gulf Syndrome.' To honor this thing with some name is ridiculous." Although Young later asked that the comments not be printed, the American Legion, the most powerful GWS lobbying group, got hold of them and complained to the VA. The VA unceremoniously yanked Young from his position, later citing his lack of compassion. As Shays staffer Robert Newman told me, "Nobody wants to go against vets; it's a very strong lobby." Amen.

Yet it's an oversimplification to say that vets are having exactly the same symptoms as anybody else. They appear to suffer more from illnesses commonly associated with stress—that is, psychosomatic ones.

Doctors have long understood that one can induce symptoms in many people by giving them reasons they *should* feel sick. David Murray, now with the Statistical Assessment Service in Washington, D.C., used to demonstrate this by telling his social anthropology students they might have suffered minor food poisoning at lunch and that, if so, they should go to the nurse's office. "Within five minutes there would be shifting of seats and belching and one or two people would walk out the door," says Murray. "Eventually a third of the class would have left or be complaining of illness."

Nothing enrages activists—or many sick vets—like suggesting that Gulf War vets are suffering psychosomatic illness. Responding to the Presidential Advisory Commission's conclusion, Denise Nichols told *The New York Times*, "I am appalled that after five years [the government] is still busy denying physical damage... this is not stress."

But "psychosomatic" does not refer to the symptom; it refers to its origin. You can get diarrhea because you're worried about tomorrow's final exam or because you ate a week-old taco. In the first case it is psychosomatic; in the second it is organic, meaning it came from some source other than stress. In either case, you're sick. Telling someone their symptoms are probably psychosomatic isn't an insult; it's just an explanation. Nor is there anything exotic about it; stress-induced symptoms—often more severe than organic ones—have been experienced by nearly everyone.

What is the source of this GWS stress? That has been muddled by the misapplication of the term, *post-traumatic stress disorder* (PTSD), coined to explain psychological (including psychosomatic) problems of Vietnam vets who had trouble adjusting to civilian life. *Nightline*, in October, said GWS couldn't possibly be PTSD because this wouldn't explain why vets' wives were sick.

Exactly right. What the vets and their wives are suffering is what I call *current traumatic stress disorder*. It isn't their experience in the Gulf that is haunting them, but rather what they're seeing on *Nightline* and other TV shows, what they're reading in the papers, what they're hearing from congressional demagogues and from activists, and finally what they hear from their fellow vets in conversations and Internet chatter. The Gulf War vets are sick for the same reason Murray's students became sick. They are bombarded with the message that they *ought* to be sick.

## EPIDEMIC HYSTERIA

Medical historian Edward Shorter of the University of Toronto calls related cases of psychosomatic illness "epidemic hysteria." As a historian, he finds the GWS phenomenon tragic yet "fascinating." Says Shorter, "Just as cholera is spread by water droplets, epidemic hysteria is spread by the media."

In his 1992 book on epidemic hysteria, *From Paralysis to Fatigue*, Shorter recounts the similar history of a 19th-century syndrome called "spinal irritation," originally diagnosed by a handful of British doctors. Once informed they had this mysterious ailment, the patients, usually young women, would present an often bizarre array of symptoms, including temporary blindness, paralysis (of the sort Brian Martin appears to suffer), constant vomiting, dribbling saliva, and painful menstruation. Doctors used a wide array of treatments, including leeching, putting caustic agents on the skin, and applying magnets. "The more convincing and resolute the treatment," wrote Shorter, "the greater the success in cases of psychosomatic illness." "Spinal irritation" eventually spread to the United States, where it continued to afflict Americans for decades.

In November, the CDC announced that a study to be published in 1997 showed that Gulf vets from a Pennsylvania National Guard unit were three times more likely than comparable troops who didn't deploy to the Gulf to complain of such symptoms as chronic diarrhea, joint pain, skin rashes, fatigue, and memory loss. "This is absolutely a breakthrough study," said Matt Puglisi, an official with the American Legion. "For those who were more skeptical" than the Legion, he said, "and wanted scientific proof, now we've got it." *The New York Times*'s Shenon also played the story this way, in several articles with titles like, "The Numbers Support Gulf War Syndrome Claims." But this was far from the smoking gun GWS activists were hoping for and claimed to have found. All of these are classic psychosomatic symptoms. Combined with studies showing the Gulf vets have no higher rates of things not generally related to psychosomatic illness, such as cancer and death, the symptoms are actually further evidence that GWS reflects epidemic hysteria. Lost in the fuss over the CDC study was the statement from one of the authors to the Associated Press that "we have found there is nothing unique to the Persian Gulf, other than having gone there."

The GWS epidemic appears to have begun in mid-1992 as true PTSD among reservists who had such complaints as "hair loss, joint aches, severe bad breath, and fatigue." As reservists they were not as psychologically prepared to fight as were the active-duty soldiers; moreover, the reservists had to return to civilian jobs almost as if nothing had happened. At that point *USA Today*—the same newspaper that launched what proved to be the phony black church-burning epidemic of 1996—went into action, dubbing the symptoms "Gulf War Syndrome" and broadcasting them throughout the country.

A study of reservists found no extraordinary health problems, just illnesses attributed to stress. But Gulf Lore Syndrome was up and running. That's when the active-duty soldiers began to fall ill. By late 1993, CNN and others were seizing upon the alleged Mississippi birth defect cluster to say that GWS could be inherited. Gulf Lore Syndrome now included children.

By early 1994 some vets were linking their spouses' illnesses—including such things as irregular menstruation—to GWS. The media ran headlines like, "Gulf War Syndrome Spreading to Veterans' Families," and suddenly complaints about GWS symptoms began increasing among vets' wives. By late 1996 GWS had reached a point where people were contracting it from *objects* that had been in the Gulf. *Nightline* said Brian Martin's daughter got it from his military gear. CNN did a spot in November about a woman who contracted it from an Army surplus duffel bag.

For a year and a half, GWS remained strictly an American problem. By December 1993, however, *The Guardian* was reporting British cases. Eventually, GWS crossed to the continent. In a February 1996 article, Hanchette and Brewer began, "As recently as 15 months ago, asking the military about [GWS] often triggered this response: If there really is a sickness emanating from that war, why are our allies free of all symptoms?" To which the Gannett reporters responded: "Not any more. Well, here's a question for Hanchette and Brewer. Pick your favorite cause of GWS—chemical weapons, Scud fuel, sand flies, MCS—and explain why it would affect Americans three years before hitting soldiers in other countries.

"It's absolutely unmistakable" that "the symptoms are thoroughly psychosomatic," Shorter says. "The syndrome has no scientific status. It's entirely driven by political needs and the media's needs for sensationalism."

That's not entirely fair. Reporters like John Hanchette and Ed Bradley have probably convinced themselves they're doing vets a favor. They're not. Nor are the demagogic congressmen or the angry activists. You don't do people a favor by terrorizing them over their own health and that of their spouses and children. You don't do people a favor by replacing science with nonsense and reality with rumors.

It's been almost six years since the men and women who served us honorably in the Gulf War survived assault. They're still under assault, only now their enemy is more insidious, and, judging from the fear I saw in them, more successful.

# POSTSCRIPT

## Is the Gulf War Syndrome Real?

In *Hystories: Hysterical Epidemics and Modern Media* (Columbia University Press, 1997), author Elaine Showalter places the Gulf War Syndrome in the same category as tales of alien abduction and abuse by satanic cults; in other words, hysterias. She states that stress is capable of causing genuine illnesses but that people feel shameful about sickness with an emotional or psychological cause. Instead, they search for another explanation, such as the chemical weapons that produce anxiety attacks. Not everyone agrees with Showalter; see "Walking Wounded," *Esquire* (May 1994).

The U.S. government has tried to deny ill veterans disability pay because it maintains that there is no proof that these illnesses are connected with service in the gulf. Articles that question the legitimacy of the syndrome include "Studies Find No Medical Evidence of Syndrome," *Disease Weekly Plus* (January 6, 1997); "Research Is Incomplete and Inadequate," *Chemistry and Industry* (January 16, 1995); and "Pentagon Study Finds No Clinical Evidence for a Single Cause of Gulf War Syndrome," *Chemical and Engineering News* (December 19, 1994). In "The Truth About Health Scares," *Health Confidential* (May 1993), Michael Fumento discusses several media-hyped environmental causes of death.

Many people feel that the government's denial of any relationship between environmental factors present in the Persian Gulf and subsequent health concerns among Gulf War veterans is similar to the government's original denial of the adverse effects of Agent Orange on Vietnam veterans. See "Congress Cites Agent Orange Coverup," *Science* (August 31, 1990).

Other articles calling for more and better research into the Gulf War Syndrome and Agent Orange include "The Gulf War and Its Syndrome," *Washington Quarterly* (Spring 1998); "Gulf War's Syndrome," *The Nation* (December 1, 1997); "Darkness at Noon," *The Economist* (January 11, 1997); "The Gulf War Syndrome," *British Medical Journal* (vol. 310, 1995); "Institute of Medicine Calls for Coordinated Studies of Gulf War Veterans' Health Complaints," *Journal of the American Medical Association* (February 8, 1995); and "The Persian Gulf Experience and Health," *Journal of the American Medical Association* (August 3, 1994).

Readings that support the existence of the Gulf War Syndrome include "A Lingering Sickness," *The Nation* (January 23, 1995) and "Mal de Guerre," *The Nation* (March 7, 1994). Although the final word is not out on whether or not troops who served in the Persian Gulf War were exposed to environmental agents that triggered illnesses, many Americans are concerned that a Vietnam-style cover-up of the cause of these illnesses may exist.

# ISSUE 17

# Is Pesticide Exposure Harmful to Human Health?

**YES: Martha Honey,** from "Pesticides: Nowhere to Hide," *Ms.* (July/August 1995)

**NO: Bruce Ames,** from "Too Much Fuss About Pesticides," *Consumers' Research* (April 1990)

### ISSUE SUMMARY

**YES:** Martha Honey, a research fellow at the Institute for Policy Studies, asserts that pesticides in the food chain are building up in animals and humans and are disrupting the immune system, causing cancers, and creating birth defects.

**NO:** Bruce Ames, a professor of biochemistry and molecular biology, argues that any risks from pesticides in foods are minimal and that fears are greatly exaggerated.

Throughout history, farmers and other food growers have fought with insect and weed pests that invade the food supply and cause disease and discomfort. Early attempts to reduce pest damage included purely physical attacks—burning and stepping on the pests—as well as saying prayers and performing ritual dances. A few more effective measures were discovered before modern times. These included sulfur compounds, plant extracts, wood ashes, and natural pest enemies.

For the past 50 years, the battle against pests has escalated, and some of the most lethal and sophisticated chemicals ever invented have been used against them. When modern pesticides, such as DDT, were first introduced in the late 1940s, scientists proclaimed total victory against crop destruction and diseases carried by insects. Many dispute this victory, but the evidence of these chemical weapons is present in streams, rivers, and soils—and in our bodies. Most of us carry traces of several chemical pesticides in our body tissues. Moreover, although pesticides are used specifically to kill insect pests, many of them are quite toxic to humans as well. Pesticides are responsible for an estimated 25 million human poisonings each year, mostly of children under 10.

To cause harm to humans, a pesticide must be taken internally through the mouth, skin, or respiratory system. Eating unwashed fruit or vegetables that were recently sprayed with pesticides or entering a field too soon after pesticide application are ways in which pesticides may enter the body. Symptoms of acute or one-time exposure include headache, fatigue, abdominal pain, coma, and death. Long-term exposure may cause cancer, mutations, or birth defects.

Pesticide poisoning from sprayed fruit and vegetables became a national issue when reports of the contamination of apple crops made headlines. Since 1968 some red varieties of apples have been sprayed with a chemical growth regulator that prevents the apples from dropping off trees before they ripen, improves color and firmness, and extends shelf life. The chemical, known as daminozide, is marketed under the trade name Alar. Alar penetrates the pulp of the apple and cannot be washed, cooked, or peeled off. In 1986 processors and stores in the United States, bowing to consumer pressure, vowed not to accept apples treated with the chemical. It was reported that a breakdown product of Alar, which is formed when treated apples are heated, is a low-level cancer-causing agent.

A report released in spring 1987 by the National Academy of Sciences asserted that pesticides may be responsible for as many as 20,000 cases of cancer a year. In its report, the academy identified 15 foods (tomatoes, beef, potatoes, oranges, lettuce, peaches, pork, wheat, soybeans, beans, carrots, chicken, corn, grapes, and apples) treated with a small group of pesticides that pose the greatest risk of cancer. Although these figures are certainly frightening, many scientists believe that too much fuss is being raised about pesticides. They point out that many foods contain natural cancer-causing agents, and they argue that people are still better off with a high intake of fruits and vegetables—ironically because they contain nutrients that may help prevent cancer.

In the following selections, Martha Honey contends that a lot of the food that is sold in supermarkets is not safe and that the government does not adequately test the fruit and vegetables that are sold to the public. Bruce Ames maintains that it is good for consumers to be concerned about what they eat, but the hysteria about pesticide residues may not be warranted by the actual risk they pose.

# YES

## Martha Honey

# PESTICIDES: NOWHERE TO HIDE

Walk into almost any supermarket these days, any month of the year, and feast your eyes: towering pyramids of grapefruit, baskets of unblemished tomatoes and cucumbers, heaping bins of avocados and kiwifruit, stacks of ripened strawberries. Nowadays, the health-conscious U.S. consumer, transcending the inconveniences of the season, is serviced 12 months of the year by fruit and vegetable growers the world over. But if you're concerned that the produce section at your local market has come to resemble a wax museum, you have good reason. The abundance and variety of fresh, picture-perfect produce is brought to you and your family at a price—and not just at the cash register.

More than 30 years have passed since Rachel Carson called world attention to the health and environmental hazards of DDT and other pesticides in her landmark book, *Silent Spring.* "If we are going to live so intimately with these chemicals—eating and drinking them, taking them into the very marrow of our bones," Carson wrote, "we had better know something about their nature and their power." There is now ample proof that Carson's early warning was well founded: at least 136 active ingredients in pesticides have been found to cause cancer in humans or animals. But global pesticide use continues to escalate as farmers and food companies look for increasingly efficient methods to expand their markets. While Carson's book paved the way for the creation of the Environmental Protection Agency (EPA) in 1970, government efforts to protect the nation's food and water supply have moved at a snail's pace—of the 136 aforementioned carcinogenic chemicals, 79 are still being used on U.S. food crops. And the few, hard-won legislative gains that have been made by consumer, labor, and environmental advocates are currently being torpedoed in the Republican-controlled Congress.

The U.S. is one of the world's largest users of pesticides, and it's the top exporter. Sales in the U.S. total close to $8 billion. With annual overseas sales of $2.4 billion, or 44 billion pounds of chemicals, U.S. companies export more than 25 tons of pesticides *every hour.* In what has been dubbed the "circle of poison," at least one third of the pesticides exported have been banned or limited for use in this country—but they often return to consumers as residue on imported produce. While the U.S. imports only 9 percent of its vegetables, more than a quarter of the fruit sold here is imported; in winter, 40 to 60 percent of produce comes from abroad.

In the mid-1980s, the U.S. government made a major push to get many Latin American and Caribbean countries to grow new "designer" crops—strawberries, melons, and asparagus—all intended for the U.S. market and most, as they are not native to the region, heavily dependent on chemical fertilizers and pesticides. As a result, Latin America leads the Southern Hemisphere in pesticide use per acre and it supplies nearly 80 percent of U.S. fruit and vegetable imports. Not surprisingly, U.S. agricultural experts in Costa Rica, who conducted a survey of pesticide residues on strawberries in the late 1980s, refused to release their results. "But I can tell you one thing," confided one official involved in the study. "I won't eat the strawberries."

But while consumers are subject to long-term, low-level pesticide exposure from both domestic and imported produce, agricultural workers' concerns are more immediate. Each year 25 million people, primarily in the Southern Hemisphere, are poisoned through occupational exposure to pesticides; of those, 220,000 die, according to the World Health Organization (WHO). In the U.S., 300,000 farmworkers are poisoned each year.

Pesticides fall into three main categories—insecticides, herbicides, and fungicides—and they are designed to control or eliminate unwanted insects, weeds, and plant-killing fungi; each contains an "active ingredient," or the poison that kills the pest, and an "inert" carrying or spreading compound. When first developed after World War II, pesticides were hailed as miracle chemicals that would protect crops and homes, make food more plentiful and safe, and wipe out world hunger. Erika Rosenthal, Latin America Program Coordinator with the San Francisco-based Pesticides Action Network (PAN), has a late-1940s poster advertising DDT hanging in her office. The text at the bottom reads: "The great expectations held for DDT have been realized. During 1946, exhaustive scientific tests have shown that, when properly used, DDT kills a host of destructive insect pests and is a benefactor of all humanity."

But by the late 1950s, scientific evidence was already mounting that DDT was not only a potent carcinogen, but it also posed a serious threat to the environment—it is now cited as the cause of the near-extinction of the bald eagle, brown pelican, and condor. Despite its prominence in *Silent Spring* it wasn't until 1972 that DDT was finally banned in the U.S., and it is still manufactured in Mexico, India, and Indonesia and used in some developing countries. "DDT had the dubious fame of being one of the most widespread contaminants of the ecosystem," says PAN's Rosenthal. "Dangerously high concentrations have been found in the breast milk of mothers in Central America. It's also been found in the fat of Arctic polar bears. So it's covered the globe," she says. DDT remains in the food chain as a result of soil and water contamination. As recently as 1993, a study found higher levels of DDE (which is formed when DDT breaks down) in U.S. women who had developed breast cancer than in women who had not.

Pesticides are now everywhere—in our food, drinking water, homes, yards, and air. But it's difficult to rate the worst pesticides. "It's Russian roulette. Pick your poison: acutely toxic, chronically hazardous, cancer-causing, or effect unknown," says Sandra Marquardt, pesticide consultant at Consumers Union in Washington, D.C. Most often, we are exposed simultaneously to a variety of types, although the EPA sets safety levels by testing only one active ingredient at a time. And even when pesticides are banned, they are often used illegally by U.S. growers. Lax enforcement of EPA regulations by the Food and Drug Administration (FDA) makes it possible for many farmers to continue to use their pesticides of choice.

In addition to breast cancer, cancers of the reproductive system have been linked to pesticides. Infants and young children are especially vulnerable to pesticides. "Millions of children in the United States receive up to 35 percent of their entire lifetime dose of some carcinogenic pesticides by age five," reports a study by the Washington, D.C.-based Environmental Working Group (EWG). There is growing evidence that pesticides also cause a variety of birth defects and genetic mutations. And one of the newest and most worrisome findings is that some pesticides—known as "hormone imitating" chemicals or "endocrine disrupters" —are building up in animals and humans and disrupting reproduction, immunity, and metabolism. In a recent National Wildlife Federation study, "Fertility on the Brink," University of Florida zoologist Louis Guillette writes: "We've released endocrine disrupters throughout the world that are having fundamental effects on the immune system and the reproductive system.... Should we be upset? I think we should be screaming in the streets."

Neither the government nor the pesticide industry has responded with much urgency to the long-term health risks faced by consumers—or the daily risks faced by farmworkers. On the evening of November 14, 1989, a few miles outside Tampa, Florida, the insecticide mevinphos was sprayed on Goodson Farms' 16 acres of cauliflower. Early the next morning, farm managers sent migrant laborers into the dewy fields to tie up the plants. Within several hours, scores were complaining of headaches, dizziness, blurred vision, slurred speech, and breathing difficulties. They began vomiting, having convulsions, and staggering out of the field; several passed out. By late afternoon an estimated 112 farmworkers were treated at the scene or at area hospitals. Thirteen were admitted to hospitals. In the following months, dozens of the workers continued to suffer symptoms, and one pregnant woman miscarried.

Florida doctors called this one of the worst cases of pesticide poisonings they had ever seen. Goodson Farms managers were fined by state authorities for sending workers into the field too soon after spraying and not giving them proper protective gear. But Goodson's fine was later reduced from $12,600 to only $7,000. And the president of Amvac Chemical Corporation, which makes mevinphos under the brand name Phosdrin, continues to praise the product: Eric Wintemute describes it as "a neat compound" and "100 percent clean" because, he says, it leaves no permanent residue on crops; its "acute toxicity" simply means it must be applied with care.

"Even if this chemical is applied as directed it can still poison the workers," remarks Michael Hancock, executive director of the Washington, D.C.-based Farmworker Justice Fund. He calls mevinphos "the single most harmful pesticide to farmworkers." For years, labor advocates have urged the EPA to speed up its pesticide review process and ban chemicals like mevinphos, which is used on some 50 crops. Finally, in June 1994, the EPA made the unusual decision to issue an "emergency suspension order" that would have taken mevinphos off the market immediately.

But the day before the order was to be implemented, the EPA received a call from Amvac's lawyer, Steven Schatzow, saying the company had decided to "voluntarily" withdraw the pesticide from the U.S. market. Schatzow was no stranger to the EPA: he had been the agency's director of pesticide programs under Ronald Reagan. This was classic Washington revolving-door politics. Despite current EPA administrator Carol Browner's pledge to "break the gridlock on pesticide reform," Schatzow and the EPA struck a deal: Amvac agreed to stop producing mevinphos for use in the U.S., but the company was given until the end of 1994 to sell off its supply. And then after the Republicans' congressional sweep last November, the EPA agreed to give Amvac until the end of November 1995 "for sale, distribution, and use of existing stocks of mevinphos products."

Environmentalists are furious. "It's ridiculous. The EPA caved in," says Marquardt at Consumers Union. "It gave Amvac another year to dump this poison on the American people," adds Hancock, who sees the EPA's handling of mevinphos as a sign of the chilling effect the Republicans' Contract with America is having on the Clinton administration. "The EPA got the message not to do anything that would create headlines saying REGULATORY ACTION FORCES COMPANY OUT OF BUSINESS."

Amvac has continued to sell mevinphos overseas, in such countries as Thailand and South Africa. Under U.S. law, the 43 active ingredients in pesticides that the EPA has deemed too dangerous for use in the U.S.—along with the hundreds of pesticide ingredients that haven't been registered by the EPA— can be exported. Dr. Robert McConnell, a World Health Organization pesticides expert, says he is most worried about unregistered pesticides exported to the Southern Hemisphere because "there is virtually no data on them." And the FDA doesn't monitor imported produce any better than domestic. Although FDA border inspectors are supposed to examine a "representative sample" of produce entering the country, few fruits and vegetables are screened. "Ninety-nine percent sail through untouched," says Marquardt. "There are so few inspectors out there, and they are more concerned with testing cosmetic appearance than pesticide residues." And about one third of the shipments detected with hazardous pesticide residues reach U.S. supermarkets anyway, due to halfhearted enforcement efforts and bureaucratic delays. "It is as if we were selling bombs around the world that come back and explode in our own backyards," Congressman Sam Gejdenson (D.-Conn.) testified at 1994 hearings on pesticide exports.

Ironically, as more humans are sickened or killed by pesticides, more strains of insects, mites, weeds, and rodents are developing immunity to these chemicals. In *Silent Spring*, Carson found that 137 species of insects and mites had already become pesticide-resistant; today it is more than 500. According to Cornell University Professor David Pimentel, the amount of crops lost to insects in the U.S. "has almost doubled during the last 40 years, despite a more than tenfold increase in the amount and toxicity of synthetic insecticides used."

Nevertheless, growers, both in the U.S. and abroad, are becoming increasingly reliant on pesticides. "My greatest concern is the expanded use of pesticides—the doubling [in the U.S.] over the last 30 years—and the effect it can have on our children, our water, air, and land," says the EPA's Browner. "And it's outrageous," she adds, "that a product banned here can be sold in other countries." But Browner, a longtime environmental activist, has not been able to "end the cycle of compromise" at the EPA, says Jay Feldman of the National Coalition Against the Misuse of Pesticides. She got points in early 1994 for proposing legislation that would create stricter safety standards for both domestic and imported produce, as well as stop the export of banned pesticides. But the administration's proposal never even made it out of the House agricultural committee last year, and this year it will not be reintroduced. It was "blocked by the pesticide lobby," which wields "tremendous power," says Browner, particularly in the current Republican-controlled Congress. "Now legislation is being written by the [pesticide industry] lobbyists." But labor advocates like Michael Hancock contend that the Clinton administration pressured the EPA to bow out too soon: "The agency seems to be in full retreat. They just surrender when they should stand and put up a fight over principle."

Behind the current antiregulatory fervor is the benign-sounding American Crop Protection Association, or ACPA (formerly the National Agricultural Chemical Association), the pesticide industry's main lobby. Comprised of 83 chemical companies, including such giants as DuPont, DOW, Monsanto, Velsicol, and American Cyanimid, this Washington, D.C.-based trade association commands enormous political clout, in part through campaign contributions to key members of the House and Senate agricultural committees. ACPA member companies constitute a global pesticide supermarket, selling to virtually every country in both the Northern and Southern Hemispheres. And ACPA members have done little to ensure that workers—especially in the South—use their products safely. Scores of studies and press accounts show that workers often are given little or no training in handling the chemicals. Many cannot read labels, frequently mix pesticides with their bare hands, and carry home the poisons on their bodies and clothing. Hazardous chemicals spill or are dumped into fields, rivers, or ponds, and the poison-laced containers are reused for storing food, water, or seeds. "It's very difficult to have safe use under tropical conditions, by small farmers wearing backpacks. The packs leak and it's too hot and too expensive to wear protective clothing," says WHO's McConnell. Four years ago, DOW was sued by male Costa Rican banana workers who were showing up sterile after years of exposure to the highly toxic pesticide DBCP; women workers and family members who were also exposed were left out of the suit but are currently documenting their high rates of miscarriages, birth defects, and cancer in preparation for a suit of their own.

In 1991, ACPA opened its first "safe use" project to train growers in Guatemala, Thailand, and Kenya. "We recognized we had to roll up our sleeves and get involved," says John McCarthy of ACPA's international division. The association's commitment to "safe use" is minuscule: $400,000 a year and one staff person in each country. But it makes good PR—as ACPA President Jay Vroom told

Congress, these projects show industry's "advances" in "product stewardship and worker safety." "Three pilot projects four decades too late—how dare [they] make such claims?" says one health expert who has worked on pesticide safety programs in the Southern Hemisphere. "This 'safe use' is about buying companies another ten years" to export their goods, he says.

Little will change for either workers or consumers until farmers move away from an "agrochemical-intensive model of production," says PAN's Rosenthal. The right direction, say activists, is toward organic farming. The EPA's Browner agrees: "We know how to grow food with fewer chemicals, and that should be our goal." EWG's Richard Wiles, who directed a National Academy of Sciences' study of alternative farming methods, says, "It's possible to grow an affordable, abundant food supply using few or no synthetic chemicals. For all major field crops—corn, soybean, wheat, barley—the science is there. You can eliminate pesticides that pose serious health risks and maintain current levels of production." What's missing, Wiles explains, is the incentive. "American farmers have very minimal regulatory or market incentive to cut back on pesticides. They see the chemicals as legal, loosely regulated, and a low-cost form of insurance, and farmers don't pay any of the cost of the environmental consequences. So what the hell? Why change?"

Contract with America Republicans are hell-bent on pushing through more deregulation and corporate perks. But they may be misreading the mood of the country. A poll commissioned by the National Wildlife Federation just after the 1994 elections found that 41 percent of people in the U.S. believe that existing regulations "don't go far enough

in protecting the environment," that 46 percent agree that laws "do not require businesses to do enough to protect the environment," and that 64 percent say that government should pay subsidies to farmers for pesticide reduction.

The public's increasing health consciousness is reflected in organic food sales, which have skyrocketed over the past five years. And the emerging market is attracting a number of big food companies, a few of which have opened up organic divisions. Such rapid expansion—involving pesticide-happy companies—has prompted calls among some activists for federal regulation for the largely self-regulated organic food industry.

The growth of the organic market confirms what Betsy Lydon, of the New York City-based group Mothers and Others for a Livable Planet, has long maintained: "Change has to happen in the marketplace. Your food dollars *can* be very powerful." Her group, which has a mailing list of 25,000, is sponsoring a nationwide "shoppers' campaign" for healthier food choices. Members in Kentucky, Illinois, and New York are working with supermarket chains like D'Agostino's and Dominick's to encourage them to offer more organic food—which in many cases, Lydon says, is just slightly more expensive than nonorganic. When there is a real disparity, she says, "people need to talk to their retailer about price gouging. They should not be selling organic food as gourmet food." Lydon's group also spearheaded a project in Lexington, Kentucky, called a "buying club," involving 26 organic farmers and 100 families. The families give the farmers money in the early part of the season for seeds and supplies; come harvest, the farmers deliver their organic produce to the families at below-market rates.

Other groups, like the New York City-based Women's Environment and Development Organization (WEDO), are focusing on political action. WEDO is planning a series of nationwide "hearings" ... on the links between environmental factors, like pesticides, and breast cancer. WEDO is working in coalition with groups like One in Nine, a Long Island breast cancer awareness organization that is campaigning to get New York State to establish a pesticide registry that would be open to the public. "We found out that farmers have to register what they use and that information is supposed to go to the government. But they put the records into cartons and no one has access to them," says Geri Barish, head of One in Nine's Pesticide Project. "We want to know how much is used, where it's used, and what the studies say." A bill mandating such a registry made it through the state assembly [in 1994], but the farm lobby killed it in the senate. Barish is determined to get it reintroduced. Although "we're just volunteers and many of us are not well," says Barish, "we decided we're not going to go away."

Internationally, the pesticide industry is running into roadblocks—many countries in the south have banned importation of the most deadly chemicals. And there are other advances: a United Nations-sponsored rice farmer training program in Southeast Asia has cut pesticide use in the region by 90 percent; in Sweden, pesticide use was reduced by 50 percent between 1985 and 1990; in Colombia, sugar growers use beneficial insects instead of pesticides; and some Cuban farmers, forced to go organic because of trade sanctions, now say that they don't want to go back to chemicals. "The global movement against pesticide misuse has grown fantastically in the last 10 to 15 years," says PAN's Rosenthal. "Today we have thousands of organizations around the world pushing for sustainable and healthy agricultural techniques." But only the combined efforts of activists and consumers, working against official indifference to the public's health, can hope to one day repel the "chemical barrage that has been hurled against the fabric of life," in the words of Rachel Carson. Although life is "delicate and destructible," Carson wrote, it is also "tough and resilient, and capable of striking back in unexpected ways."

# NO

Bruce Ames

# TOO MUCH FUSS ABOUT PESTICIDES

In the wake of the Alar-in-apples scare last year [1989], consumers have become highly concerned about the threat posed to their health by the ingestion of trace amounts of man-made pesticides. While it is good for consumers to be concerned about what they eat, the hysteria about pesticide residues may not be warranted by the actual risk they pose. In helping consumers develop a fuller picture of the true risk of man-made pesticides (or other chemical additives to food), we present below an excerpt of a letter from Dr. Bruce Ames to *Consumer Reports* magazine. The letter was in response to an article run in that magazine (October 1989), which, according to Dr. Ames, "distorts my views and misstates facts." ...

—Ed. [of Consumers' Research.]

*Consumer Reports'* four-page attack on my scientific work both distorts my views and misstates the facts on which they are based. Good scientists are committed to challenging assumptions rigorously, and this is particularly important in the prevention of cancer, a murky, complex, multidisciplinary field to which I have devoted much of my scientific career. Sound public policy should be based on sound science, and new data or theory may require altering some prevailing assumptions.

In our efforts to prevent human cancer, it makes no sense to apply a double standard for human exposures to natural vs. synthetic chemicals. My colleagues and I have therefore attempted to provide an overview of possible carcinogenic hazards.

The following points clarify my views and their factual and theoretical basis:

**1) Discovering the Causes of Cancer.** Epidemiologists are continually coming up with clues about the causes of different types of human cancer, and these hypotheses are then refined by animal and metabolic studies. This approach will, in my view, lead to the understanding of the causal factors for the major human cancers during the next decade. Current epidemiologic data point to the major risk factors for human cancer as cigarette smoking (which is responsible for 30% of cancer), dietary imbalances, hormones, viruses, and lifestyle factors—not to such factors as water pollution or synthetic pesticide residues.

For example, epidemiologists in many countries have identified excessive salt as a risk factor for stomach cancer, one of the major types of cancer. Extensive experimental work in rodents on salt as a co-carcinogen supports the epidemiology. Yet *Consumer Reports* unfairly criticized Edith Efron for saying that salt is a carcinogen.

*Consumer Reports* criticized me for calling alcohol a carcinogen, yet alcoholic beverages, of numerous types, are carcinogenic in humans at a level of 5 drinks/day. Alcohol itself was positive in one rat test and also was co-carcinogenic in other tests. Acetaldehyde, the main metabolite of alcohol, is a carcinogen in rodents. Most of the leading scientists in the field believe that the active ingredient in alcoholic beverages is alcohol itself. I think that chronic high doses of alcohol are active by causing cell proliferation and inflammation and that, therefore, low doses are not of much interest.

**2) Animal Cancer Tests.** There are three fundamental problems with the use of animal cancer tests in trying to prevent human cancer from low-dose human exposures.

a) There are millions of chemicals in the world that we are exposed to in low or moderate doses, 99.9+% of which are natural. To identify significant risks, we need to identify the right chemicals to test in rodents.

b) About half of the chemicals tested in long-term bioassays in both rats and mice have been found to be carcinogens at the high doses administered, the maximum tolerated dose (MTD). Synthetic industrial chemicals account for almost all (82%) of the chemicals (427) tested in both species. However, despite the fact that humans eat vastly more natural than synthetic chemicals, only a small number (75) of *natural* chemicals have been tested in both rats and mice. For the 75 natural chemicals the proportion of positive results (47%) is similar, also about *half*. While some synthetic or natural chemicals were selected for testing precisely because of suspect structures, most chemicals were tested because they were natural or synthetic food additives, colors, high volume industrial compounds, pesticides, or natural or synthetic drugs. Thus, the high proportion of carcinogens among synthetic test agents in rodent studies is not simply due to selection of suspicious chemical structures, and the natural world of chemicals has never been looked at systematically. Recent research into the mechanism of carcinogenesis (see #4 below) supports the idea that when tested in rodents at the MTD, a high proportion of all chemicals we test in the future, whether natural or synthetic, will prove to be carcinogenic.

c) The problem of knowing whether there is any risk at all from the very low doses of human exposure to chemicals causing tumors in rodents at very high doses has been argued by toxicologists and regulators for years, precisely because one cannot measure effects at low doses. Regulators have opted for worst-case estimates, using assumptions that increasing scientific evidence suggests may be incorrect.

Because conventional risk assessment is focused mainly on man-made chemicals and is based on worst-case assumptions that we believe are proving to exaggerate hazard greatly, many leading scientists have argued that it is misleading to the public to try to present estimates of "worst-case risk" from animal studies in terms of expected numbers of human cancers. Our HERP [Human Exposure/Rodent Potency, Dr. Ames's index for estimating carcinogenic risk] uses essentially the same information as that in conventional risk assessment, but is explicitly intended as a relative scale. We have attempted to achieve some perspective on the plethora of possible hazards to humans from exposure to known rodent carcinogens by establishing a scale of the possible hazards for the amounts of various common carcinogens to which humans might be chronically exposed. We view the value of our calculations not as providing a basis for absolute human risk assessment, but as a guide for priority setting.

Carcinogens clearly do not all work in the same way, and as we learn more about the mechanisms, HERP comparisons can be refined, as can risk assessments.

Thus, if the public is told that the possible hazard of the UDMH residue [the breakdown product of Alar] in a daily glass of apple juice (about 30 parts per billion) is 1/18 that of aflatoxin (a mold carcinogen) in a daily peanut butter sandwich (the Food and Drug Administration [FDA] allows 10 times that residue level), 1/50 that of a daily mushroom, and 1/1,000 that of a daily beer, it puts these items in perspective. The possible relative hazard of a daily apple is at least 10× less than the apple juice. This is quite different from showing a witch's hand holding an apple [as was depicted on the May 1989 *Consumer Reports* cover on Alar—Ed].

**3) Pesticides, 99.99% All Natural.** All plants produce toxins to protect themselves against fungi, insects, and animal predators such as man. Tens of thousands of these natural pesticides have been discovered, and every species of plant contains its own set of different toxins, usually a few dozen. In addition, when plants are stressed or damaged, such as during a pest attack, they increase their natural pesticide levels many fold, occasionally to levels that are acutely toxic to humans. We estimate that Americans eat about 1,500 mg/day of natural pesticides, 10,000 times more than man-made pesticide residues, which FDA estimates at a total of 0.15 mg/day. Their concentration is usually measured in parts per thousand or million, rather than parts per billion (ppb), the usual concentration of synthetic pesticide residues and pollutants in water. We estimate that Americans are ingesting 5,000 to 10,000 different natural pesticides and their breakdown products, a subset of the tremendous number of natural chemicals we ingest. For example, there are 49 different natural pesticides (and breakdown products) ingested in eating cabbage.

Surprisingly few plant pesticides have been tested in animal cancer bioassays, but among those tested, again about *half* (25 out of 47) are carcinogenic. A search for the presence of just these 25 carcinogens in foods indicates that they occur naturally in the following (those at levels over 50,000 ppb are listed in parentheses); anise, apples (50,000+ ppb), bananas, basil (4 million ppb), broccoli, Brussels sprouts (500,000 ppb), cabbage (100,000 ppb), cantaloupe, carrots (50,000+ ppb), cauliflower, celery (50,000+ ppb), cinnamon, cloves, cocoa, coffee (brewed) (90,000 ppb), comfrey tea, fennel (3 million ppb), grapefruit juice, honeydew melon, horseradish (4 million ppb), kale, lettuce (300,000 ppb), mushrooms, mustard (black) (40 million ppb), nutmeg (5 million ppb), orange juice (30,000 ppb), parsley, parsnips (30,000 ppb), peaches, black pepper (100,000 ppb), pineapples, potatoes (50,000+ ppb), radishes, raspberries, strawberries, tarragon (1 million ppb), and turnips.

There is every reason to expect that we will continue to find mutagens and carcinogens among nature's pesticides if we ever test them systematically. In short-term tests for detecting mutagens, the proportion of natural pesticides that turn up positive is just as high as for synthetic industrial chemicals. In a compendium on the ability of 950 chemicals to break chromosomes in animal tests, there were 62 natural pesticides: half of them were positive. Thus, it seems highly probable that almost every plant product in the supermarket will contain natural carcinogens at much higher levels than those of man-made pesticides. We have suggested that many more natural pesticides (and chemicals from cooking of food) be tested in long-term bioassays.

Additionally, there is a fundamental trade-off between nature's pesticides and man-made pesticides. We can easily breed out many of nature's pesticides to protect our crops from being eaten by insects. In contrast, growers are currently breeding some plants for insect resistance and unwittingly raising the levels of natural pesticides. A new variety of insect-resistant celery that is being widely sold is almost 10× higher in carcinogens (6,200 ppb) than standard celery.

**4) Mechanisms of Carcinogenesis.** In the rapidly advancing field of mechanisms of carcinogenesis, there is now evidence to suggest that cell proliferation is extremely important. A large number of the major human carcinogens such as hormones, chronic viral infection, salt, asbestos, and alcohol are likely to be primarily active through causing cell proliferation. A cell is at considerably greater genetic risk during division, so chronic cell proliferation in itself is a mutagenic and carcinogenic stress. Cancers induced in animal cancer tests done at high doses seem to be primarily caused by cell proliferation, in part due to chronic cell killing, and inflammation that results from high toxic doses. This would be in agreement with the high proportion of all chemicals that are turning out to be carcinogens at high doses and the relation of toxicity to carcinogenic potency. The induction of cell proliferation is restricted to high doses, and this strongly suggests that low doses of carcinogens are of no risk, or are very much less hazardous than has been assumed.

In addition, humans, who live in a world of natural toxins, are well protected by many layers of inducible general defenses against low doses of toxins—defenses that do not distinguish between synthetic and natural toxins. Therefore, even the high levels of natural plant pesticides may not be of much concern in a balanced diet.

**5) Trade-offs.** Identifying and controlling the major causes of human cancer are not a matter of blame. We have tried in our scientific work to put into perspective the tiny exposures to pesticide residues by comparing them to the enormous background of natural substances. Minimizing pollution is a separate issue, and is clearly desirable, aside from any effect on public health, but it involves economic trade-offs. As a society, efforts to regulate pesticides or other synthetic rodent carcinogens down to the ppb level inevitably involve understanding these trade-offs. Synthetic pesticides (and chemicals such as Alar) have markedly lowered the cost of our food, a major advance in nutrition and, thus, health. Every complex mixture from gasoline to cooked food to orange juice contains rodent carcinogens. When people drive to work, put logs on a fire, or make a barbecue they are putting carcinogens into the air. There are costs and benefits to all of these. Exaggerating the risks from man-made substances, ignoring the natural world, and converting the issue to one of blaming U.S. industry does not advance our public health efforts. If we spend all our efforts on minimal, rather than important, hazards, we hurt public health. The Environmental Protection Agency (EPA) is trying to prevent hypothetical risks of 1 in a million at enormous economic cost. Yet the leading scientists trying to prevent cancer are working on numerous possible carcinogenic risks in the 1 in a 100 to 1 in 10 range: my lab is working on 4 that we think are in this range.

# POSTSCRIPT

## Is Pesticide Exposure Harmful to Human Health?

Increased consumer fear of pesticide residues on food has encouraged many activists to push for a ban on pesticide use. Although doing so might provide some health benefits, Ronald Knutson, director of the Agricultural and Food Policy Center at Texas A & M University, believes that such a ban would cause a significant rise in food prices. In "Pesticide-Free Equals Higher Food Prices," *Consumers' Research* (November 1990), Knutson and his colleagues argue that if there were a complete ban on the use of pesticides, food bills would rise at least 12 percent, crop yields would fall, and there would need to be a 10 percent increase in cultivated acreage, which would result in a corresponding rise in soil erosion.

An investigation by Constance Matthiessen challenges the opinions of Knutson and others. Matthiessen, writing in *Mother Jones* (March/April 1992), takes the position that despite the widespread use of pesticides, insects and weeds seem to be doing as much damage as ever. The reason: insects and weeds have the ability to adapt and evolve to become pesticide-resistant. As a result, the share of crop yields lost to pests has almost doubled over the last 40 years. Environmentalist Shirley A. Briggs agrees that pesticides have failed to decrease crop losses while causing widespread environmental damage. In "Silent Spring: The View from 1990," *The Ecologist* (March/April 1990), Briggs argues that we must find ways to reduce pesticide dependence. Other articles that support this viewpoint include "Organic: A Four-Letter Word," *Vegetarian Times* (March 1996) and "Breasticides," *Earth Island Journal* (Fall 1996), which discusses the relationship between pesticides and breast cancer.

Robert J. Scheuplein, a scientist with the Office of Toxicological Sciences at the Food and Drug Administration, shares the opinions of Ames. In "The Risk from Food," *Consumers' Research* (April 1990), Scheuplein argues that the public has an unrealistic view of pesticides and that other factors, particularly overall diet, contribute much more to the development of different cancers than pesticide-treated foods.

Most scientists agree that pesticide residues can affect human health to *some* degree. Many experts, however, maintain that current levels of residues are insignificant and that our food supply is safe. The articles "Ban All Plants —They Pollute," *Forbes* (October 24, 1993); "Proposed Food Safety Laws Are Starved for Scientific Merit," *Insight on the News* (November 1, 1993); "Are People Too Worried About Carcinogens for Their Own Good?" *Business Week* (October 19, 1992); and "Do Pesticides Cause Cancer?" *Consumers' Research*

(December 1991) argue that people are overly concerned about low levels of man-made chemicals in food when there are numerous natural carcinogens present. Dennis Avery, the director of global food issues at the Hudson Institute, believes that it is habitat loss, not chemicals, that we should be most worried about. In his book *Biodiversity: Saving Species With Biotechnology* (Hudson Institute, 1993), Avery states that the "judicious use of modern pesticides can increase agricultural yields without creating any significant increase in the risk of developing cancer." Environmental journalist Ronald Bailey, writing in "Once and Future Farming," *Garbage: The Independent Environmental Quarterly* (Fall 1994), argues that pesticides and fertilizers are needed to feed the world population. An overall analysis of the pesticide risk/benefit relationship can be found in "EPA Begins Initial Approval," *Chemical Week* (February 12, 1997) and "Regulating Pesticides," *CQ Researcher* (January 28, 1994). Others argue that pesticides pose health risks, are environmentally unsound, and do not work in the long run, because many pests have become resistant to them. For an overview of the National Research Council of the National Academy of Science report on safety of current levels of pesticides in foods and the health of children, see "Pesticides and Kids' Risks," *Newsweek* (June 1, 1998); "Some Good News on Pesticide Risks from Produce," *Child Health Alert* (January 1998); and "Pesticide Risks from Produce Judged Slight," *Pediatric Alert* (December 11, 1997). Researching alternatives to pesticides, as described in "Organics: Hot Debate," *Vegetarian Times* (August 1993) and "Could Marigolds Stop Killer Mosquitoes?" *New Scientist* (July 17, 1993), may be a safer, more ecologically sound, and ultimately more successful approach to limiting pest damage than is maintaining a total reliance on chemicals.

# ISSUE 18

## Public Policy and Health: Is Global Warming a Real Threat?

**YES: Ross Gelbspan,** from "The Heat Is On," *Harper's Magazine* (December 1995)

**NO: Arthur B. Robinson and Zachary W. Robinson,** from "Science Has Spoken: Global Warming Is a Myth," *The Wall Street Journal* (December 4, 1997)

### ISSUE SUMMARY

**YES:** Journalist Ross Gelbspan contends that we need to act now to prevent future catastrophic climatic changes that may result from global warming.

**NO:** Chemists Arthur B. Robinson and Zachary W. Robinson argue that even though carbon dioxide levels have increased during the past 20 years, global temperatures have decreased.

For the past several hundred million years, the relative concentrations of the four major gases in the atmosphere—nitrogen, oxygen, argon, and carbon dioxide ($CO_2$)—have remained constant. Within recent decades, however, scientists have been concerned that an increase in the amount of atmospheric $CO_2$ may be occurring due to the rapid rise in the burning of fossil fuels and the global slashing and burning of forests. When fossil fuels are burned, $CO_2$ is released. The natural processes that absorb excess $CO_2$ are currently being overwhelmed by the huge volume being released from industry, automobiles and other forms of transportation, and the burning of tropical forests. As a result, the concentration of $CO_2$ is rising at the rate of .05 percent per year, or a 12 percent increase since 1960.

Although $CO_2$ is not toxic to human beings, there is concern over its effect on global temperatures, a phenomenon known as the greenhouse effect. Carbon dioxide in the atmosphere appears to act as a blanket around the Earth, increasing the absorption of heat from the sun. This blanketing has already appeared to affect the Earth's average temperature. In 1988 a team of researchers from NASA found that the global mean temperature is now almost one degree Fahrenheit warmer than it was a century ago. A scientific panel made up of several hundred eminent researchers working under the sponsorship of the United Nations and the International Panel on Climate Change (IPCC) concluded that the reality of global warming cannot be ignored. In a 1990 report, the IPCC claimed that the projected increases in $CO_2$ would result in the average global temperature rising three to eight degrees within the next 100 years, making the Earth warmer than ever before in recorded history.

Although a warmer Earth may not seem to be a crisis, several health and environmental effects could be disastrous. The increasing frequency of excessive heat waves will have an impact on human illness and death rates. Extreme heat will cause deaths due to heart attacks and stroke, and certain diseases spread by mosquitoes and other vectors, such as malaria, may spread from warmer to colder climates. Hotter weather could affect crop yields and the long-term survival of certain plants and animals. The most dramatic consequence of global warming will be a worldwide rise in sea level related to the melting of the Antarctic and Greenland ice caps. This could mean flooding of low-lying coastal areas and loss of coastal wetlands.

For the past 25 years, climatologists have been warning about the rise in global temperatures. They have urged policymakers to take action to prevent a doomsday scenario. Since 1980 the 10 hottest summers on record have added urgency to demands that the government launch efforts to reduce the emission of greenhouse gases. Although $CO_2$ is the primary greenhouse gas, several other gases (methane, nitrous oxide, and chlorofluorocarbons) are further enhancing the greenhouse effect by absorbing waves of heat. A call for action, however, is easier than actually implementing change. At the Earth Summit in Brazil in 1992, representatives from 12 countries agreed to stabilize concentrations of greenhouse gases at 1990 levels. In 1993 President Bill Clinton vowed that the United States would comply. Unfortunately, even if all nations who signed the pact were to move immediately to cap emissions, global temperatures would continue to rise. Only if emissions were *slashed* would there be a genuine decline in atmospheric $CO_2$ levels. Because of the economic impact, no nation is currently contemplating this action.

Can anything be done to reduce the greenhouse gases? Several policy options, including improving energy efficiency, switching to alternative sources such as solar and wind energy, and replanting forests are possible. Green plants remove $CO_2$ from the air during photosynthesis. The worldwide cutting and burning of forests has removed this $CO_2$ consumer, contributing to a rise in atmospheric $CO_2$.

Many eminent scientists believe that global warming will have a catastrophic effect on human health and the well-being of the planet. In the following selections, Ross Gelbspan argues that although the energy industry claims otherwise, the Earth's temperature continues to climb, and this will have a catastrophic effect. Arthur B. Robinson and Zachary W. Robinson state that there is no evidence that humans have been responsible for increasing worldwide temperatures. They also assert that carbon dioxide emissions have actually improved the environment.

# YES

Ross Gelbspan

# THE HEAT IS ON

After my lawn had burned away to straw last summer, and the local papers announced that the season had been one of the driest in the recorded history of New England, I found myself wondering how long we can go on pretending that nothing is amiss with the world's weather. It wasn't just the fifty ducks near my house that had died when falling water levels in a creek exposed them to botulism-infested mud, or the five hundred people dead in the Midwest from an unexpected heat wave that followed the season's second "one-hundred-year flood" in three years. It was also the news from New Orleans (overrun by an extraordinary number of cockroaches and termites after a fifth consecutive winter without a killing frost), from Spain (suffering a fourth year of drought in a region that ordinarily enjoys a rainfall of 84 inches a year), and from London (Britain's meteorological office reporting the driest summer since 1727 and the hottest since 1659).

The reports of changes in the world's climate have been with us for fifteen or twenty years, most urgently since 1988, when Dr. James Hansen, director of NASA's Goddard Institute for Space Studies, declared that the era of global warming was at hand. As a newspaper correspondent who had reported on the United Nations Conferences on the environment in Stockholm in 1972 and in Rio in 1992, I understood something of the ill effects apt to result from the extravagant burning of oil and coal. New record-setting weather extremes seem to have become as commonplace as traffic accidents, and three simple facts have long been known: the distance from the surface of the earth to the far edge of the inner atmosphere is only twelve miles; the annual amount of carbon dioxide forced into that limited space is six billion tons; and the ten hottest years in recorded human history have all occurred since 1980. The facts beg a question that is as simple to ask as it is hard to answer. What do we do with what we know?

The question became more pointed in September, when the 2,500 climate scientists serving on the Intergovernmental Panel on Climate Change [IPCC] issued a new statement on the prospect of forthcoming catastrophe. Never before had the IPCC (called into existence in 1988) come to so unambiguous a conclusion. Always in years past there had been people saying that we didn't yet know enough, or that the evidence was problematical, or our system of computer simulation was subject to too many uncertainties. Not this year. The panel flatly announced that the earth had entered a period of climatic instability likely to cause "widespread economic, social and environmental dislocation over the next century." The continuing emission of greenhouse gases would create protracted, crop-destroying droughts in continental interiors, a host of new and recurring diseases, hurricanes of extraordinary malevolence, and rising sea levels that could inundate island nations and low-lying coastal rims on the continents.

I came across the report in the *New York Times* during the same week that the island of St. Thomas was blasted to shambles by one of thirteen hurricanes that roiled the Caribbean this fall. Scientists speak the language of probability. They prefer to avoid making statements that cannot be further corrected, reinterpreted, modified, or proven wrong. If its September announcement was uncharacteristically bold, possibly it was because the IPCC scientists understood that they were addressing their remarks to people profoundly unwilling to hear what they had to say.

That resistance is understandable, given the immensity of the stakes. The energy industries now constitute the largest single enterprise known to mankind. Moreover, they are indivisible from automobile, farming, shipping, air freight, and banking interests, as well as from the governments dependent on oil revenues for their very existence. With annual sales in excess of one trillion dollars and daily sales of more than two billion dollars, the oil industry alone supports the economies of the Middle East and large segments of the economies of

Russia, Mexico, Venezuela, Nigeria, Indonesia, Norway, and Great Britain. Begin to enforce restriction on the consumption of oil and coal, and the effects on the global economy—unemployment, depression, social breakdown, and war —might lay waste to what we have come to call civilization. It is no wonder that for the last five or six years many of the world's politicians and most of the world's news media have been promoting the perception that the worries about the weather are overwrought. Ever since the IPCC first set out to devise strategies whereby the nations of the world might reduce their carbon dioxide emissions, and thus ward off a rise in the average global temperature on the order of 4 or 5 degrees Celsius (roughly equal in magnitude to the difference between the last ice age and the current climatic period), the energy industry has been conducting, not unreasonably, a ferocious public relations campaign meant to sell the notion that science, any science, is always a matter of uncertainty. Yet on reading the news from the IPCC, I wondered how the oil company publicists would confront the most recent series of geophysical events and scientific findings. To wit:

- A 48-by-22 mile chunk of the Larsen Ice Shelf in the Antarctic broke off last March, exposing rocks that had been buried for 20,000 years and prompting Rodolfo del Valle of the Argentine Antarctic Institute to tell the Associated Press, "Last November we predicted the [ice shelf] would crack in ten years, but it has happened in barely two months."

- In April, researchers discovered a 70 percent decline in the population of zooplankton off the coast of southern California, raising questions about the survival of several species of fish that feed on it. Scientists have linked the change to a 1 to 2 degree C increase in the surface water temperature over the last four decades.

- A recent series of articles in *The Lancet*, a British medical journal, linked changes in climate patterns to the spread of infectious diseases around the world. The *Aedes aegypti* mosquito, which spreads dengue fever and yellow fever, has traditionally been unable to survive at altitudes higher than 1,000 meters above sea level. But these mosquitoes are now being reported at 1,150 meters in Costa Rica and at 2,200 meters in Colombia. Ocean warming has triggered algae blooms linked to outbreaks of cholera in India, Bangladesh, and the Pacific coast of South America, where, in 1991, the disease infected more than 400,000 people.

- In a paper published in *Science* in April, David J. Thomson, of the AT&T Bell Laboratories, concluded that the .6 degree C warming of the average global temperature over the past century correlates directly with the buildup of atmospheric carbon dioxide. Separate findings by a team of scientists at the National Oceanic and Atmospheric Administrations's National Climatic Data Center indicate that growing weather extremes in the United States are due, by a probability of 90 percent, to rising levels of greenhouse gases.

- Scientists previously believed that the transitions between ice ages and more moderate climatic periods occur gradually, over centuries. But researchers from the Woods Hole Oceanographic Institution, examining deep ocean sediment and ice core samples, found that

these shifts, with their temperature changes of up to 7 degrees C, have occurred within three to four decades—a virtual nanosecond in geological time. Over the last 70,000 years, the earth's climate has snapped into radically different temperature regimes. "Our results suggest that the present climate system is very delicately poised," said researcher Scott Lehman. "Shifts could happen very rapidly if conditions are right, and we cannot predict when that will occur." His cautionary tone is underscored by findings that the end of the last ice age, some 8,000 years ago, was preceded by a series of extreme oscillations in which severe regional deep freezes alternated with warming spikes. As the North Atlantic warmed, Arctic snowmelts and increased rainfall diluted the salt content of the ocean, which, in turn, redirected the ocean's warming current from a northeasterly direction to one that ran nearly due east. Should such an episode occur today, say researchers, "the present climate of Britain and Norway would change suddenly to that of Greenland."

These items (and many like them) would seem to be alarming news—far more important than the candidacy of Colin Powell, or even whether Newt Gingrich believes the government should feed poor children—worthy of a national debate or the sustained attention of Congress. But the signs and portents have been largely ignored, relegated to the environmental press and the oddball margins of the mass media. More often than not, the news about the accelerating retreat of the world's glaciers or the heat- and insect-stressed Canadian forests comes qualified with the observation that the question of global warming never can be conclusively resolved. The confusion is intentional, expensively gift wrapped by the energy industries.

* * *

Capital keeps its nose to the wind. The people who run the world's oil and coal companies know that the march of science, and of political action, may be slowed by disinformation. In the last year and a half, one of the leading oil industry public relations outlets, the Global Climate Coalition, has spent more than a million dollars to downplay the threat of climate change. It expects to spend another $850,000 on the issue next year. Similarly, the National Coal Association spent more than $700,000 on the global climate issue in 1992 and 1993. In 1993 alone, the American Petroleum Institute, just one of fifty-four industry members of the GCC, paid $1.8 million to the public relations firm of Burson-Marsteller partly in an effort to defeat a proposed tax on fossil fuels. For perspective, this is only slightly less than the combined yearly expenditures on global warming of the five major environmental groups that focus on climate issues—about $2.1 million, according to officials of the Environmental Defense Fund, the Natural Resources Defense Council, the Sierra Club, the Union of Concerned Scientists, and the World Wildlife Fund.

For the most part the industry has relied on a small band of skeptics—Dr. Richard S. Lindzen, Dr. Pat Michaels, Dr. Robert Balling, Dr. Sherwood Idso, and Dr. S. Fred Singer, among others— who have proven extraordinarily adept at draining the issue of all sense of crisis. Through their frequent pronouncements in the press and on radio and television, they have helped to create the illusion that the question is hopelessly mired in unknowns. Most damaging has been their influence on decision makers; their contrarian views have allowed conservative Republicans such as Representative Dana Rohrabacher (R., Calif.) to dismiss legitimate research concerns as "liberal claptrap" and have provided the basis for the recent round of budget cuts to those government science programs designed to monitor the health of the planet.

Last May, Minnesota held hearings in St. Paul to determine the environmental cost of coal burning by state power plants. Three of the skeptics—Lindzen, Michaels, and Balling—were hired as expert witnesses to testify on behalf of Western Fuels Association, a $400 million consortium of coal suppliers and coal-fired utilities.[1]

An especially aggressive industry player, Western Fuels was quite candid about its strategy in two annual reports: "[T]here has been a close to universal impulse in the trade association community here in Washington to concede the scientific premise of global warming... while arguing over policy prescriptions that would be the least disruptive to our economy.... We have disagreed, and do disagree, with this strategy." "When [the climate change] controversy first erupted... scientists were found who are skeptical about much of what seemed generally accepted about the potential for climate change." Among them were Michaels, Balling, and S. Fred Singer.

Lindzen, a distinguished professor of meteorology at MIT, testified in St. Paul that the maximum probable warming of the atmosphere in the face of a doubling of carbon dioxide emissions over the next century would amount to no more than a negligible

.3 degrees C. Michaels, who teaches climatology at the University of Virginia, stated that he foresaw no increase in the rate of sea level rise—another feared precursor of global warming. Balling, who works on climate issues at Arizona State University, declared that the increase in emissions would boost the average global temperature by no more than one degree.

At first glance, these attacks appear defensible, given their focus on the black holes of uncertainty that mark our current knowledge of the planet's exquisitely interrelated climate system. The skeptics emphasize the inadequacy of a major climate research tool known as a General Circulation Model, and our ignorance of carbon dioxide exchange between the oceans and the atmosphere and of the various roles of clouds. They have repeatedly pointed out that although the world's output of carbon dioxide has exploded since 1940, there has been no corresponding increase in the global temperature. The larger scientific community, by contrast, holds that this is due to the masking effect of low-level sulfur particulates, which exert a temporary cooling effect on the earth, and to a time lag in the oceans' absorption and release of carbon dioxide.

But while the skeptics portray themselves as besieged truth-seekers fending off irresponsible environmental doom-sayers, their testimony in St. Paul and elsewhere revealed the source and scope of their funding for the first time. Michaels has received more than $115,000 over the last four years from coal and energy interests. World Climate Review, a quarterly he founded that routinely debunks climate concerns, was funded by Western Fuels. Over the last six years, either alone or with colleagues, Balling has received more than $200,000 from coal and oil interests in Great Britain, Germany, and elsewhere. Balling (along with Sherwood Idso) has also taken money from Cyprus Minerals, a mining company that has been a major funder of People for the West—a militantly anti-environmental "Wise Use" group. Lindzen, for his part, charges oil and coal interests $2,500 a day for his consulting services; his 1991 trip to testify before a Senate committee was paid for by Western Fuels, and a speech he wrote, entitled "Global Warming: the Origin and Nature of Alleged Scientific Consensus," was underwritten by OPEC. Singer, who last winter proposed a $95,000 publicity project to "stem the tide towards ever more onerous controls on energy use," has received consulting fees from Exxon, Shell, Unocal, ARCO, and Sun Oil, and has warned them that they face the same threat as the chemical firms that produced chlorofluorocarbons (CFCs), a class of chemicals found to be depleting atmospheric ozone. "It took only five years to go from . . . a simple freeze of production [of CFCs]," Singer has written, " . . . to the 1992 decision of a complete production phase-out—all on the basis of quite insubstantial science."[2]

The skeptics assert flatly that their science is untainted by funding. Nevertheless, in this persistent and well-funded campaign of denial they have become interchangeable ornaments on the hood of a high-powered engine of disinformation. Their dissenting opinions are amplified beyond all proportion through the media while the concerns of the dominant majority of the world's scientific establishment are marginalized. By keeping the discussion focused on whether there is a problem in the first place, they have effectively silenced the debate over what to do about it.

Last spring's IPCC conference in Berlin is a good example. Delegations from 170 nations met to negotiate targets and timetables for reducing the world's carbon dioxide emissions. The efforts of the conference ultimately foundered on foot-dragging by the United States and Japan and active resistance from the OPEC nations. Leading the fight for the most dramatic reductions—to 60 percent of 1990 levels—was a coalition of small island nations from the Caribbean and the Pacific that fear being flooded out of existence. They were supported by most western European governments, but China and India, with their vast coal resources, argued that until the United States significantly cuts its own emissions, their obligation to develop their own economies outranked their obligation to the global environment. In the end, OPEC, supported by the United States, Japan, Australia, Canada, and New Zealand, rejected calls to limit emissions, declaring emission limits premature.

*   *   *

As the natural crisis escalates, so will the forces of institutional and societal denial. If, at the cost of corporate pocket change, industrial giants can control the publicly perceived reality of the condition of the planet and the state of our scientific knowledge, what would they do if their survival were truly put at risk? Billions would be spent on the creation of information and the control of politicians. Glad-handing oil company ads on the op-ed page of the *New York Times* (from a quarter-page pronouncement by Mobil last September 28: "There's a lot of good news out there") would give way to a new stream of selective finding by privatized scientists. Long before the planet itself collapsed, democracy would break apart under the stress of "natural" disasters. It is not difficult to foresee that in an ecological state of emergency our political liberties would be the first casualties.

Thus, the question must be asked: can civilization change the way it operates? For 5,000 years, we have thought of ourselves as dependent children of the earth, flourishing or perishing according to the whims of nature. But with the explosion of the power of our technology and the size of our population, our activities have grown to the proportion of geological forces, affecting the major systems of the planet. Short of the Atlantic washing away half of Florida, the abstract notion that the old anomalies have become the new norm is difficult to grasp. Dr. James McCarthy of Harvard, who has supervised the work of climate scientists from sixty nations, puts it this way: "If the last 150 years had been marked by the kind of climate instability we are now seeing, the world would never have been able to support its present population of 5 billion people." We live in a world of man-size urgencies, measured in hours or days. What unfolds slowly is not, by our lights, urgent, and it will therefore take a collective act of imagination to understand the extremity of the situation we now confront. The lag time in our planet's ecological systems will undoubtedly delay these decisions, and even if the nations of the world were to agree tomorrow on a plan to phase out oil and coal and convert to renewable energies, an equivalent lag time in human affairs would delay its implementation for years. What too many people refuse to understand is that the global economy's existence depends upon the global environment, not the other way around. One cannot negotiate jobs, development, or rates of economic growth with nature.

What of the standard list of palliatives —carbon taxes, more energy-efficient buildings, a revival of public transportation? The ideas are attractive, but the thinking is too small. Even were the United States to halve its own carbon dioxide contribution, this cutback would soon be overwhelmed by the coming development of industry and housing and schools in China and India and Mexico for all their billions of citizens. No solution can work that does not provide ample energy resources for the development of all the world's nations.

So here is an informal proposal—at best a starting point for a conversation—from one man who is not an expert. What if we turned the deserts of the world into electricity farms? Let the Middle East countries keep their oil royalties as solar royalties. What if the world mobilized around a ten-year project to phase out all fossil fuels, to develop renewable energy technologies, to extend those technologies to every corner of the world? What if, to minimize the conflict of so massive a dislocation, the world's energy companies were put in charge of the transition—answering only to an international regulatory body and an enforceable timetable? Grant them the same profit margins for solar electricity and hydrogen fuel they now receive for petroleum and coal. Give them the licenses for all renewable energy technologies. Assure them the same relative position in the world's economy they now enjoy at the end of the project.

Are these ideas mere dream? Perhaps, but here are historical reasons to have hope. Four years ago a significant fraction of humanity overturned its Communist system in a historical blink of an eye. Eight years ago the world's governments joined together in Montreal to regulate CFCs. Technology is not the issue. The atomic bomb was developed in two and a half years. Putting a man on the moon took eleven. Surely, given the same sense of urgency, we can develop new energy systems in ten years. Most of the technology is already available to us or soon will be. We have the knowledge, the energy, and the hunger for jobs to get it done. And we are different in one unmeasurable way from previous generations: ours is the first to be educated about the larger world by the global reach of electronic information.

The leaders of the oil and coal industry, along with their skeptical scientists, relentlessly accuse environmentalists of overstating the climatic threat to destroy capitalism. Must a transformation that is merely technological dislodge the keystone of the economic order? I don't know. But I do know that technology changes the way we conceive of the world. To transform our economy would oblige us to understand the limits of the planet. That understanding alone might seed the culture with a more organic concept of ourselves and our connectedness to the earth. And corporations, it is useful to remember, are not only obstacles on the road to the future. They are also crucibles of technology and organizing engines of production, the modern expression of mankind's drive for creativity. The industrialist is no less human than the poet, and both the climate scientist and the oil company operator inhabit the same planet, suffer the same short life span, harbor the same hopes for their children.

# NOTES

1. In 1991, Western Fuels spent an estimated $250,000 to produce and distribute a video entitled "The Greening of Planet Earth," which was shown frequently inside the Bush White House as well as within the governments of OPEC. In near-evangelical tones, the video promises that a new age of agricultural abundance will result from increasing concentrations of carbon dioxide. It portrays a world where vast areas of desert are reclaimed by the carbon dioxide-forced growth of new grasslands, where the earth's diminishing forests are replenished by a nurturing atmosphere. Unfortunately, it overlooks the bugs. Experts note that even a minor elevation in temperature would trigger an explosion in the planet's insect population, leading to potentially significant disruptions in food supplies from crop damage as well as to a surge in insect-borne diseases. It appears that Western Fuels' video fails to tell people what the termites in New Orleans may be trying to tell them now.

2. Contrary to his assertion, however, virtually all relevant researchers say the link between CFCs and ozone depletion is based on unassailably solid scientific evidence. As if to underscore the point, in May the research director of the European Union Commission estimated that last winter's ozone loss will result in about 80,000 additional cases of skin cancer in Europe. This fall, the three scientists who discovered the CFC-ozone link won the Nobel Prize for Chemistry.

# NO

Arthur B. Robinson and
Zachary W. Robinson

# SCIENCE HAS SPOKEN: GLOBAL WARMING IS A MYTH

Political leaders are gathered in Kyoto, Japan, working away on an international treaty to stop "global warming" by reducing carbon dioxide emissions. The debate over how much to cut emissions has at times been heated—but the entire enterprise is futile or worse. For there is not a shred of persuasive evidence that humans have been responsible for increasing global temperatures. What's more, carbon dioxide emissions have actually been a boon for the environment.

The myth of "global warming" starts with an accurate observation: The amount of carbon dioxide in the atmosphere is rising. It is now about 360 parts per million, vs. 290 at the beginning of the 20th century. Reasonable estimates indicate that it may eventually rise as high as 600 parts per million. This rise probably results from human burning of coal, oil and natural gas, although this is not certain. Earth's oceans and land hold some 50 times as much carbon dioxide as is in the atmosphere, and movement between these reservoirs of carbon dioxide is poorly understood. The observed rise in atmospheric carbon dioxide does correspond with the time of human release and equals about half of the amount released.

Carbon dioxide, water, and a few other substances are "greenhouse gases." For reasons predictable from their physics and chemistry, they tend to admit more solar energy into the atmosphere than they allow to escape. Actually, things are not so simple as this, since these substances interact among themselves and with other aspects of the atmosphere in complex ways that are not well understood. Still, it was reasonable to hypothesize that rising atmospheric carbon dioxide levels might cause atmospheric temperatures to rise. Some people predicted "global warming," which has come to mean extreme greenhouse warming of the atmosphere leading to catastrophic environmental consequences.

## Careful Tests

The global-warming hypothesis, however, is no longer tenable. Scientists have been able to test it carefully, and it does not hold up. During the past 50 years, as atmospheric carbon dioxide levels have risen, scientists have made precise measurements of atmospheric temperature. These measurements have definitively shown that major atmospheric greenhouse warming of the atmosphere is not occurring and is unlikely ever to occur.

The temperature of the atmosphere fluctuates over a wide range, the result of solar activity and other influences. During the past 3,000 years, there have been five extended periods when it was distinctly warmer than today. One of the two coldest periods, known as the Little Ice Age, occurred 300 years ago. Atmospheric temperatures have been rising from that low for the past 300 years, but remain below the 3,000-year average.

Why are temperatures rising? The first chart nearby shows temperatures during the past 250 years, relative to the mean temperature for 1951–70. The same chart shows the length of the solar magnetic cycle during the same period. Close correlation between these two parameters—the shorter the solar cycle (and hence the more active the sun), the higher the temperature—demonstrates, as do other studies, that the gradual warming since the Little Ice Age and the

large fluctuations during that warming have been caused by changes in solar activity.

The highest temperatures during this period occurred in about 1940. During the past 20 years, atmospheric temperatures have actually tended to go down, as shown in the second chart, based on very reliable satellite data, which have been confirmed by measurements from weather balloons.

Consider what this means for the global-warming hypothesis. This hypothesis predicts that global temperatures will rise significantly, indeed catastrophically, if atmospheric carbon dioxide rises. Most of the increase in atmospheric carbon dioxide has occurred during the past 50 years, and the increase has continued during the past 20 years. Yet there has been no significant increase in atmospheric temperature during those 50 years, and during the 20 years with the highest carbon dioxide levels, temperatures have decreased.

In science, the ultimate test is the process of experiment. If a hypothesis fails the experimental test, it must be discarded. Therefore, the scientific method requires that the global warming hypothesis be rejected.

Why, then, is there continuing scientific interest in "global warming"? There is a field of inquiry in which scientists are using computers to try to predict the weather—even global weather over very long periods. But global weather is so complicated that current data and computer methods are insufficient to make such predictions. Although it is reasonable to hope that these methods will eventually become useful, for now computer climate models are very unreliable. The second chart shows predicted temperatures for the past 20

*Figure 1*

**What Warms the Earth?**

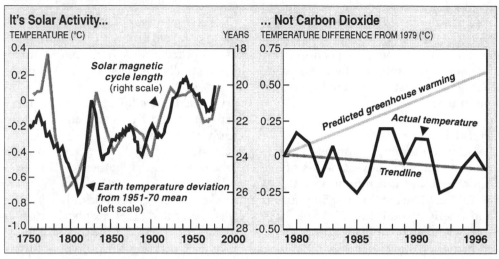

Source: Astrophysical Journal

Source: Marshall Institute

years, based on the computer models. It's not surprising that they should have turned out wrong—after all the weatherman still has difficulty predicting local weather even for a few days. Long-term global predictions are beyond current capabilities.

So we needn't worry about human use of hydrocarbons warming the Earth. We also needn't worry about environmental calamities, even if the current, natural warming trend continues: After all the Earth has been much warmer during the past 3,000 years without ill effects.

But we should worry about the effects of the hydrocarbon rationing being proposed at Kyoto. Hydrocarbon use has major environmental benefits. A great deal of research has shown that increases in atmospheric carbon dioxide accelerate the growth rates of plants and also permit plants to grow in drier regions. Animal life, which depends upon plants, also increases.

Standing timber in the United States has already increased by 30% since 1950. There are now 60 tons of timber for every American. Tree-ring studies further confirm this spectacular increase in tree growth rates. It has also been found that mature Amazonian rain forests are increasing in biomass at about two tons per acre per year. A composite of 279 research studies predicts that overall plant growth rates will ultimately double as carbon dioxide increases.

**Lush Environment**

What mankind is doing is moving hydrocarbons from below ground and turning them into living things. We are living in an increasingly lush environment of plants and animals as a result of the carbon dioxide increase. Our children will enjoy an Earth with twice as much plant and animal life as that with which we now are blessed. This is a wonderful and unexpected gift from the industrial revolution.

Hydrocarbons are needed to feed and lift from poverty vast numbers of people across the globe. This can eventually allow all human beings to live long, prosperous, healthy, productive lives. No other single technological factor is more important to the increase in the quality, length and quantity of human life than the continued, expanded and unrationed use of the Earth's hydrocarbons, of which we have proven reserves to last more than 1,000 years. Global warming is a myth. The reality is that global poverty and death would be the result of Kyoto's rationing of hydrocarbons.

# POSTSCRIPT

## Public Policy and Health: Is Global Warming a Real Threat?

In 1987, geochemist Wallace S. Broecker of Columbia University claimed, "The inhabitants of Planet Earth are quietly conducting a gigantic environmental experiment. So vast and so sweeping will be the impacts of this experiment that, were it brought before any responsible council for approval, it would be firmly rejected as having potentially dangerous consequences. Yet, the experiment goes on with no significant interference from any jurisdiction or nation. The experiment in question is the release of carbon dioxide and other so-called greenhouse gases to the atmosphere." The vast majority of researchers agree with Broecker, but in 1991 the Science and Environmental Policy Project circulated a statement to over 300 atmospheric scientists in the United States. Approximately 50 have signed this statement, which states that policies to tax fossil fuels and environmental regulations are based on unsupported assumptions that catastrophic global warming is caused by the burning of fossil fuels. The scientists who signed the statement also maintain that the theoretical climate models used to predict a future warming trend are not valid.

There is obvious disagreement among scientists about the risks of global warming, or even if there is a problem, and some researchers believe that global warming will actually benefit the environment. They contend that longer growing seasons will be beneficial to crops and that humans will be able to live in greater numbers in arctic areas. They argue that the United States should not make major policy changes regarding fossil fuel emissions and taxation before all the data are available. See "The Great Climate Flip-flop," *The Atlantic Monthly* (January 1998). Other scientists argue that if we wait until all available information is processed, it may be too late. Articles that support this viewpoint include "Copout in Kyoto," *Sierra* (March/April 1998); "Can We Stop Global Warming?" *USA Today Magazine* (March 1997); and "Stormy Weather," *Rolling Stone* (March 20, 1997). "Global Warming May Cause Epidemics," *Malaria Weekly* (January 6, 1997) supports the theory that as the Earth's temperature rises, vector-borne diseases such as dengue fever will move north.

Readings that deny that there are problems associated with global warming include "Globalist Heart-Warming," *National Review* (December 8, 1997); "Global Warmers," *American Spectator* (November 1997); "It's Time to Reconsider Global Climate Change Policy," *USA Today Magazine* (March 1997); and "Global Warming Chills Out," *National Review* (March 24, 1997).

# On the Internet . . .

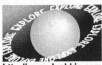

### American Dietetics Association
This official site of the American Dietetics Association offers FAQs, resources on nutrition and dieting, and a section on hot topics. *http://www.eatright.org*

### The Homeopathy Home Page
The Homeopathy Home Page provides links to resources on homeopathy. This site includes discussion groups and a reference library on homeopathy and alternative medicine. *http://www.homeopathyhome.com*

### The USDA's Food and Nutrition Information Center
The Web site of the USDA's Food and Nutrition Information Center supplies publications and databases on topics such as foodborne illness, dietary guidelines for Americans, and a comprehensive index of food and nutrition information on the Internet. *http://www.nalusda.gov/fnic*

### Global Vaccine Awareness League
The Global Vaccine Awareness League Web site is dedicated to the education of parents and concerned citizens regarding vaccination. This site includes a live, interactive message board and a list of related links and articles that reflect both pro-vaccine and pro-choice opinions. *http://pages.prodigy.com/gval/*

# PART 6

## Consumer Health and Nutrition Decisions

*A shift is occurring in medical care toward informed self-care. People are starting to reclaim their autonomy, and the relationship between doctor and patient is changing. Many patients are asking more questions of their physicians, considering a wider range of medical options, and becoming more educated about what determines their health. Although most physicians support dietary changes and moderate exercise, critics claim that many people who follow diet and nutrition fads may actually develop nutritional deficiencies and increase their risk of physical complications from their diet. Some individuals are rejecting traditional medicine altogether and seeking alternative health providers, while others are rejecting only some aspects of traditional medicine such as immunizations. This section debates some of the choices consumers may make regarding their health care and diets.*

■ Should a Low-Fat, High-Carbohydrate Diet Be Recommended for Everyone?

■ Should All Children Be Immunized Against Childhood Diseases?

■ Are Homeopathic Remedies Legitimate?

# ISSUE 19

## Should a Low-Fat, High-Carbohydrate Diet Be Recommended for Everyone?

**YES: William E. Connor and Sonja L. Connor,** from "The Case for a Low-Fat, High-Carbohydrate Diet," *The New England Journal of Medicine* (August 21, 1997)

**NO: Martijn B. Katan, Scott M. Grundy, and Walter C. Willett,** from "Beyond Low-Fat Diets," *The New England Journal of Medicine* (August 21, 1997)

### ISSUE SUMMARY

**YES:** Physician William E. Connor and registered dietitian Sonja L. Connor argue that a low-fat, high-carbohydrate diet has many health benefits, including the reduction of disease risk factors.

**NO:** Nutritionist Martijn B. Katan and physicians Scott M. Grundy and Walter C. Willett maintain that a low-fat, high-carbohydrate diet does not reduce the risk of heart disease, cancer, or obesity.

Dieting has become a way of life for many in the United States. Close to 50 million Americans are currently dieting, but most will not lose as much weight as they want. Many, within a short period of time, will regain the weight they have lost. Despite the fact that Americans have reduced their fat intake by 17.5 percent since 1977, the rate of obesity has increased 25 percent during the same period.

Obesity is linked with an increased risk of diseases, including diabetes, heart disease, and some cancers. In 1957 the American Heart Association (AHA) advised Americans to restrict their dietary fat intake to reduce the risk of heart disease. In the early 1970s the AHA recommended a diet in which no more than 30 percent of total calories comes from fat. This recommendation is still endorsed today.

Since the 1950s the national average fat intake has declined from more than 40 percent of calories to approximately 33 percent. As Americans are reaching the 30 percent recommendation, there is a growing debate among experts. Some argue that 30 percent is still too high. Others counter that most people can eat more fat as long as it is not saturated fat, which clogs arteries and increases the risk of heart disease.

Advocates of reducing total fat state that the level of saturated fat decreases as the level of overall fat intake decreases. Reducing fat intake also helps to control weight since fat contains more calories per ounce than carbohydrates or protein. In addition, some cancers, notably colon cancer, may be prevented by restricting fat consumption. Physician Dean Ornish recommends an extremely low-fat diet to his patients. His research has shown that a diet in which only 10 percent of total calories comes from fat reverses heart disease by reducing arterial blockage, lowering blood pressure, and decreasing serum cholesterol. Although Ornish and other physicians and researchers believe that the AHA recommendation is not low enough, others believe that the 30 percent limit could be higher. They argue that there is a low rate of heart disease among people living in the Mediterranean region. These people typically consume a diet high in total fat but low in saturated fat. The fat in their diet is obtained mainly from olive oil, fish, nuts, and seeds. The Mediterranean diet is also high in fruits and vegetables and low in artificially hardened fats called trans fats (TFAs). TFAs have the same effect on cholesterol levels as saturated fats.

A number of Americans have reduced the total fat in their diets. Unfortunately, many have replaced fat with refined carbohydrates, such as sugar and white flour products, rather than with more nutritious sources of carbohydrates, such as fruits, vegetables, and whole grains. The food industry accommodates the demand for low- and fat-free versions of potato chips, cookies, and other snack foods. Consumers may become confused. Many state that they are on a low-fat diet and still cannot lose weight. Others are not seeing a reduction in their risk of heart disease. The fat free products are usually lower in calories than the full-fat versions, but the calorie reduction is often minimal. Thus, many people have reduced their fat intake but not their caloric intake.

During his research physician Walter C. Willett found that a low-fat, high-carbohydrate diet contributes to obesity. He asserts that people eat too much rice and pasta, believing that complex carbohydrates will not cause weight gain. They neglect to eat healthy fats that are found in foods such as olive and canola oils. The risk for heart disease increases when these fats are eliminated from the diet.

In the following selections, William E. Connor and Sonja L. Connor argue that Americans have improved their health by lowering their intake of fat. They contend that serum cholesterol levels and heart disease rates have lowered since Americans began consuming less fat. Martijn B. Katan, Scott M. Grundy, and Willett counter that the focus on total fat intake distracts people from the lifestyle changes that can have a genuine health benefit. These changes include eating less saturated and trans fats and eating more fruits, vegetables, and whole grains.

# YES

William E. Connor and
Sonja L. Connor

# THE CASE FOR A LOW-FAT, HIGH-CARBOHYDRATE DIET

The association between the dietary intake of fat and cholesterol and the extent of atherosclerosis and coronary heart disease has been recognized since 1907, when de Langen found little atherosclerosis in native Javanese but extensive atherosclerosis in the Dutch settlers in Java.[1] As might be expected, the diets of the two groups of people differed greatly in fat content. At almost the same time in Russia, Anitschkow produced extensive atherosclerosis in rabbits by feeding them cholesterol and fat.[2] In both humans and animals fed high-fat, high-cholesterol diets, serum cholesterol levels greatly increased. Subsequently, after World War II, Keys emphasized that mortality from coronary disease in various countries was directly related both to the amount of dietary fat consumed and to serum cholesterol levels. An extensive data base on this subject was reported in the Seven Countries Study.[3] Mortality from coronary disease also correlated well with dietary cholesterol intake in another analysis of data from 35 countries.[4]

Exceptions to these associations were observed, however. The intake of saturated fat and animal fat correlated better with the incidence of coronary disease than did total fat intake, as is now widely recognized. It was subsequently shown that saturated fats, as well as dietary cholesterol, elevate plasma total and low-density lipoprotein (LDL) cholesterol by down-regulating the LDL receptors in the liver.[5] Another exception was observed in Crete, where there was a high intake of olive oil (a monounsaturated fat) but a low rate of death due to coronary disease in a population adapted to a frugal lifestyle.[3] The Greenland Eskimos also had a low incidence of coronary disease despite a diet rich in fat and cholesterol. The Eskimo diet was protective against coronary disease because it contained n–3 fatty acids from fish and seal.[6] These fatty acids are antithrombotic and lower serum lipid levels.

Experiments in monkeys and other animals confirmed these epidemiologic observations. Feeding fat and cholesterol (e.g., eggs and butterfat) to rhesus monkeys produced high serum cholesterol levels and severe coronary atherosclerosis,[7] even myocardial infarction. That these conditions were

From William E. Connor and Sonja L. Connor, "The Case for a Low-Fat, High-Carbohydrate Diet," *The New England Journal of Medicine*, vol. 337, no. 8 (August 21, 1997). Copyright © 1997 by The Massachusetts Medical Society. Reprinted by permission.

largely reversible was documented when a low-fat, cholesterol-free diet was subsequently fed to the monkeys, proving that a drastic reduction in serum cholesterol levels would ultimately be followed by considerable reversal of coronary atherosclerotic lesions (from 60 percent to 20 percent occlusion).[7] Years later, angiographic evidence of improvement in lesions was found in humans treated with low-fat diets alone or with diet plus lipid-lowering drugs.

Various scientific bodies, including the American Heart Association[8] and the National Heart, Lung, and Blood Institute,[9] have recommended reductions in dietary fat intake to treat or prevent coronary disease. The suggested level of dietary fat is 30 percent or less of total energy intake, reduced from the previous high population intake of 40 percent in the 1960s. Even the American Cancer Society has suggested a 50 percent reduction in fat intake (from 40 to 20 percent of energy intake) to prevent cancer of the colon and breast and other cancers.[10] There is universal agreement that the dietary level of saturated fat should be greatly reduced, from the current intake of 11 percent to 6 to 8 percent of energy intake, along with a reduction in dietary cholesterol. Most recommendations have specified that the saturated fat eliminated from the diet be replaced by carbohydrates from grains, vegetables, legumes, and fruits. This change would diversify the diet and add protective constituents from plant sources.

If the saturated fat were replaced by monounsaturated or polyunsaturated fat, as some have suggested, the fasting serum total and LDL cholesterol levels would be decreased without significantly decreasing total fat intake. Is this an appropriate idea? The strategy of replacing fat with fat does not take into account the disadvantages of a high-fat diet. First, postprandial lipemia is atherogenic and directly reflects the amount of dietary fat ingested.[11] A lower-fat diet would reduce postprandial lipemia composed of chylomicrons and atherogenic remnants that circulate in the plasma after the ingestion of dietary fat. Second, although obesity remains an unsolved problem, there is good evidence that Americans who follow a low-fat diet high in plant foods lose weight more easily than those whose fat intake is higher.[12] Third, the energy cost of metabolizing a dense nutrient like fat is lower than the energy needed to metabolize carbohydrate from plants. Finally, the advantages of a lower-fat diet in the prevention of cancer and the control of hypertension are lost when saturated fat is replaced by other fats, rather than by vegetable foods.

Since 1980, the recommendations of scientific bodies have been translated for the public by the Department of Agriculture (USDA) and the Department of Health and Human Services and published every five years as "Dietary Guidelines for Americans,"[13] and both the public and the food industry have attempted to follow them. According to the USDA's Continuing Survey of Food Intakes by Individuals,[14] dietary fat intake has decreased to about 33 percent of energy intake from a previous 40 percent, and dietary carbohydrate has increased from 45 to 52 percent of energy intake from the 1960s to 1995. These changes bring the average diet close to the goal of obtaining no more than 30 percent of energy intake from fat and 55 percent from carbohydrate. However, dietary fiber intake is still low at 15 g per day (the goal is 20 to 35 g per day).

The plethora of "fat-free" foods has offered people the opportunity to consume more sugar in, for example, sweet rolls, cookies, and frozen yogurt. According to recent USDA food-consumption data,[15] the intake of sugar and other refined sweeteners increased from about 55 kg (120 lb) per person per year in 1970 to 68 kg (150 lb) per person per year in 1995. There has been a small increase in the consumption of plant foods containing protective factors such as antioxidants, soluble fibers, and saponins from grains, legumes, vegetables, and fruits and in the intake of the n–3 fatty acids found in seafood, dark green vegetables, nuts, and oils, but all are short of the recommended goals.

Table 1 shows which of the recommended dietary changes for optimal health throughout life the U.S. population has adopted, as well as recommended changes not yet made. Although there has been progress, further steps need to be taken to achieve a more healthful diet.

There is little doubt that Americans have improved their health by lowering their dietary intake of fat and cholesterol. Serum cholesterol levels are lower, and mortality due to coronary disease is 20 to 30 percent lower than 25 years ago. The directions for change are clear, and further implementation of the currently recommended dietary goals is indicated.

\* \* \*

Although there is refreshing agreement about increasing the consumption of plant-derived foods, we suggest that a greater amount be consumed, to provide optimal intake of fiber, antioxidants, and other protective factors. In the study cited by Katan et al.,[16] subjects were fed a high-fat diet (41 percent of total energy), most

*Table 1*

**Recommended Dietary Changes.***

| ADOPTED BY THE PUBLIC | NOT YET ADOPTED BY THE PUBLIC |
|---|---|
| Consume leaner meats | Consume less sugar in foods and beverages |
| Eat more chicken | Eat more seafood |
| Use oils for cooking | Reduce intake of added fats |
| Eat fewer egg yolks | Use low-fat cheeses |
| Drink less whole milk | Drink skim milk |
| Eat frozen yogurt | Double intake of grains, legumes, vegetables, and fruits |

*Recommendations are adapted from Department of Agriculture data.[15]

of this from olive oil, which would dilute the effect of grains, beans, vegetables, and fruits. We emphasize that Americans have already cut fat intake to 33 percent of total energy consumption, but the fat has been replaced largely with sugar, not complex carbohydrates and fiber. Fat intake should be reduced further. A low-fat diet (27 percent of energy intake from fat) is even advantageous for blood-pressure reduction.[17]

There are no data showing that the physiologic reduction of HDL cholesterol levels with a low-fat diet is detrimental. Diet-induced lowering of HDL cholesterol does not confer the same risk of atherosclerosis as do low HDL cholesterol levels in Americans consuming a high-fat diet.[18] Lowering HDL cholesterol levels by the consumption of a low-fat diet results in more rapid clearance of HDL and decreased transport of HDL apoproteins.[18] Populations eating a low-fat diet that have low HDL cholesterol levels do not have an increased incidence of coronary disease.[19,20] Neither do patients with some forms of inherited low plasma HDL cholesterol levels, including

Tangier disease, in which HDL is virtually absent.[21]

Finally, the recommendations of Katan et al. invite the American public to increase fat intake when all health agencies are advocating the consumption of less fat and more complex carbohydrates and fiber. Such conflicting recommendations only compound public confusion about health and nutrition. Ninety years of research should permit the scientific community to speak with a consistent voice about diet and the prevention of coronary disease. The public deserves the opportunity to implement fully the current, scientifically sound recommendations.

## REFERENCES

1. de Langen C. Het cholesteringegehalte van het bloed in Indie. Geneeskd Tijdschr Ned Indie 1922;62;1–4.
2. Anitschkow N. Experimental arteriosclerosis in animals. In: Cowdry EV, ed. Arteriosclerosis. New York: MacMillan, 1933:271–322.
3. Keys A. Seven Countries: a multivariate analysis of death and coronary heart disease. Cambridge, Mass.: Harvard University Press, 1980.
4. Connor WE. Dietary cholesterol and the pathogenesis of atherosclerosis. Geriatrics 1961;16:407–15.
5. Spady DK, Dietschy JM. Interaction of dietary cholesterol and triglycerides in the regulation of hepatic low density lipoprotein transport in the hamster. J Clin Invest 1988;81:300–9.
6. Bang HO, Dyerberg J. Lipid metabolism and ischemic heart disease in Greenland Eskimos. In: Draper HH, ed. Advances in nutrition research. Vol. 3. New York: Plenum Press, 1980:1–22.
7. Armstrong ML, Warner ED, Connor WE. Regression of coronary atheromatosis in rhesus monkeys. Circ Res 1970;27:59–67.
8. American Heart Association. Dietary guidelines for healthy American adults: a statement for physicians and health professionals by the Nutrition Committee, American Heart Association. Circulation 1988;77:721A–724A.
9. Expert Panel on Detection, Evaluation, and Treatment of High Blood Cholesterol in Adults. Summary of the Second Report of the National Cholesterol Education Program (NCEP) Expert Panel on Detection, Evaluation, and Treatment of High Blood Cholesterol in Adults (Adult Treatment Panel II). JAMA 1993;269:3015–23.
10. The American Cancer Society 1996 Advisory Committee on Diet, Nutrition, and Cancer Prevention. Guidelines on diet, nutrition, and cancer prevention: reducing the risk of cancer with healthy food choices and physical activity. CA Cancer J Clin 1996;46:325–41.
11. Zilversmit DB. Atherogenesis: a postprandial phenomenon. Circulation 1979;60:473–85.
12. Schaefer EJ, Lichtenstein AH, Lamon-Fava S, et al. Body weight and low-density lipoprotein cholesterol changes after consumption of a low-fat ad libitum diet. JAMA 1995;274:1450–5.
13. Kennedy E, Meyers L, Layden W. The 1995 dietary guidelines for Americans: an overview. J Am Diet Assoc 1996;96:234–7.
14. Department of Agriculture, Agricultural Research Service. Data tables: results from USDA's 1995 continuing survey of food intakes by individuals and 1995 diet and health knowledge survey: CSFI/DHKS 1995. Riverdale, Md.: Food Surveys Research Group, 1995 (CD-ROM).
15. Department of Agriculture, Economic Research Service. Food consumption, prices, and expenditures, 1995. Stat Bull (in press).
16. Mensink RP, Katan MB. Effect of monounsaturated fatty acids versus complex carbohydrates on high-density lipoproteins in healthy men and women. Lancet 1987;1:122–5.
17. Appel LJ, Moore TJ, Obarzanek E, et al. A clinical trial of the effects of dietary patterns on blood pressure. N Engl J Med 1997;336:1117–24.
18. Brinton EA, Eisenberg S, Breslow JL. A low-fat diet decreases high density lipoprotein (HDL) cholesterol levels by decreasing HDL apolipoprotein transport rates. J Clin Invest 1990;85:144–51.
19. Connor WE, Cerqueira MT, Connor RW, Wallace RB, Malinow MR, Casdorph HR. The plasma lipids, lipoproteins, and diet of the Tarahumara Indians of Mexico. Am J Clin Nutr 1978;31:1131–42.
20. Knuiman JT, West CE, Burema J. Serum total and high density lipoprotein cholesterol concentrations and body mass index in adult men from 13 countries. Am J Epidemiol 1982;116:631–42.
21. Rader DJ, Ikewaki K, Duverger N, et al. Very low high-density lipoproteins without coronary atherosclerosis. Lancet 1993;342:1455–8.

# NO

## Martijn B. Katan, Scott M. Grundy, and Walter C. Willett

# BEYOND LOW-FAT DIETS

Excess intake of fat is considered an important cause of chronic diseases, but will a reduction in total dietary fat intake provide the health benefits implied by supporters of this strategy? We are concerned that popular belief and scientific evidence on this question have diverged to an alarming extent.

Studies in the 1950s and 1960s showed that replacing saturated fat with polyunsaturated fats lowered serum total cholesterol levels,[1] and clinical trials subsequently suggested that this dietary change may reduce the incidence of coronary heart disease.[2] Consequently, diets high in polyunsaturated fats were widely recommended for the prevention of coronary heart disease. However, concern developed about the safety of polyunsaturated fats, whereas the perception grew that carbohydrates were innocuous. The focus of recommendations therefore shifted to diets low in fat and high in carbohydrates. Interest in monounsaturated fat also increased,[3] but at present the dominant dietary advice is to replace foods high in total or saturated fat and cholesterol with high-carbohydrate foods such as pasta, potatoes, rice, and bread.

### High-Carbohydrate Diets and Cholesterol Levels

Diets that lower serum total cholesterol levels are believed to lower the risk of coronary heart disease. This belief is justified if the cholesterol being lowered is LDL cholesterol; high LDL cholesterol levels cause coronary heart disease, and treatments that lower LDL cholesterol reduce the incidence of coronary heart disease. Replacement of saturated fats by unsaturated oils reduces mainly LDL cholesterol.[4] However, as illustrated in Figure 1, low-fat, high-carbohydrate diets lower not only LDL cholesterol but also high-density lipoprotein (HDL) cholesterol levels.[4] HDL cholesterol levels are lowered by both sugars and complex carbohydrates (starch),[5] and the depression of HDL cholesterol lasts for as long as the low-fat diet is eaten.[6,7]

This effect of carbohydrates on HDL cholesterol is a cause for concern. Low HDL cholesterol levels are strongly associated with coronary heart disease, and many factors that produce lower HDL cholesterol levels increase

From Martijn B. Katan, Scott M. Grundy, and Walter C. Willett, "Beyond Low-Fat Diets," *The New England Journal of Medicine*, vol. 337, no. 8 (August 21, 1997). Copyright © 1997 by The Massachusetts Medical Society. Reprinted by permission.

the risk of coronary heart disease; examples are smoking, obesity, lack of physical activity, abstinence from alcohol, and male sex. Premature coronary heart disease is seen in most genetic HDL deficiency syndromes,[8] especially in those in which LDL cholesterol levels are normal or high. In trials of lipid-lowering agents, drug-induced changes in HDL cholesterol levels independently predicted changes in the risk of coronary heart disease. Also, the induction of high HDL cholesterol levels in animals retards atherogenesis, and the infusion of HDL protein retards the development of fatty streaks.[8] Thus, lowering HDL cholesterol levels usually increases the risk of coronary heart disease, and diets that lower HDL cholesterol levels must be viewed with concern.

People in China and rural Japan have both low total dietary fat intake and low rates of coronary heart disease. However, such populations are also highly active and extremely lean—both factors that raise HDL cholesterol levels and reduce plasma triglyceride levels, thus offsetting the adverse changes caused by low-fat diets. The low rates of coronary heart disease in the Chinese and other rural populations may therefore be due largely to their high levels of physical activity and low body fat, plus their low intake of saturated and trans fats, rather than to low total fat intake. (Trans fats are created during the partial hydrogenation of oils; they raise LDL cholesterol and lower HDL cholesterol levels.)

## Obesity

A major argument for low-fat diets is that they should promote weight reduction. Fat is calorically dense and often is hidden in food products. Theoretically, high-fat diets could facilitate the overcon-

### Figure 1

**Effects on Blood Lipids of a Diet High in Olive Oil as Compared with a Diet High in Carbohydrates and Fiber and Low in Fat in 48 Healthy Volunteers**

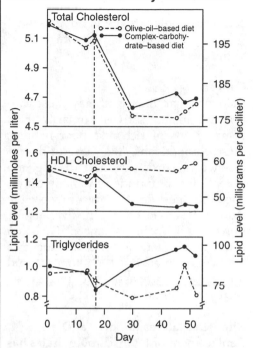

Note: Subjects received a Western-type diet for 17 days (dashed vertical line). Subsequently, half were randomly assigned to an olive-oil–based diet low in saturated fats, which provided 41 percent of calories from fat, and the other half to a diet high in bread, legumes, vegetables, potatoes, fruits, and jam, which provided 22 percent of calories from fat. Reprinted from Mensink and Katan,[5] with the permission of the publisher.

sumption of calories and promote weight gain; however, controlled trials have not supported this idea. In a free-living population, when calories from fat are intentionally restricted, they appear to be largely replaced by carbohydrate. A limited weight reduction is seen after people start a fat-restricted diet, but weight loss stops after a few months, and the long-term net weight loss is only 0.8 to 2.6 kg

(Fig. 2).[9] The prevalence of obesity has increased by one third in the United States since 1976, whereas the percentage of total energy intake from fat has declined. Thus, fat restriction does not invariably produce weight reduction; obesity is a complex problem that will not be solved solely by reducing the percentage of fat in the diet.[15]

## Cancer

Evidence that dietary fat may cause cancer in humans derives primarily from comparisons of rich and poor nations; these comparisons, like those of the incidence of coronary heart disease, are potentially confounded by many differences in lifestyle. In large prospective studies, fat intake has had no overall relation to the risk of breast cancer.[16] For colon cancer, more detailed evidence suggests a role of red meat but not of total fat, and for prostate cancer associations have been seen with animal but not vegetable fat.[16]

## The Alternatives to Low-Fat Diets

Replacement of fat by carbohydrates has not been shown to reduce the risk of coronary heart disease,[2] and benefits are unlikely, because this change similarly lowers HDL and LDL cholesterol[4] and reduces the intake of vitamin E and essential fatty acids. Beneficial effects of high-carbohydrate diets on the risk of cancer or on body weight have also not been substantiated. Alternatively, the replacement of fats high in saturated and trans fatty acids by unhydrogenated unsaturated oils improves the ratio of HDL to LDL cholesterol. Overweight persons can decrease their intake of saturated and trans fat by reducing their consumption of fat from dairy products, meats, and partially hydrogenated oils; they should also eat less sugar and highly refined starch. Carbohydrates should be consumed mainly in the form of fruits, vegetables, legumes, and whole grains. In people who are close to their ideal weight, saturated and trans fats could be replaced largely by unsaturated vegetable oils and highly refined carbohydrates by fruits, vegetables, and whole grains.

Everything we know about lipoproteins and heart disease tells us that such diets will reduce the risk of coronary heart disease. For oils high in polyunsaturated fats, this effect is supported by controlled clinical trials.[2] However, studies in animals have aroused concern about a relation between polyunsaturated fats and cancer, even though observations in humans are reassuring. At present it appears prudent to replace the majority of saturated and trans fats by oils high in monounsaturated fats such as rapeseed (canola) oil and olive oil. The experience in Mediterranean countries shows that diets high in monounsaturated fats can be attractive and that they are associated with longevity and a low incidence of coronary heart disease and cancer.

Finally, the intense focus on total fat intake not only is unlikely to be beneficial but also distracts people from lifestyle changes that can have real benefits. These include specific dietary reductions in saturated and trans fat, increases in the consumption of fruits, vegetables, and whole grains, and the prevention of excessive weight by greater physical activity and reductions in overall caloric intake.

*　*　*

We agree that the intake of fruits, vegetables, and high-fiber foods should be increased and that the high amounts of saturated and trans fatty acids consumed by Americans in the 1950s were unhealth-

## Figure 2

### Effects of Dietary Fat Reduction on Body Weight in Long-Term Randomized, Controlled Trials

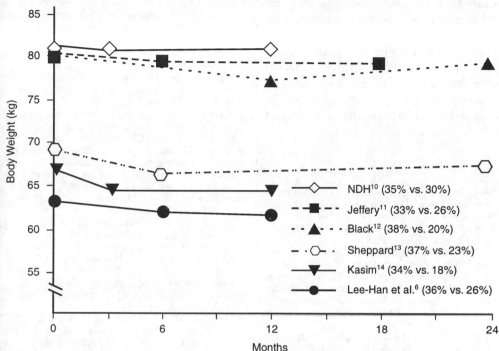

Note: The studies are those reviewed by Willett.[9] Values for the fat-reduction group have been corrected for weight changes in the concurrent control group. Values in parentheses are the percentages of energy from fat in the control group and the fat-reduction group, respectively. NDH denotes National Diet–Heart Study.

ful. However, one cannot generalize from those fats to all fats, because unsaturated fats, which make up the majority of fats in the current U.S. diet, lower LDL cholesterol levels.[17] Reductions in saturated fat and cholesterol in the diet cannot by themselves account for the decline in mortality due to coronary heart disease since the 1950s; increases in the consumption of unsaturated vegetable oils may have been important as well.[18]

Connor and Connor object to substituting unsaturated fats for unhealthful fats because fats produce postprandial lipemia. However, long-term substitu-tion of carbohydrate, instead, does not reduce postprandial lipemia,[19,20] probably because high carbohydrate intake increases the levels of endogenous triglycerides that delay postprandial clearance of lipoproteins. HDL cholesterol levels are also reduced. In the study cited by Connor and Connor, a low-fat, high-fiber diet reduced weight after 12 weeks, but this effect was transient in longer studies (see our Fig. 2). There is no good evidence that reducing total dietary fat will prevent cancer or hypertension.[21]

Like Connor and Connor, we lament the plethora of fat-free products high in sugar and the avoidance of foods such as nuts and oil-based salad dressing that provide n–3 fatty acids. However, the failure to distinguish among types of fat and the emphasis on total fat reduction are the very causes of these problems.

Lower consumption of saturated and trans fats is desirable, but nonspecific recommendations to reduce total fat consumption have no strong scientific basis and could be harmful if unsaturated fats are avoided.

## REFERENCES

1. Keys A, Anderson JT, Grande F. Prediction of serum-cholesterol responses of man to changes in fats in the diet. Lancet 1957;2:959–66.

2. Sacks FM. Dietary fats and coronary heart disease. J Cardiovasc Risk 1994;1:3–8.

3. Grundy SM. Comparison of monounsaturated fatty acids and carbohydrates for lowering plasma cholesterol. N Engl J Med 1986;314:745–8.

4. Mensink RP, Katan MB. Effect of dietary fatty acids on serum lipids and lipoproteins: a meta-analysis of 27 trials. Arterioscler Thromb 1992;12:911–9.

5. Idem. Effect of monounsaturated fatty acids versus complex carbohydrates on high-density lipoproteins in healthy men and women. Lancet 1987;1:122–5.

6. Lee-Han H, Cousins M, Beaton M, et al. Compliance in a randomized clinical trial of dietary fat reduction in patients with breast dysplasia. Am J Clin Nutr 1988;48:575–86.

7. Ernst N, Fisher M, Smith W, et al. The association of plasma high-density lipoprotein cholesterol with dietary intake and alcohol consumption. Circulation 1980;62:Suppl IV:IV-41–IV-52.

8. Vega GL, Grundy SM. Hypoalphalipoproteinemia (low high density lipoprotein) as a risk factor for coronary heart disease. Curr Opin Lipidology 1996;7:209–16.

9. Willett WC. Is dietary fat a major determinant of body fat? Am J Clin Nutr (in press).

10. National Diet-Heart Study Research Group. Body weight changes. Circulation 1968;37:Suppl I:I-170–I-180.

11. Jeffery RW, Hellerstedt WL, French SA, Baxter JE. A randomized trial of counseling for fat restriction versus calorie restriction in the treatment of obesity. Int J Obes Relat Metab Disord 1995;19:132–7.

12. Black HS, Herd JA, Goldberg LH, et al. Effect of a low-fat diet on the incidence of actinic keratosis. N Engl J Med 1994;330:1272–5.

13. Sheppard L, Kristal AR, Kushi LH. Weight loss in women participating in a randomized trial of low-fat diets. Am J Clin Nutr 1991;54:821–8.

14. Kasim SE, Martino S, Kim PN, et al. Dietary and anthropometric determinants of plasma lipoproteins during a long-term low-fat diet in healthy women. Am J Clin Nutr 1993;57:146–53.

15. Willett WC. Diet and health: what should we eat? Science 1994;264:532–7.

16. Idem. Cancer prevention: diet and risk reduction: FAT. In: DeVita V, Hellman S, Rosenberg S, eds. Cancer: principles and practice of oncology. 5th ed. New York: Lippincott-Raven, 1997:559–66.

17. Mensink RP, Katan MB. Effect of dietary fatty acids on serum lipids and lipoproteins: a meta-analysis of 27 trials. Arterioscler Thromb 1992;12:911–9.

18. Hetzel BS, Charnock JS, Dwyer T, McLennan PL. Fall in coronary heart disease mortality in U.S.A. and Australia due to sudden death: evidence for the role of polyunsaturated fat. J Clin Epidemiol 1989;42:885–93.

19. Blades B, Garg A. Mechanisms of increase in plasma triacylglycerol concentrations as a result of high carbohydrate intakes in patients with non-insulin-dependent diabetes mellitus. Am J Clin Nutr 1995;62:996–1002.

20. Chen YD, Coulston AM, Zhou MY, Hollenbeck CB, Reaven GM. Why do low-fat high-carbohydrate diets accentuate postprandial lipemia in patients with NIDDM? Diabetes Care 1995;18:10–6.

21. Morris MC. Dietary fats and blood pressure. J Cardiovasc Risk 1994;1:21–30.

# POSTSCRIPT

## Should a Low-Fat, High-Carbohydrate Diet Be Recommended for Everyone?

American weight gain has increased despite the fact that consumption of dietary fat has decreased. "Epidemic Obesity in the United States: Are Fast Foods and Television Viewing Contributing?" *American Journal of Public Health* (February 1998) concludes that the combination of physical inactivity and the consumption of high-calorie fast foods are contributing to obesity in America. Contrary to theories in many books on dieting, calories count. However, in *The T-Factor Diet* (Bantam Books, 1993), psychologist Martin Katahn states, "You can't get fat except by eating fat." Katahn encourages consumers to only count fat grams and to disregard total calories. Some may believe that they can eat whatever they want as long as it does not contain fat. In one study 17 subjects were given meals made from a variety of low-calorie, low-fat foods. When the subjects were told that the meals were low in fat and calories, they consumed more than when they were told that the meals were high in fat and calories. A 1996 survey found that one-third of consumers believe that it is okay to overeat if the food is low-fat or has no fat.

Food manufacturers accommodate consumers who believe that fat-free foods will help achieve better health and weight loss. Sales of fat-free foods surpassed $30 billion in 1997. Unfortunately, fat is replaced by sugar in many fat-free foods, particularly cookies. Thus, calories may be minimally reduced at best. In addition, fat-free snacks and desserts often lack nutrients. Many experts assert that the emphasis on fat reduction distracts people from the real issues. Many Americans consume too many calories for the level of physical activity they perform. Many are also not eating enough fruits, vegetables, and whole grains. These foods are naturally low in fat and calories, and high in fiber and other nutrients.

Many experts argue that the fat content of a diet is not a good gauge of nutritional quality. It is not correct to abandon a varied diet in order to consume more pasta, white rice, and fat-free cookies. These foods do not supply the fiber and nutrients found in fruits, vegetables, and whole grains.

Further readings on diets, fat intake, and diet books include "Good Fats, Bad Fats," *Self* (August 1998); "The Latest Skinny on Fat," *Harvard Heart Letter* (April 1998); "Healer of Heart," *Newsweek* (March 16, 1998); "Living Off the Fat of the Land," *The Washington Monthly* (January/February 1998); "Top Selling Diets," *Consumer Reports* (January 1998); "Busting the Low-Fat Dieting Myth," *Consumers' Research Magazine* (October 1997); and "How Little Fat Should We Really Eat?" *Consumer Reports on Health* (October 1997).

# ISSUE 20

## Should All Children Be Immunized Against Childhood Diseases?

**YES: Arthur Allen,** from "Injection Rejection," *The New Republic* (March 23, 1998)

**NO: Richard Moskowitz,** from "Vaccination: A Sacrament of Modern Medicine," *The Homoeopath* (March 1992)

### ISSUE SUMMARY

**YES:** Freelance writer Arthur Allen states that parental refusal to immunize children could trigger disease outbreaks.

**NO:** Physician Richard Moskowitz argues that compulsory vaccination undermines the development of a healthy, functioning immune system.

A number of infectious diseases are almost completely preventable through childhood immunization. These diseases include diphtheria, meningitis, pertussis (whooping cough), tetanus, polio, measles, mumps, and rubella (German measles). Largely as a result of widespread vaccination, these once-common diseases have become relatively rare. Before the introduction of the polio vaccine in 1955, polio epidemics occurred each year. In 1952 a record 20,000 cases were diagnosed, as compared to the last outbreak in 1979, when only 10 cases were identified.

The incidence of measles, which can cause serious complications or death, has also declined considerably since the measles vaccine became available. In 1962 there were close to 500,000 cases in the United States, as compared to 138 confirmed cases in 1997. However, in some parts of the United States, particularly urban areas, measles epidemics occur among nonimmunized children.

Many diseases that were thought to be nearly eradicated are making a comeback. In 1983 an outbreak of whooping cough in Oklahoma affected over 300 people. By 1988 nearly 3,000 cases nationwide had been diagnosed. Whooping cough is a serious and sometimes fatal disease, especially among infants. Although the risks of whooping cough and other childhood diseases are serious, many children have not been vaccinated. Currently, between 37 percent and 56 percent of preschool children in the United States have not received immunization. Some parents either cannot afford vaccination or are unaware of the dangers of childhood diseases. Others believe that the risks of vaccination outweigh the benefits—the last of these reasons is the basis for this debate.

The whooping cough vaccine has been the subject of more concern than any other immunization. Although almost all of the 18 million doses administered each year cause little or no reaction, approximately 50 to 75 children who receive the vaccine suffer serious neurological injury. In a few cases the vaccine has been fatal. Some consider this risk to be too high, but before the vaccine was available, nearly 8,000 children died annually from whooping cough. Still, many parents who are concerned about the dangers of the vaccine have chosen not to immunize their children, and an antivaccine movement has grown in the United States and other developed countries. This movement may prove to be dangerous, as indicated in "Impact of Anti-Vaccine Movements on Pertussis Control: The Untold Story," *The Lancet* (January 31, 1998). This study reports that whooping cough is 10–100 times less prevalent in countries with high vaccination rates compared to countries with low vaccination rates due to antivaccine movements.

In the following articles, Arthur Allen states that the growing antivaccine movement is dangerous and may trigger disease outbreaks. Richard Moskowitz disagrees and maintains that vaccines depress the immune system and increase the risk of disease.

# YES

Arthur Allen

# INJECTION REJECTION

President Clinton's ongoing initiative to immunize every American child against infectious disease seems like the kind of safe-as-milk, baby-step health policy that everyone should love. The ultimate motherhood issue. But Clinton, presumably, didn't consult Len Horowitz. A former dentist-turned-"healthcare motivational speaker," Horowitz is carving out a new niche in the history of the paranoid style in American politics. His message: The AIDS and Ebola epidemics resulted from the contamination—possibly intentional —of common vaccines by the military-medico-industrial complex. The Rockefeller Foundation, the Centers for Disease Control, famed AIDS researcher Dr. Robert Gallo, and—yes—Henry Kissinger all figure in Horowitz's gallery of germ-warfare conspirators. Horowitz, who apparently honed his expertise on such matters by drilling teeth in Gloucester, Massachusetts, has urged the government to stop immunizing children until independent researchers can determine if the shots are spreading disease. He charges up to $3,500 to share his theories with holistic-medicine groups, survivalist conventions, and other pockets of suspiciousness. During the past couple of years, he has rarely lacked for speaking engagements.

The pronouncements of Len Horowitz might safely be filed away next to the *Protocols of the Elders of Zion* and the Roswell alien snapshots were it not for the fact that they are reaching an audience that has few antibodies to quackery. Most distressing to the Centers for Disease Control and the Food and Drug Administration, and to public health experts more generally, Horowitz and Louis Farrakhan have found each other.

According to a Nation of Islam official, Farrakhan heard Horowitz last year on a talk-radio program in Phoenix and invited him to dinner. A joint news release followed from Horowitz and Dr. Abdul Alim Muhammad, Farrakhan's "minister of health and human services," calling for a moratorium on the immunization of Nation of Islam children. (Muhammad was already notorious in public health circles for having race-baited the National Institutes of Health into conducting a clinical study of Kemron, a drug he has dispensed to AIDS patients at his D.C. clinic. The study, begun in 1996, quickly closed for lack of patients.) Alarmed that already underimmunized ghetto populations were about to get goaded into forgoing vaccinations altogether, the National Medical Association—a mainstream professional group for black physicians—hastily arranged for public health officials to meet with Muhammad at a Washington hotel last summer. Afterward, Muhammad agreed to shelve the moratorium, at least temporarily. Solicitous CDC and FDA officials later accepted his invitation to debate Horowitz in a panel discussion at the Nation of Islam's annual Savior's Day festival on February 20 in Chicago.

It appears unlikely that the Nation of Islam will truly dispense with immunizations, but, as it happens, Horowitz and Muhammad are merely the most baroque figures in a widespread and growing anti-vaccination movement. Its adherents range from clueless paranoids to parents and physicians with more or less genuine concerns about the safety of vaccinations and more or less solid scientific evidence to back them up. The movement poses a counterweight to what is arguably among the most encouraging developments in medicine: a generation of new vaccines for everything from AIDS and dengue fever to common childhood ear and gut infections.

* * *

For years, vaccination has been a basic tenet of public health and one of its unqualified successes. The elimination of polio and diphtheria along with the decline of such potential killers as measles, mumps, whooping cough, and rubella are well-documented triumphs. A less known and more recent success story is that of the HIB vaccine, which inoculates children against the Haemophilus influenza type B bacteria, the main cause of bacterial meningitis. In 1984, the year before HIB was introduced, the disease struck about 20,000 Americans, mostly children, killing about 1,000 and causing brain damage or permanent hearing loss in a few thousand others. In 1997, only 150 cases of bacterial meningitis were reported.

Notwithstanding its achievements, vaccination is a counterintuitive biological process. Dead or weakened forms of a fearsome microorganism are injected into a healthy person, provoking an immune response—and often a few symptoms of the disease in question. The immune system's antibodies in turn protect the inoculated person from future attack from the "wild" forms of the germ. Since Edward Jenner smeared his first patient with cowpox to shield him from the more dangerous smallpox germs in 1796, immunization has inspired anxiety. The turn-of-the-century American anti-vaccinationist movement spread across the country and set off riots in Milwaukee. The "state quackery" of "compulsory blood poisoning" is an "abomination against God and human nature itself, and every intelligent, conscientious person regards it accordingly," a physiology professor wrote in a 1902 edition of The Vaccination Inquirer, the mouthpiece of the anti-vaccination movement (which was funded by a mail-order patent medicine company in Battle Creek, Michigan).

For the early anti-vaccinationists, immunization was a crime against hygiene and a get-rich scheme for doctors. But they didn't see it, exactly, as a political issue. Today, in contrast, some of the loudest opponents draw their support and arguments from left-meets-right anti-governmentalism. Horowitz, for example, has appeared at survivalist conventions cheek-by-jowl with right-wing militiamen and as a guest on Gary Null's

"Natural Living," a holistic health program that airs several times a week on left-wing Pacifica radio stations in Washington and New York.

Null himself is a florid example of the new conspiracy thinking about public health. In a voice that suggests Mister Rogers with a hangover, Null warns that fluoridation kills (the John Birch Society made similar claims during the early 1960s) and denies that HIV causes AIDS. He hosts everyone from right-wing media critic Reed Irvine to JFK assassination obsessive Robert Morningstar—with a lot of chiropractors in between. Antivaccination guests have included Viera Scheibner, a shrill Australian who insists that vaccines suppress immunity. (Scheibner obfuscated so wildly during a speaking tour of Australia last year that *The Skeptic* magazine honored her with its annual Bent Spoon Award for Australia's biggest charlatan.) One Null show that aired last December 17 on WPFW in Washington featured a Brooklyn "researcher" named Curtis Cost, who shared the following pearls of wisdom: "If you take the measles vaccine, you have a sixty, sixty-five percent chance of getting measles. If you take polio vaccine, you have a roughly eighty, eighty-seven percent chance you will get polio."

\* \* \*

This is, of course, pure rubbish. Nevertheless, if you follow the foolishness to its source, you find that there are some real problems with vaccines.

In a sense, mass childhood immunization has become a victim of its own success. Infant mortality rates in the U.S. are a quarter of what they were in 1950. The average child's risk of contracting polio, measles, or diphtheria is vanishingly low. No one questioned whether Nor-

mandy had been worth it after Hitler was crushed. But, the more the killer germs of the century (with the exception of HIV) fade from memory, the more the public's attention focuses on the adverse reactions vaccines themselves inevitably, if only occasionally, cause.

Take the polio scourge. "Polio was such a frightening specter that a few people's bad reactions to the vaccine simply didn't register," says Dr. Edgar Marcuse, chair of the National Vaccine Advisory Committee. "But the diseases that terrified our grandparents are no longer part of anyone's experience." While "wild" polio struck 21,269 people in 1952, it has not been reported in the United States since 1979. Since then, however, oral polio vaccines have given about 200 people the crippling disease. While that's awful enough if one of the 200 happens to be your child, it's still just one in 2.4 million doses—pretty good odds by any measure.

Another illustrative case study is the controversy over the whole-cell pertussis vaccine—the P in the DPT shot. In 1982, a group of parents who were convinced that the vaccine had harmed their children began organizing to press the government to do something about it. Barbara Loe Fisher is the president of the group, the National Vaccine Information Center, which is run out of a second-story office in a strip mall in suburban Vienna, Virginia. Fisher's oldest child, now 20, suffered a seizure and became learning-disabled after his fourth DPT shot in 1979. "The afternoon after the shot I went up to his room, and he was sitting in his little chair, staring straight ahead," she says in an interview. "I held him, and he pitched forward, with his eyes rolling around in his head. Later that night he had terrible diarrhea and then he slept, and I couldn't wake him. He's never been the same."

To be sure, Fisher's group has had at least some salutary impact: its pressure helped spur development of the even safer acellular pertussis vaccine, which became widely available last year. And, in 1986, after thousands of lawsuits against vaccine manufacturers threatened the supply of cheap vaccines, Fisher's group, the vaccine industry, and the CDC pushed Congress to pass the National Childhood Vaccine Injury Act. That act created a no-fault claims court, funded by a levy on vaccines, where the parents of sickened or dead children could collect compensation.

The vaccine court has handed out cash to more than 2,600 people whose children died or were seriously injured after vaccination—with DPT, in a large majority of the cases. Yet, while that number must be read as a tacit admission that vaccines carry some risk, neither it nor the 63,000 vaccine reactions (including 1,094 deaths) recorded in the past seven years by an FDA-CDC vaccine injury reporting system are necessarily proof of widespread vaccine failures. As CDC officials explain it, the reactions the system records are rarely distinctive enough for doctors to be sure a particular vaccine caused them. Babies suffer terrible illnesses, and since babies are often vaccinated it is likely that illness will occur not long after some immunization or another. In a 1994 report on vaccine safety, the Institute of Medicine reported that "the vast majority of deaths reported... are temporally but not causally related to vaccination." A later report amended that finding to acknowledge that the whole-cell pertussis vaccine could lead to permanent brain damage, but the bottom line, as one institute official puts it, remains that "a lot of

bad things happen to small children that we don't understand."

The problem, in any event, is not the cases for which the government implicitly accepts responsibility, but the thousands—even millions—more that advocates like Fisher claim go unrecorded. "Kids get shots, something happens to them, and nobody makes the connection," says Fisher. "Why can't we do a better job of admitting we've got a problem here? Why can't they do the science to figure out what's going on?" Her group has trumpeted some recent studies that suggest vaccination may trigger autoimmune problems, in which the body attacks itself, and may be responsible for the increased incidence of diseases like asthma and diabetes and, for that matter, Gulf war syndrome. "You have to ask whether we're simply trading childhood sickness for chronic diseases," Fisher says.

This is a fascinating thought—and a rather disturbing one, particularly since it's so easy to disseminate. Although few scientists share it, there have been enough widely disparate studies on vaccine safety over the years that anybody —well, anyone with computer access to MEDLINE—can document anything he or she wants to say on his or her personal website, with all the sites hyperlinking back and forth in a frenetic group grope. Vaccine anxiety is the perfect symptom of what British medical writer Paul Hodgkin describes as postmodern medicine. "Utterly unquestioned biological givens are disintegrating all around us: the stability of the climate, the immutability of species... the unchangeable genetic makeup of one's unborn children," Hodgkin wrote recently in the *British Medical Journal*. With certainties fading, it is easy for people who feel medically vulnerable to build seductive hints and fragments into a coherent, if warped, belief system. "Trust is fragile," says Regina Rabinovich, chief of clinical studies in microbiology at the National Institute for Allergy and Infectious Diseases, "and in science we're not very good at proving the negative."

* * *

In 1994, Heather Whitestone became the first Miss America with a disability. She went deaf at the age of only 18 months, the initial news reports said, after suffering an adverse reaction to a DPT shot. In fact, as Whitestone's pediatrician later confirmed, it was not DPT but a bout of bacterial meningitis —the disease now nearly eliminated by the HIB vaccine—that cost Whitestone her hearing. The Whitestone case helped spur public health officials to begin an initiative last month to improve vaccine-safety information. They chose to run the project under the auspices of the Infectious Disease Society of America rather than the federal CDC. "There's too much anti-government, anti-industry sentiment out there," says one physician involved in the effort.

One of the major concerns of the project is the relatively low vaccination rate among poor blacks. In 1996, the CDC's National Immunization Survey found only 63 and 65 percent compliance with a recommended vaccination regimen for children in majority-black Newark and Detroit, respectively, compared to the U.S. average of 79 percent and the high of 88 percent in the state of Connecticut. Since vaccinations can be had for free, the major reasons for these low rates are clearly social— family disorganization and high dropout

rates on the one hand, suspicion of the government on the other.

Meanwhile, Barbara Loe Fisher recently embarked on a new crusade to win parents the federally guaranteed right to enroll their children in school without vaccinations if they don't believe in them. "It is not in the best interest of the citizens of this free society, or of public health officials in positions of authority, to use the heel of the boot of the state to crush all dissent to mandatory vaccination laws," she said in a recent speech. Fisher may not be Horowitz, but her position on mandatory vaccination worries public health officials —for good reason.

About half of one percent of all parents in the United States currently take advantage of religious exemptions from immunization, permitted in all states except for Mississippi and West Virginia, or of variously defined philosophical exemptions, which are allowed in 17 states. While public health officials generally see families who exempt their children as free-riders enjoying "herd immunity" without participating in the risk, they're usually willing to grant exemptions to any family that whines insistently enough, if only because a crackdown could provoke a more serious backlash. But with Fisher and others stirring up more support, public health officials worry that the anti-vaccination movement will gain footholds in the socially isolated groups that have distorted views of reality—and are, already, at greater risk of disease. Farrakhan's dalliance with Horowitz, for example, enraged many black physicians because they fear the target population's reliance on urban legends. "It's one thing to talk about AIDS as genocide and a whole different thing to fan the flames of mistrust and fear about immunizations," says Stephen Thomas, director of the Institute for Minority Health Research at Emory University's school of public health. "We know [vaccines] save lives."

There's no evidence that current exemptions are causing major disease outbreaks in the United States—at least for now. But infectious diseases have a way of finding the chinks in a society's immunological armor. In the January 31 issue of *The Lancet*, epidemiologists led by Eugene Gangarosa of Emory University charted the return of whooping cough after a decline of DPT shots in countries that had vaccination scares during the late 1970s. In Japan, after the deaths of two children who had gotten DPT shots in 1974, the percentage of school-age children receiving the pertussis vaccine fell from 80 percent to ten percent. Whooping cough, which had nearly disappeared, returned with a vengeance: in 1979, there were 13,000 cases and 41 deaths. Similar outbreaks followed declining vaccine coverage in Australia, Britain, and Sweden. The most crushing evidence of the continued need for vaccines comes from Russia, where crumbling public health services and Rasputin-like antivaccinationists have led to a collapse of immunizations in many areas and an explosion of long-dormant infectious diseases. In 1995, to cite the most tragic statistic, 1,700 Russians died of diphtheria, a disease of the 1920s.

\* \* \*

In the United States, officials have gotten some sense of the opportunism of infectious diseases by studying small outbreaks. Of the 508 measles cases reported in 1996, 107 occurred in and around the town of St. George, Utah. In a fascinating study of that outbreak, CDC epidemiologists were able to demonstrate just how risky a few unvaccinated children could be. The St. George area has a high rate of school-children with religious and philosophical exemptions from vaccination. Of the 107 measles cases, 48 were in exempted, unvaccinated children who played the key role in spreading the disease. Measles takes two weeks to incubate, so officials were able to track six successive generations of the outbreak. According to Daniel Salmon, a fellow at the CDC, two of the three children in the first generation were unvaccinated. The measles vaccine is thought to be 95 percent effective, which accounts for the 59 vaccinated children who contracted the disease. As the outbreak slowly spread through successive generations, exposing more and more children, the germs eventually found the small percentage of kids whose vaccinations had failed.

Whooping cough has increased slightly in the United States since Fisher's movement got underway. No one has linked the two, but, as it happens, no one is more aware of the risks than Fisher herself. After her son's episode with the DPT shot, Fisher decided not to vaccinate her two younger children. And, in a peculiarly bitter twist of fate, of the several thousand U.S. cases of pertussis in 1992, two were Fisher's children. "I watched as my five-year-old daughter's face turned white," she recalled in a recent speech. "Her lips turned blue, and her eyes bulged out of her head during a paroxysm of whooping cough that I thought would take her life."

# NO

Richard Moskowitz

# VACCINATION: A SACRAMENT OF MODERN MEDICINE

Vaccines have become sacraments of our faith in biotechnology in the sense that 1) their efficacy and safety are widely seen as self-evident and needing no further proof; 2) they are given automatically to everyone, by force if necessary, but always in the name of the public good; and 3) they ritually initiate our loyal participation in the medical enterprise as a whole. They celebrate our right and power as a civilization to manipulate biological processes ad libitum and for profit, without undue concern for or even any explicit concept of the total health of the populations about to be subjected to them.

. . . I have mostly a lot of questions to offer, questions so thorny and difficult that decades of careful investigation will be needed to disentangle them. But they seem so basic and important that it would be reckless indeed to require vaccination of every newborn child without adequate measures being taken to address them. Until then, my position remains simply to make vaccines optional and freely available to all at the discretion of their parents, as is now the rule in the UK and other European countries.

I want to begin with a brief history of the measles vaccine, because its dramatic career highlights so many of the issues pertaining to the others as well.

In its natural state, the measles virus enters the body of a susceptible person through the nose and mouth and incubates silently for about 14 days in the lymphoid tissues of the nasopharynx, the regional lymph nodes, and finally in the liver, spleen, bone marrow, and the lymphocytes and macrophages of the peripheral blood. The illness known as the measles is the process by which the virus is expelled from the blood, through the same orifices that it came in, and involves a concerted and massive effort of the entire immune system. Once specific antibodies have succeeded in targeting the virus, the ability to synthesize them on short notice remains as a coded "memory" of the whole experience, a virtual guarantee that people who have recovered from the measles will never get it again, no matter how many times they are re-exposed.

In addition to conferring this specific immunity, the process of recovering from the natural disease also "primes" the organism nonspecifically to respond promptly and efficiently to other microorganisms in the future. A crucial step in the maturation of a healthy immune system, the ability to mount a vigorous, acute response to infection unquestionably represents a major ingredient of optimum health and well-being in general.

Finally, measles is about 20% fatal in populations exposed to it for the first time. It has taken us centuries of adaptation and "herd immunity" to convert it into an ordinary childhood disease, such that, when I first encountered it at the age of 6, nonspecific mechanisms were already in place to help me deal with it effectively. In that historical sense, the permanent immunity acquired by recovery from the natural disease represents an absolute net gain for the total health of the race as well. However the vaccines act inside the human body, true natural immunity or any other qualitative benefit cannot be ascribed to them: their effectiveness is a mere statistic, and the resulting "immunity" a narrowly defined technicality.

Thus, in contrast with the natural disease, the vaccine virus produces no local sensitization at the portal of entry, no incubation, no massive outpouring, and no acute disease of any kind. It can elicit long-term antibody production solely by surviving in latent form in the lymphocytes and macrophages of the blood. But then the vaccinated individual would have no way to get rid of it, and the technical feat of antibody synthesis could at most represent the memory of this chronic infection. Nobody would be foolish enough to argue that vaccines render us "immune" to viruses if in fact they merely weakened our ability to expel them and forced us to harbor them permanently instead. On the contrary, such a carrier state would tend to compromise our ability to respond to other infections as well, and would have to be regarded as immunosuppressive in that sense.

The laws mandating vaccination against the measles were enacted in the early 1960's, when the disease was limited almost entirely to children in elementary school, and both deaths and surface complications had already reached an all-time low. There was very little public debate, and the decision appears to have been made purely as a matter of policy, almost as soon as the vaccine became available. With very few people requesting exemptions, the compliance rate averaged well over 95 per cent. From an average of over 400,000 cases annually in the prevaccine era, the incidence of the measles in the United States dropped to less than 5000 in the early 1980's (1), and it looked as though the disease would soon be eliminated.

In the 1980's, however, this comforting mythology began to unravel, as measles began to reappear even in fully vaccinated populations, and public health authorities began to grapple with the mysterious phenomenon of "vaccine failure."

Thus in 1984, 27 cases of measles were reported at a high school in Waltham, Mass., where over 98% of the students had documentary proof of vaccination (2). In 1985, 157 cases were reported over a 3-month period in Corpus Christi, Texas, and the surrounding Nucces County, despite a vaccination rate of over 99% and significant antibody levels in over 95% (3). In 1989, an Illinois high school with vaccination records for 99.7%

of the students reported 69 cases over a 3-week period (4).

In all of these outbreaks, the authors concentrated on the documented vaccination rates of the target populations, and curiously neglected to mention the number of actual cases that had not been vaccinated. But they all implicitly refuted the hypothetical "reservoir" of the disease in the unvaccinated, an argument still popular with health departments for frightening wavering parents into compliance.

As the data from these various outbreaks were collected and analyzed, tentative generalizations were made and new strategies formulated. A survey of over 15,000 Canadian cases in 1985–86 indicated that 60% of the patients had documented vaccination records, with 28% "unvaccinated," and the status of the other 12% "unknown" (5). Since the "unvaccinated" group would also have been identifiable only by their own statements, the category "unknown" presumably refers to those who claimed to have been vaccinated but could no longer prove it.

A comparable American survey (6) of 152 separate outbreaks comprising over 9000 cases in 1985–86 yielded similar results:

1. A large majority of cases (69%) were children of school age, i.e., 5 to 19 years of age.
2. Of these, 60% had been "appropriately vaccinated," i.e., at 15 months or more (the schedule then currently in vogue), and another 20% "inappropriately vaccinated" (at 12–19 months, the schedule recommended before 1979), with the number of unvaccinated cases again omitted.
3. A significant minority of cases (26%) were children less than 5 years old, most of them unvaccinated and belonging to black, Hispanic, or other indigent minorities in urban ghettos.

All of these data indicated a resurgence of the disease mainly in older children and adolescents of high-school and college age, groups with much higher rates of serious complications. The usual explanation was that vaccine-mediated immunity was time-limited, and "wore off" with increasing age, presumably leaving the child otherwise unaffected and susceptible as before. This usually unstated assumption also formed the principal rationale for mandatory revaccination at a later date.

Unfortunately, this assumption had already been disproved by an earlier study, which demonstrated that previously vaccinated children with declining antibody titers responded minimally and for an unacceptably short time to booster doses of the measles vaccine (7).

Another refutation came from a sustained outbreak of 235 cases in Dane County, Wisconsin, over a 9-month period in 1986, although the authors of the study declined to take it seriously. As in earlier studies, they found that the vast majority of the cases were in the school-age group (5 to 19 years), but that only 6% of these had not been vaccinated (8). Their most unexpected finding was that "mild measles," with typical rash but minimal fever, was much more likely in children who lacked vaccine-specific antibodies than in either the unvaccinated or those whose vaccinations had "taken" properly. This apparent reversal suggested some kind of inapparent or latent activity of the virus that had not been suspected before and did not show up on routine serological investigation.

Yet, despite these warnings, none of these investigators dared consider the possibility that the "immunity" conferred by the measles vaccine might not be genuine. Much as in the peak years of the Vietnam War, or the chemotherapy of advanced cancer patients after the initial round has failed, the purely quantitative redefinition of immunity cleared the way for the simple escalation of force as needed to approximate the desired goal.

In the last three years, the theologians of revaccination have generally carried the day in the face of all logical, scientific, and ethical considerations. Ironically, the major historical development in their favor has been the increasing progress of the disease among unvaccinated minority infants.

Thus over 500 cases were reported for Los Angeles County in 1988, over 17% of the total nationwide; and of these about 65% were under 5 years of age, 77% were Hispanic, and 38% were actually less than 16 months old, the age at which the vaccine is usually given (9)! These data have been used effectively to browbeat state legislatures into allocating more funds and local officials into tighter enforcement of vaccination laws in minority districts.

As a result, lowering the vaccination age to 9 months has been recommended for certain high-incidence areas, an idea which brings us back full circle to the pre-1979 era, when large numbers of kids were "inappropriately vaccinated" according to similar guidelines. These absurd vacillations have nevertheless caught millions of innocent children in their web, and even the most sanctimonious faith and piety will no longer suffice to excuse them.

Although only the measles vaccine has been implicated, the medical and public health authorities are currently advocating revaccination with the mumps and rubella vaccine as well, but cannot even agree on the proper age, while the various state legislatures are left to try to figure out which of them if any to pay attention to. Thus the American Academy of Family Practice currently advocates a second MMR booster at 4 to 6 years of age (10), and a bill now before the Ohio legislature mandates documented proof of MMR revaccination before entering the seventh grade (11). The general idea seems to be that the extra dose can't possibly hurt, and therefore it makes sense to throw in the mumps and rubella vaccines as well.

This same generic faith continues to bless the pharmaceutical industry in its endless and immensely profitable quest of new vaccines, seemingly for no other reason that its technical capacity to make them.

In the late 1980's, a vaccine was introduced against Hemophilus influenzae Type B, associated with scattered outbreaks of meningitis in crowded day-care facilities. At first purely optional for the preschool-age group (2 to 4 years), it was eventually made compulsory for all infants, even those who never need day care, and is presently given at or before 18 months, in some cases before the first birthday.

Always primarily a disease of adult IV drug users, hepatitis B quickly found its way into blood banks and has become a more or less institutionalized risk of patients requiring transfusion and other blood products. As with chicken pox, the hepatitis B vaccine was developed in the 1970's; it is now being marketed only because the medical authorities have never figured out how to approach or "target" the drug subculture in a useful way. Once again, when all else fails, the favored solution is simply to vaccinate everybody.

In the past few months, the CDC and the American Academy of Pediatrics have decided to mandate Hepatitis B vaccination for all newborn babies (12), and are still trying to decide whether to give it at birth or with the DPT at 2 months of age. It remains to be seen whether the American public, already increasingly upset about the vaccination issue, will simply acquiesce in this latest baptism of its newly born, explicitly intended as their very first immunological experience.

Although still technically optional, comparable transubstantiations are also available at the other end of life. Originally intended for the entire adult population, the influenza and pneumococcus vaccines have never been popular, and several studies have shown them to be ineffective as well (13, 14). When the swine flu "epidemic" of 1978 never materialized, and thousands of vaccines developed crippling Guillain-Barre syndrome, the American public began to question the concept of vaccination openly for the first time. Yet the elderly and infirm continue to be pressured heavily to accept these "rejects" on a yearly basis as a form of extreme unction against both diseases.

Seemingly without limit, the search goes on, now indissolubly linked to the technology of genetic engineering. Currently in the works are vaccines against the Group A streptococcus, the common cold, and bronchiolitis, all of which are being bred into the gene pool of mice, rats, baboons, and other experimental animals without any discernible caution or restraint (15). A fitting denouement not far off is the AIDS vaccine, monstrous even in principle, since those at risk are already seriously immunocompromised:

a suppressive vaccine would not only increase their chances of getting it, but help to soften up the general population as well.

Next I want to reconsider the DPT story, presently the major battleground of the vaccine controversy in the United States, and the area in which most of my own experience with vaccine related illness has been concentrated. Thanks to consumer organizations like Dissatisfied Parents Together (DPT), and books like Harris Coulter and Barbara Fisher's A Shot in the Dark, the plight of vaccine-injured children is beginning to be recognized and taken seriously by the general public.

In 1986, despite intensive lobbying by the AMA and other vested interests, Congress belatedly enacted the National Childhood Vaccine Injury Act, which requires the Public Health Service to investigate all reports of vaccine injury and formulate guidelines for compensation (16). Unfortunately, the Public Health Service and its subsidiary agency, the Center for Disease Control (CDC), can usually be counted on to look the other way, since a large part of their budget is earmarked for advocating and enforcing the same compulsory vaccination programs.

Thus the new DPT compensation guidelines rule out every condition other than the few already identified (collapse, anaphylaxis, and brain damage), and everything chronic unless it appears less than 7 days after the vaccination (17). Even these massive exclusions are insufficient for many vaccine proponents, who still deny the encephalopathy charge as well (18, 19).

So the battle continues, with no end in sight: the unit cost of the DPT vaccine has skyrocketed, as have the number and size of personal injury awards against manufacturers, and many pediatricians are privately willing to give the DT alone if the parents insist. Meanwhile, pertussis has made a slight comeback in the years 1986–88, when the CDC reported a 3-year total of roughly 10,500 cases (20).

As in the case of the measles, the bureaucratic language effectively conceals the true demographics. Thus, of those cases with "known vaccination status," 63% had been "inappropriately immunized," and 34% had not been vaccinated at all. We are meant to infer that the vaccine is nearly 100% effective, with very few cases in the vaccinated group. Only by reading the fine print do we learn that those whose vaccination status was "unknown" (7,700 cases) actually comprise more than 70% of the total. Since even its chief proponents concede the DPT to be the least effective of all the vaccines, my bet once again is that most or all the "unknown" 70% were simply vaccines without documentation acceptable to the Inquisitorial authorities.

Indeed, after reporting several cases in infants less than 2 months old, a Philadelphia pediatrician recently advocated that the DPT be given even earlier, ideally "as early in life as possible" (21). The sacramental status of vaccines is widely interpreted by public health officials as prior authorization for vaccinating almost anyone against anything at any time....

In conclusion, I want to address the most important and difficult problems of all: the research that will have to be done in the future, and the political will that will be needed to carry it out. Both questions are inseparably connected, and both will need radically new models to succeed.

Because current studies ignore and indeed preclude any concept of the total health picture over time, they cannot provide unambiguous information about how vaccines act. At the same time, controlled scientific investigations based on the totality of symptoms will require a large population of unvaccinated kids, just what the existing laws are designed to prevent. To those parents who decide not to vaccinate we therefore owe a considerable debt of gratitude.

Similarly, the accusation that unvaccinated children help propagate the various diseases and thus threaten the rest of the population cuts both ways. For the extent to which this argument is true also admirably quantifies the ineffectiveness of the vaccines: if the "immunity" they conferred were genuine and lasting, the unvaccinated kids would pose a threat only to themselves.

Furthermore, it will not be possible to study each vaccine independently unless we legally authorize parents to choose some vaccines but not others. At present, even the most liberal states allow parents to refuse all vaccinations across the board, on religious or philosophical grounds, but not to make informed medical decisions for their children. Once the vaccines are made totally optional, as in the UK, the experimental and control groups can become purely self-selecting for each vaccine, with those receiving it matched as closely as possible to those exempted.

Once these groups are in place, it will be necessary to follow them prospectively for at least a generation, if not a lifetime. For the present, pilot studies could also be done retrospectively, using older kids with known vaccination histories.

But by far the most difficult and important questions are the inextricably connected theoretical one of what to measure and the technical one of how to measure it....

In studying large populations, we will eventually need to select a few key variables sufficiently broad and inclusive to reflect the most fundamental aspects of human functioning, yet also flexible enough to accommodate the infinite richness and diversity of real people. Which ones we choose will then further determine and be determined by the techniques with the requisite detail and precision for measuring them.

Probably this means that we won't really know what we need to measure until we've followed a much smaller pilot group more extensively for a shorter period of time, perhaps four or five years, and just see what happens. In any case, the homeopathic agenda—the total health picture over time—remains the best available methodology for such an investigation; and any progress we can make toward it will automatically contribute to research design in biomedicine generally.

How, then, is one to investigate the total health picture of large populations over time? Clearly, we need to look at the elements of the standard medical history, and to follow the incidence and severity of the usual acute and chronic diseases. Regular physical and laboratory examinations might also suggest persistent or subclinical changes of a more "constitutional" or chronic type, such as swollen nodes for rubella, abnormal white cell and differential counts for pertussis, and nonspecific developmental criteria (height and weight, dentition, gross and fine motor co-ordination, vision, hearing, etc.) for all the vaccines.

Other important variables lying outside the medical history per se would include intelligence, language, socialization in family and school settings, and other demographic, socioeconomic, and psychological factors (poverty, race, learning disabilities, behavior and emotional problems, school attendance and performance).

On the other hand, pilot studies of the pneumococcus and influenza vaccines might need only a few simple variables, because they are given primarily to elderly people at high risk or in nursing homes, when their chronic disease structure is already more or less firmly established. Under these circumstances, a reasonable first approximation of how these vaccines act might be simply to measure their effect on the life span, the sheer ability to survive, compared to that of their unvaccinated friends and neighbors.

Finally, I want to explain why, in spite of the very considerable dangers I have been talking about (and innumerable others we all could mention), I remain strangely optimistic about the future of the healing arts. The principal reason has to do with the growing awareness of ordinary people taking more responsibility for their own health and more control over their transactions with the medical system as a whole.

In the United States, the movement for free choice in health care now includes not only such groups as DPT, but also the supporters of midwifery, home birth, homeopathy and other forms of alternative or "complementary" medicine, and even of the right to die. Within the last 20 years, all of these groups have already achieved major changes in the conventional doctor-patient relationship. Now that the American economy is manifestly unable to afford the personal health care system, no matter how it is organized, it is virtually certain that these changes will continue to accelerate, and that organized medicine will face further repudiation until it accepts them.

# NOTES

1. Cherry, J., "The New Epidemiology of Measles and Rubella," Hospital Practice, July 1980, p. 49, and Markowitz, L., et al., "Patterns of Transmission in Measles Outbreaks in the U.S.," New England Journal of Medicine 320. 77, Jan. 12, 1989.

2. Nkowane, B., et al., American Journal of Public Health 77: 434–38, 1987.

3. Gustafson, T., et al., "Measles Outbreak in a Fully Immunized Secondary-School Population," New England Journal of Medicine 316: 771–74, March 26, 1987.

4. Chen, R., et al., American Journal of Epidemiology 129: 17382, 1989.

5. Medical Tribune, Aug. 26, 1987, p. 2.

6. Markowitz, et al., op.

7. Cherry, op. cit. 1980, p. 52. Cit. 1989, pp. 75–81.

8. Edmondson, M., et al., "Mild Measles and Secondary Vaccine Failure During a Sustained Outbreak in a Highly Vaccinated Population," Journal of the AMA 263: 2467–71, May 9, 1990.

9. "Measles: Los Angeles County, 1988," MMWR Report, Journal of the AMA 261: 1111f., Feb. 24, 1989.

10. Family Practice News, April 1, 1990, p. 3.

11. LSC 119 0911-1, Sub. H. B. 168, Ohio General Assembly, 1991 1992.

12. Boston Globe, June 11, 1991, p. lf.

13. "Medical World News, April 14, 1986, p. 53.

14. Simberkoff, M., et al., "Efficacy of Pneumococcal Vaccine in High-Risk Patients," New England Journal of Medicine 313. 1318–27, Nov. 20, 1986.

15. "Medical News and Perspectives," Journal of the AMA 262: 2055, Oct. 20, 1989.

16. Vaccine Adverse Event Reporting System (VAERS), Public Health Service, 1986.

17. "Reportable Events Following Vaccination," VAERS op. cit., Table 1.

18. Griffin, R., et al., "Risk of Seizures and Encephalopathy after Immunization with the DTP Vaccine," Journal of the AMA 263: 1641–45, March 23, 1990.

19. Cherry, J., "Pertussis Vaccine Encephalopathy: It's Time to Recognize It as the Myth that It Is," Editorial, Journal of the AMA 263: 1679–80, March 23, 1990.

20. "Pertussis Surveillance: U.S., 1986–1988," MMWR Report, Journal of the AMA 263: 1058–69, Feb. 23, 1990.

21. Family Practice News, Nov. 15, 1990, p. 6.

# POSTSCRIPT

## Should All Children Be Immunized Against Childhood Diseases?

Currently, all 50 states require children to be vaccinated before enrolling in school. Exemptions apply for children whose parents' religious beliefs prohibit vaccinations. Some children are exempt for medical reasons, which must be certified by their doctors. Almost all children are vaccinated by the time they enter school. However, the safety of various vaccines, particularly the diphtheria, pertussis, and tetanus (DPT) vaccine, continues to be the subject of debate. Although both the American Academy of Pediatrics and the U.S. Public Health Service continue to endorse the DPT vaccine, many parents and health providers believe that the risks associated with it are too high. Steven Black, codirector of the Kaiser-Permanente Pediatric Vaccine Study Center, contends that the DPT vaccine is far from ideal. Newer vaccines, particularly a new pertussis vaccine, reduce the risk of injury by a significant percentage. See "The Perils of Pertussis," *American Health* (June 1991). Unlike the current DPT vaccine, which uses whole, killed bacteria cells to trigger the formation of antibodies, the new, acellular pertussis vaccine contains only a part of the bacteria cells. This new vaccine, currently available in Japan but not yet in the United States, causes fewer local and systemic reactions, such as high fever and swelling. However, studies have raised concerns that the acellular vaccines may cause more severe side effects, such as brain damage, than the DPT vaccine.

Widespread publicity about the genuine but extremely rare adverse effects of the pertussis vaccine is causing concern among drug manufacturers. Fewer companies are willing to produce vaccines due to expensive lawsuits brought by parents of injured children. This will lead to vaccine shortages and higher costs (which will be passed on to the consumer). The following articles discuss cost factors in relation to the low rates of immunizations: "Persistent Low Immunization Coverage Among Inner City Children," *Pediatrics* (April 1998); "Shots in the Dark," *Reason* (November 1994); "Why Haven't Millions of Youngsters Gotten All Their Shots?" *CQ Researcher* (June 18, 1993); "Cheap Shots," *The New Republic* (October 26, 1992); and "Unprotected Children," *The Atlantic Monthly* (March 1993).

Vaccines other than the DPT vaccine are also thought to be harmful. "Epidemiology of Smallpox Vaccine-Related Granulocytopenia," *Mutation Research* (February 1980) indicates that children who had smallpox vaccinations in Czechoslovakia showed harmful changes in their white blood cells. "Changing Concepts of Epstein-Barr Syndrome: An Immunization Reaction?" *Medical Hypothesis* (January 1988) reports a study of 200 patients who contracted Epstein-Barr syndrome when vaccinated with a live rubella (German measles) virus. Other articles discussing the risks of vaccination include "Juvenile Diabetes and Vaccination: New Evidence for a Connection," *The Vaccine Reaction* (February 1998); "Experts Forum," *Mothering* (Summer 1996); "Immunizations: Do You Know the Risks?" *Second Opinion* (May 1994); "Mean Vaccines: For the Record," *Vegetarian Times* (February 1993); "A New 'P' in DPT," *Vegetarian Times* (July 1992); and "Who Calls the Shots?" *East West Journal* (November 1988). For information on the antivaccine movement, see "Anti-Vaccine Movements and Whooping Cough: The Controversy Continues," *Vaccine Weekly* (February 16, 1998).

The medical community's endorsement of vaccination is evident in "U.S. Measles Cases at Record Low," *Health Letter on the CDC* (May 4, 1998); "Safety of Vaccinations," *Journal of the American Medical Association* (December 18, 1996); and "The War We Thought We Had Won," *Medical Update* (April 1996). For a comprehensive update on vaccine safety, see "Update: Vaccine Side Effects, Adverse Reactions, Contraindications, and Precautions," *Morbidity and Mortality Weekly Report* (September 6, 1996).

# ISSUE 21

# Are Homeopathic Remedies Legitimate?

**YES: Nancy Bruning,** from "The Mysterious Power of Homeopathy," *Natural Health* (January/February 1995)

**NO: Stephen Barrett,** from "Homeopathy," *Nutrition Forum* (May/June 1998)

### ISSUE SUMMARY

**YES:** Author Nancy Bruning asserts that neither skeptics nor believers can exactly explain how homeopathy works but that it can successfully treat a wide range of health problems.

**NO:** Physician and health consumer advocate Stephen Barrett argues that homeopathic remedies are so dilute that they are useless.

Many Americans, disillusioned with traditional medicine, are seeking alternative health providers, such as homeopaths, acupuncturists, and chiropractors. Among the various alternatives, homeopathy has recently surged in popularity. Demand for these remedies has never been greater, and consumer advocates and scientists want the Food and Drug Administration (FDA) to regulate the sale of these products, which they claim are worthless.

Americans spend over $150 million on homeopathic medicines each year. Overall, sales have climbed 25 percent per year since the late 1980s. This surprises many scientists and physicians because homeopathy has been out of fashion since the turn of the century. Interestingly, homeopathy has never lost its appeal in Europe. In England homeopathic services and remedies are even covered by the national health insurance. It has also remained popular in France and Germany.

Homeopathy is a medical theory and practice that developed over 200 years ago in response to the harsh procedures, such as bloodletting, used in those days. Samuel Hahnemann, a German doctor disenchanted with harsh treatments, developed a theory based on three principles: the minimum dose, the law of similars, and the single remedy. The word homeopathy comes from the Greek words for "like" and "suffering." With the minimum dose, or law of infinitesimals, Hahnemann believed that a substance's strength and effectiveness heightened the more it was diluted. The dilution makes the drug virtually nonexistent, but the homeopathic belief is that the substance has left its imprint or a spirit-like essence that stimulates the body to heal itself. With the law of similars, Hahnemann theorized that if a large amount of a substance causes certain symptoms in a healthy person, smaller amounts of the same substance can cure those symptoms in an ill person. Hahnemann developed this belief after a strong dose of the malaria treatment, quinine, caused his healthy body to develop symptoms similar to those experienced by malaria patients. Finally, a homeopathic practitioner generally prescribes only a single remedy to cover all symptoms that the patient is experiencing.

Although most homeopaths do not recommend that people abandon conventional treatments for AIDS, cancer, and other serious illnesses, they often advise homeopathic remedies along with traditional medications. In most states it is illegal to practice homeopathy without a license to prescribe drugs, but many people with no formal training claim to be homeopaths. The American Medical Association (AMA) does not accept homeopathy, but it does not totally reject it either. The AMA has recently stated that doctors should be aware of alternative therapies and use them if appropriate.

Do homeopathic remedies work? Supporters often point to an analysis of 107 clinical studies published in the *British Medical Journal* in 1991. The results of 81 of these studies suggested that homeopathic treatment was more effective than a placebo, while the others found no difference. There did appear to be methodological problems, however, with many of the studies. The National Center for Homeopathy, an information clearinghouse, points to research published in the *Lancet* (December 10, 1994). The rigorously conducted study showed that asthma patients improved considerably after undergoing homeopathic treatment, though the researchers were unable to explain the results. Dr. Herbert Benson, president of the Mind-Body Institute at Deaconess Hospital in Boston, Massachusetts, maintains that homeopathy's effects are consistent with the placebo effect. For the placebo effect to work, there must be "belief and expectation" that it will, both on the part of the practitioner and the patient. If homeopathy rests solely on faith and belief, sick persons can recover without homeopathic medications. So why do consumers need to spend millions of dollars a year on homeopathic remedies?

In the following selections, Nancy Bruning states that although scientists scoff at claims that homeopathy can relieve symptoms and treat disease, many people swear that it can. Stephen Barrett counters that homeopathic remedies are a fraud. He states that "if the FDA required homeopathic remedies to be proven effective in order to remain on the market . . . homeopathy would face extinction in the United States."

# YES

Nancy Bruning

# THE MYSTERIOUS POWER
# OF HOMEOPATHY

Forget the skeptics—even practitioners of homeopathy struggle to explain this bizarre but seemingly effective system of healing. This is not surprising given that homeopathy defies the known laws of chemistry, physics, and pharmacology. For starters, homeopathic medicines contain substances known to cause the symptoms you want to eliminate. Imagine taking poison ivy pills to relieve itching.

And if that isn't enough, the homeopathic preparations are made by repeatedly diluting the active ingredient—putting an ounce of the ingredient in ten ounces of water, then an ounce of that dilution in ten ounces of water, and so on—until it's unlikely that even a single molecule of the active ingredient will be present in the dose you take. Moreover, the more dilute the preparation, the more potent it is considered to be. All this combines to throw skeptic and believer alike into a baffling realm of theory and speculation where matter dissolves into pure energy, where small permutations in a system can create large changes, and where wave patterns and electromagnetic messages affect not only the body and mind but even the spirit.

Naturally, most scientists scoff at claims that homeopathy can relieve illness. What they can't do, however, is ignore the many people who swear that it can. My own experience a few years ago landed me in the ranks of the believers. When my yoga instructor recommended a popular homeopathic remedy, Calmes Forté, for my insomnia; I tried it, and it worked. Also, I had no druggy feeling the next day, as I might have had with sleeping pills. Over the next several months it continued to work more often than not. But like most people who use homeopathic medicines, I hadn't a clue as to why.

Two years later, I teamed up with a physician trained in homeopathic medicine—Corey Weinstein—and wrote a book about homeopathy. It was then that I learned that this system has an impressive track record and is supported with increasing frequency by publications in scientific journals.

In fact, homeopathy was the medicine of choice for many nineteenth-century American physicians. In the 1850s, however, the newly formed American Medical Association began to rout homeopathy from the halls of "respected" medicine. At the turn of the century there were 15,000 practicing homeopaths in the United States (15 to 20 percent of the entire medical profession), but by the 1970s fewer than 200 practitioners remained.

Now, homeopathy is on the rebound. A survey published in the *New England Journal of Medicine* found that 2.3 million Americans used homeopathy in 1990, and the National Center for Homeopathy estimates that at least 2,500 practitioners use homeopathy in the United States. Sales of homeopathic medicines in health and drug stores are rising at the rate of 25 percent annually as people use these medicines to treat themselves for a variety of problems.

## HOW HOMEOPATHY WORKS

There is a principle of homeopathy called the Law of Similars, which holds that "like cures like." This means that a substance that causes certain symptoms in a healthy person can, when given in infinitesimal doses, cure those same symptoms in a sick person. For example, consider the homeopathic remedy *Coffea*. It's made from coffee, well-known for its ability to cause jumpiness and wakefulness. As a remedy, however, *Coffea* is prescribed to calm your nerves and help you sleep. Similarly, *Allium cepa*, which is made from onions, relieves the symptoms of watery eyes and runny nose.

In homeopathy, symptoms are seen neither as enemies to be squashed nor as the disease itself. "Rather," says Dana Ullman, president of the Foundation for Homeopathic Research in Berkeley, California, "they are signs of the body's effort to deal with infection or stress, to defend and heal. Because our bodies are not always completely effective in

healing, giving a substance that mimics the body's defense helps trigger that process."

Homeopaths maintain that while suppressing symptoms outright may help you feel better temporarily, it won't help the healing process. In one of the many analogies that homeopaths use to explain their system, countering symptoms with "anti"-histamines or "anti"-biotics is said to be like smashing a beeping smoke alarm instead of looking for the fire that set it off.

Unlike a smoke alarm, however, symptoms are part of the healing process. For instance, even conventional medicine now recognizes that fever helps the body fight infection and that a runny nose clears the body of mucus and dead pathogens.

Homeopaths believe that although symptoms may be unpleasant, they play an important role in healing, and therefore should be stimulated and supported rather than suppressed. Only then can the body rid itself of disease and return to health; the symptoms will fade away naturally when they are no longer needed. Ullman likens homeopathy to "steering *into* a skid" to regain control of your car, rather than steering against the direction of the skid, which only sends you further out of control.

You can take one of two basic categories of homeopathic remedies: *combination* remedies or *single* remedies. Combination remedies include two or more of the single remedies that are most likely to alleviate specific symptoms, such as a cough, indigestion, or muscle aches. Single homeopathic remedies are specific to an individual's overall pattern of symptoms, which in the case of a cough, for example, may include whether the person feels hot or cold, what time of day the cough is worst, and how dry or wet the cough is. Since people's overall symptom patterns will differ, two people with a cough may require different single remedies. Thus, combination remedies are more likely to contain the remedy you will need. For people without experience in homeopathy, they are much easier to use than single remedies.

Combination remedies are used mainly for acute (sudden onset, short-lived) conditions which have simpler and more consistent symptom patterns than chronic (slower developing, longer-lasting) conditions. Acute conditions include minor injuries and wounds, insect bites, burns and sunburn, and muscle strains and sprains. You can also use combination remedies to treat yourself pre- and post-operatively to help deal with shock and to speed healing. And they are often used successfully to fight flus, colds, coughs, and sore throats; headaches and hangovers; digestive problems such as nausea, vomiting, diarrhea, and constipation; and kids' problems, such as earaches, teething pain, and toothaches. A correct combination remedy can even soothe acute emotional reactions such as fear and anxiety before an exam, performance, or other big event.

Brands of combination remedies vary as to the remedies they contain, and although this "shotgun" approach increases the chance a product will contain the remedy you need, it doesn't guarantee it. So if you don't get relief from one particular combination, you may need to try other brands until you find the one that works. If you still fail to see any benefits, don't give up on homeopathy altogether—the combinations you've tried may not contain the particular remedy you require. For another ailment, or at another time, the same or another prod-uct may work wonderfully. Also, you may need to find a homeopathic specialist who will help you find the correct single remedy needed for your symptoms.

## CONSTITUTIONAL REMEDIES

Single remedies (sometimes called constitutional remedies) are often necessary for chronic conditions that have endured for months, years, or your whole life, and which may be more deep-seated and complicated. Choosing the correct single remedy requires some study and perhaps a little luck on the part of the patient, or the skill and expertise of a professional homeopath.

Constitutional homeopathy can often help cure such chronic conditions as acne, allergies, migraine headaches, asthma, depression, anxiety, fatigue, premenstrual syndrome, arthritis, eczema, and psoriasis. Professionally guided constitutional therapy is also recommended if you want to go beyond self-care and cure the underlying disease that may be at the root of recurring acute symptoms.

While combination remedies tend to be easier to use, some homeopaths, such as Jennifer Jacobs, M.D., a family physician in Seattle, encourage people to at least try self-prescribing single remedies for acute conditions. If chosen correctly, they are more effective than the combinations because they are used in higher potencies and are more specific to the individual. However, you can't just wander into a store and expect to choose the right single remedy off the shelf. The playing field can be confusing to the novice, in part because manufacturers label single remedies with just a few parts of the total symptom profile. . . .

*Table 1*

## Picking the Right Remedy

| Conditions | Aconite | Apis | Arnica | Arsenicum | Belladonna | Bryonia | Carbo veg. | Chamomilla | Ferrum phos. |
|---|---|---|---|---|---|---|---|---|---|
| | | | | | Homeopathic Products | | | | |
| Acne | | | | x | | | | | |
| Anxiety | x | | | | | | | | |
| Backache | | | x | | | | | | |
| Bruises, Sprains & Strains | | | x | | | | | | |
| Coughs & Cold | x | | | | | | | | x |
| Depression | | | | | | | | | x |
| Eczema | | | | x | | | | | |
| Exhaustion | | | x | | | | x | | |
| Gas | | | | x | | | x | x | |
| Headache | x | | | | x | x | | | x |
| Indigestion | | | | | | | x | | |
| Insomnia | | | | | | | | x | |
| Irritability | | x | | | | | | | |
| Neck Stiffness | x | | | | | x | | | |
| PMS | | | | | | | | x | |
| Sinusitis | | | | | x | | | | x |
| Toothache | | | | | x | | | x | |

| Conditions | Gelsemium | Hepar sulph. | Ipecac | Mercurius | Nux vomica | Phosphorus | Pulsatilla | Rhus tox. | Sulphur |
|---|---|---|---|---|---|---|---|---|---|
| | | | | | Homeopathic Products | | | | |
| Acne | | | | x | | | | x | x |
| Anxiety | x | | | | x | | x | | |
| Backache | | | | | x | | x | x | |
| Bruises, Sprains & Strains | | | | | x | | x | x | |
| Coughs & Cold | | x | | | | | x | | |
| Depression | | | | x | | | x | x | |
| Eczema | | x | | | | | | x | x |
| Exhaustion | x | | | | x | | | | |
| Gas | | | | | x | | | | |
| Headache | | | | | | | | | |
| Indigestion | | | x | | x | | x | | |
| Insomnia | | x | | x | | | x | | |
| Irritability | | | | | x | x | x | | |
| Neck Stiffness | | | | | x | | | x | |
| PMS | | | | | x | | x | x | |
| Sinusitis | | x | | | | | x | | |
| Toothache | | | | x | | | x | | |

Source: Nancy Bruning, *Natural Health,* January/February 1995.

## RULES FOR HOMEOPATHY

Homeopathy comes with its own set of rules to follow for taking remedies. Some—such as caveats against touching the remedy or drinking coffee—may seem illogical to the average person. And, admittedly there are differences of opinion within the profession as to how strictly you need to observe these rules. However, the consensus is that to be safe and to give homeopathy the best chance of working, it's advisable to follow these guidelines:

1. The frequency of the dosage depends on the intensity of the symptoms. Severe symptoms that come on suddenly, such as earache, may require a dose every five minutes; a slowly developing flu may need the remedy every three or four hours. As the symptoms improve or disappear, increase the interval between doses or stop the medication. Start again if the same symptoms return. However, if there has been no response to the remedy after six doses, switch to another remedy.
2. Avoid touching the remedy with your hands. Instead, tip the required number of pellets into the container cap and from the cap into your mouth; if the tablets are blister-packed, pop them directly into your mouth. Homeopaths say that touching the remedy could contaminate it or inactivate it.
3. Avoid eating or drinking anything but chlorine-free water for fifteen to thirty minutes before and after taking the remedy. And allow the remedy to dissolve slowly under your tongue so it is absorbed directly into the tiny sublingual capillaries. (Some combination tablets include instructions to chew them.)
4. Store homeopathic remedies in their original containers, away from heat and sunlight. Also, keep them away from strong-smelling substances that might contaminate them, such as perfumes, camphor, and eucalyptus. (These and other aromatic substances are found in items that inhabit the medicine chest.) Some homeopaths also advise against drinking herbal teas or ingesting products containing mint (for instance, toothpaste) within a half-hour of taking remedies.
5. Avoid drinking coffee during treatment. Coffee may counteract the remedy's effect by acting as an antidote or by otherwise slowing the healing process.

Another area of debate among homeopaths is the relationship of homeopathic treatment to other forms of medicine. Some homeopaths feel that all you really need to treat an illness is the right homeopathic remedy. However, most say that other natural healing methods help when used appropriately, and that conventional medicine also has its place. Most homeopaths stress the importance of good health habits such as proper diet, exercise, rest, vacation time, satisfying social relationships, creative living, effective stress management, and spiritual nourishment. Since the goal of homeopathy is to stimulate the body's ability to heal, it makes sense to support the body's efforts with healthy living.

# NO

**Stephen Barrett**

# HOMEOPATHY

### Much Ado About Little or Nothing

Homeopathic "remedies" enjoy a unique status in the health marketplace: They are the only category of quack products legally marketable as drugs. This situation exists for two reasons. First, the 1938 Federal Food, Drug, and Cosmetic Act, which was shepherded through Congress by a homeopathic physician who was a senator, recognizes the Homeopathic Pharmacopeia of the United States. Second, the FDA has not held homeopathic products to the same standards as other drugs.

### Basic Misbeliefs

Homeopathy dates back to the late 1700s when Samuel Hahnemann (1755–1843), a German physician, began formulating its basic principles. Hahnemann was justifiably distressed about bloodletting, leeching, purging, and other medical procedures of his day that did far more harm than good. Thinking that these treatments were intended to "balance the body's 'humors' by opposite effect," he developed his "Law of similars"—a notion that symptoms of disease can be cured by extremely small amounts of substances that produce similar symptoms in healthy people when administered in large amounts. The word "homeopathy" is derived from the Greek words homoios (similar) and pathos (suffering or disease).

Hahnemann and his early followers conducted "provings" in which they administered herbs, minerals, and other substances to healthy people, including themselves, and kept detailed records of what they observed. Later these records were compiled into lengthy reference books called materia medica, which were and still are used to match a patient's symptoms with a "corresponding" drug.

Hahnemann declared that diseases represent a disturbance in the body's ability to heal itself and that only a small stimulus is needed to begin the healing process. He also claimed that chronic diseases were manifestations of a suppressed itch (psora), a kind of miasma or evil sprit.

From Stephen Barrett, "Homeopathy," *Nutrition Forum* (May/June 1998). Copyright © 1998 by Prometheus Books. Reprinted by permission. References omitted.

At first he used small doses of accepted medications. But later he used enormous dilutions and theorized that the smaller the dose, the more powerful the effect —a notion often referred to as the "law of infinitesimals." That, of course, is just the opposite of the dose-response relationship that pharmacologists have demonstrated.

The basis for inclusion in the Homeopathic Pharmacopeia is not modern scientific testing, but homeopathic "provings," many of which took place during the 1800s and early 1900s. These provings had little consistency because methods varied greatly from practitioner to practitioner. Some used a single dose, others dosed as often as three times a day for months; and potencies ranged from the undiluted original substance to dilutions so high that not one molecule of the original substance was likely to remain. The book's current (ninth) edition describes how more than a thousand substances are prepared for homeopathic use. It does not identify the symptoms or diseases for which homeopathic products should be used; that is decided by the practitioner (or manufacturer). The fact that substances listed in the Homeopathic Pharmacopeia are legally recognized as "drugs" does not mean that either the law or the FDA recognizes them as effective.

Because homeopathic remedies were actually less dangerous than those of nineteenth-century medical orthodoxy, many medical practitioners began using them. At the turn of the twentieth century homeopathy had about 14,000 practitioners and 22 schools in the United States. But as medical science and medical education advanced homeopathy declined sharply in America, where its schools either closed or converted to modern methods. The last pure homeopathic school in this country closed during the 1920s.

Many homeopaths maintain that certain people have a special affinity to a particular remedy (their "constitutional remedy") and will respond to it for a variety of ailments. Such remedies can be prescribed according to the person's "constitutional type"—named after the corresponding remedy in a manner resembling astrologic typing. The "Ignatia Type," for example, is said to be nervous and often tearful, and to dislike tobacco smoke. The typical "Pulsatilla" is a young woman, with blonde or light-brown hair, blue eyes, and a delicate complexion, who is gentle, fearful, romantic, emotional, and friendly but shy. The "Nux Vomica Type" is said to be aggressive, bellicose, ambitious, and hyperactive. The "Sulfur Type" likes to be independent. And so on.

### The 'Remedies' Are Placebos

Homeopathic products are made from minerals, botanical substances, and several other sources. If the original substance is soluble, one part is diluted with either nine or ninety-nine parts of distilled water and/or alcohol and shaken vigorously (succussed); if insoluble, it is finely ground and pulverized in similar proportions with powdered lactose (milk sugar). One part of the diluted medicine is then further diluted, and the process is repeated until the desired concentration is reached. Dilutions of 10 are designated by the Roman numeral X ($1X = 1/10$, $3X = 1/1,000$, $6X = 1/1,000,000$). Similarly, dilutions of 1 to 100 are designated by the Roman numeral C ($1C = 1/100$, $3C = 1/1,000,000$, and so on). Most remedies today range from 6X to 30X, but products of 30C or more are marketed.

A 30X dilution means that the original substance has been diluted 10[sup 30] times. Assuming that a cubic centimeter of water contains 15 drops, this number is greater than the number of drops of water that would fill a container more than 50 times the size of the Earth. Imagine placing a drop of red dye into such a container so that it disperses evenly. Homeopathy's "law of infinitesimals" is the equivalent of saying that any drop of water subsequently removed from that container will possess an essence of redness. Robert L. Park, PhD, a prominent physicist who is executive director of the American Physical Society, has noted that since the least amount of a substance in a solution is one molecule, a 30C solution would have to have at least one molecule of the original substance dissolved in a minimum of 100[sup 30] molecules of water. This would require a container more than 30 billion times the size of the Earth.

Occillococcinum, a 200C product "for the relief of colds and flu-like symptoms," involves "dilutions" that are even more far-fetched. Its "active ingredient" is prepared by incubating small amounts of a freshly killed duck's liver and heart for 40 days. The resultant solution is then filtered, freeze-dried, rehydrated, repeatedly diluted, and impregnated into sugar granules. If a single molecule of the duck's heart or liver were to survive the dilution, its concentration would be 1 in 100 [sup 200]. This huge number, which has 400 zeroes, is vastly greater than the estimated number of molecules in the universe (about one googol, which is a 1 followed by 100 zeroes). U.S. News & World Report has noted that only one duck per year is needed to manufacture the product, which had total sales of $20 million in 1996. The

magazine dubbed that unlucky bird "the $20-million duck."

Actually, the laws of chemistry state that there is a limit to the dilution that can be made without losing the original substance altogether. This limit, called Avogadro's number, corresponds to homeopathic potencies of 12C or 24X (1 part in 10[sup 24]). Hahnemann himself realized that there is virtually no chance that even one molecule of original substance would remain after extreme dilutions. But he believed that the vigorous shaking or pulverizing with each step of dilution leaves behind a "spirit-like" essence—"no longer perceptible to the senses"—which cures by reviving the body's "vital force." This notion is unsubstantiated. Moreover, if it were true, every substance encountered by a molecule of water might imprint an "essence" that could exert powerful (and unpredictable) medicinal effects when ingested by a person. Dr. Park has noted that to expect to get even one molecule of the "medicinal" substance allegedly present in 30X pills, it would be necessary to take some two billion of them, which would total about a thousand tons of lactose plus whatever impurities the lactose contained.

Many proponents claim that homeopathic products resemble vaccines because both provide a small stimulus that triggers an immune response. This comparison is not valid. The amounts of active ingredients in vaccines are much greater and can be measured. Moreover, immunizations produce antibodies whose concentration in the blood can be measured, but high-dilution homeopathic products produce no measurable response.

### 'Electrodiagnosis'

Some physicians, dentists, and chiropractors use "electrodiagnostic" devices to help select the homeopathic remedies they prescribe. These practitioners claim they can determine the cause of any disease by detecting the "energy imbalance" causing the problem. Some also claim that the devices can detect whether someone is allergic or sensitive to foods, vitamins, and/or other substances.

The procedure, called electroacupuncture according to Voll (EAV), electrodiagnosis, or electrodermal screening, was begun during the 1970s by Reinhold Voll, MD, a West German physician who developed the original device. Subsequent models include the Dermatron, Vegatest, Interro, and Omega AcuBase.

Proponents claim that these devices measure disturbances in the flow of "electro-magnetic energy" along the body's "acupuncture meridians." Actually, they are fancy galvanometers that measure electrical resistance of the patient's skin when touched by a probe. Each device contains a low-voltage source. One wire from the device goes to a brass cylinder covered by moist gauze, which the patient holds in one hand. A second wire is connected to a probe, which the operator touches to "acupuncture points" on the patient's foot or other hand. This completes a circuit, and the device registers the flow of current. The information is then relayed to a gauge that provides a numerical readout. The size of the number depends on how hard the probe is pressed against the patient's skin. Recent versions, such as the Interro, make sounds and provide the readout on a computer screen. The treatment selected depends on the scope of the practitioner's practice and may include acupuncture, dietary change, and/or vitamin supplements, as well as homeopathic products. Regulatory agencies have seized several types of "electrodiagnostic" devices but have not made a systematic effort to drive them from the marketplace.

### Unimpressive 'Research'

Since many homeopathic remedies contain no detectable amount of active ingredient, it is impossible to test whether they contain what their label says. Unlike most potent drugs, they have not been proven effective against disease by double-blind clinical testing. In fact, the vast majority of homeopathic products have never even been tested.

Homeopathy's favorite article is probably a 1994 report claiming that homeopathic treatment had been demonstrated to be effective against mild cases of diarrhea among Nicaraguan children (Pediatrics 93:719–725, 1994). The claim was based on findings that, on certain days, the "treated" group had fewer loose stools than the placebo group. However, the data were not properly interpreted. In a rebuttal article, Wallace Sampson, MD, and William London, EdD, noted that the data were oddly grouped and contained errors and inconsistencies (Pediatrics 96:961–964, 1995).

In December 1996, a lengthy report was published by the Homeopathic Medicines Research Group (HMRG), an expert panel convened by the Commission of the European Communities. The HMRG included homeopathic physician-researchers and experts in clinical research, clinical pharmacology, biostatistics, and clinical epidemiology. Its aim was to evaluate published and unpublished reports of controlled trials of homeopathic treatment. After examining 184 reports, the panelists concluded:

(1) only 17 were designed and reported well enough to be worth considering; (2) in some of these trials, homeopathic approaches may have exerted a greater effect than a placebo or no treatment; and (3) the number of participants in these 17 trials was too small to draw any conclusions about the effectiveness of homeopathic treatment for any specific condition. Simply put: Most homeopathic research is worthless, and no homeopathic product has been proven effective for any therapeutic purpose. The National Council Against Health Fraud has warned "the sectarian nature of homeopathy raises serious questions about the trustworthiness of homeopathic researchers."

Proponents trumpet the few "positive" studies as proof that "homeopathy works." Even if their results can be consistently reproduced (which seems unlikely), the most that the study of a single remedy for a single disease could prove is that the remedy is effective against that disease. It would not validate homeopathy's basic theories or prove that homeopathic treatment is useful for other diseases.

Placebo effects can be powerful, of course, but the potential benefit of relieving symptoms with placebos should be weighed against the harm that can result from relying upon—and wasting money on—ineffective products. Spontaneous remission is also a factor in homeopathy's popularity. I believe that most people who credit a homeopathic product for their recovery would have fared equally well without it.

Homeopathic practitioners claim to provide care that is safer, gentler, more "natural," and less expensive than conventional care—and more concerned with prevention. The fact is, however, that homeopathic treatments prevent nothing and many homeopathic leaders preach against immunization. Equally bad, a report on the National Center for Homeopathy's 1997 Conference described how a homeopathic physician had suggested using homeopathic products to help prevent and treat coronary artery disease. According to the article, the speaker recommended various 30C and 200C products as alternatives to aspirin or cholesterol-lowering drugs (Homeopathy Today 17(8):3, 1997).

## Greater Regulation Is Needed

If the FDA required homeopathic remedies to be proven effective in order to remain marketable—the standard it applies to other categories of drugs—homeopathy would face extinction in the United States. However, there is no indication that the agency is considering this. FDA officials regard homeopathy as relatively benign (compared, for example, to unsubstantiated products marketed for cancer and AIDS) and believe that other problems should get enforcement priority. FDA guidelines issued in 1988 permit manufacturers to sell nonprescription homeopathics for "self-limiting conditions recognizable by consumers," provided that their labeling "adequately instructs consumers in the product's safe use." But if a product doesn't work, the only truly adequate instruction for use is to avoid it.

In August 1994, 42 critics of quackery and pseudoscience petitioned the FDA to initiate a rulemaking procedure to require that all over-the-counter (OTC) homeopathic drugs meet the same standards of safety and effectiveness as nonhomeopathic OTC drugs. The petition also asked the FDA to warn the public that although the agency has permitted homeopathic products to be sold, it does not recognize them as effective. The FDA has not yet ruled on the petition. On March 3, 1998, at a symposium sponsored by Good Housekeeping magazine, former FDA Commissioner David A. Kessler, MD, JD, acknowledged that homeopathic products do not work but that he did not attempt to ban them because he felt that Congress would not support a ban.

The Federal Trade Commission could take effective action against homeopathic manufacturers that make false claims in their ads. Since no homeopathic product now advertised has been proven effective, and since few if any have even been reliably tested, it is hard to imagine how therapeutic claims for them could stand up in court. However, the FTC has shown no inclination to regulate homeopathic advertising.

If the FDA and FTC attack homeopathy too vigorously, its proponents might even persuade a lobby-susceptible Congress to rescue them. Regardless of this risk, federal agencies should not permit worthless products to be marketed with claims that they are effective. Nor should they continue to tolerate the presence of quack "electrodiagnostic" devices in the marketplace.

## Dubious Marketing

America's most blatant homeopathic marketer appears to be Biological Homeopathic Industries (BHI) of Albuquerque, New Mexico, which in 1983 sent a 123-page catalog to 200,000 physicians nationwide. Its products included BHI Anticancer Stimulating, BHI Antivirus, BHI Stroke, and 50 other types of tablets claimed to be effective against serious diseases.

In 1984, the FDA forced BHI to stop distributing several of the products and to tone down its claims for others. However, BHI has continued to make illegal claims. Its 1991 Physicians Reference ("for use only by health care professionals") inappropriately recommended products for heart failure, syphilis, kidney failure, blurred vision, and many other serious conditions. The company's publishing arm issues the quarterly Biological Therapy: Journal of Natural Medicine, which regularly contains articles whose authors make questionable claims. An article in the April 1992 issue, for example, listed "indications" for using BHI and Heel products (distributed by BHI) for more than 50 conditions—including cancer, angina pectoris, and paralysis. And the October 1993 issue, devoted to the homeopathic treatment of children, includes an article recommending products for acute bacterial infections to the ear and tonsils. The article is described as selections from Heel seminars given in several cities by a Nevada homeopath who also served as medical editor of Biological Therapy. In 1993, Heel published a 503-page hardcover book describing how to use its products to treat about 450 conditions. Twelve pages of the book cover "Neoplasia and neoplastic phases of disease." ("Neoplasm" is a medical term for tumor.) In March 1998, during an osteopathic convention in Las Vegas, Nevada, a Heel exhibitor distributed copies of the book when asked for detailed information on how to use Heel products.

# POSTSCRIPT

## Are Homeopathic Remedies Legitimate?

Why do so many Americans seek out alternative medicine such as homeopathy? In a study published in 1993, researchers at Harvard Medical School found that one out of three patients said they had used some kind of alternative treatment, while seven out of ten said they had not told their doctors. The Harvard study estimated that Americans made 425 million visits to alternative practitioners in 1990, spending over $14 billion. Much of the money was paid directly by the consumers since alternative medicine is usually not covered by health insurance. It may be that consumers are dissatisfied with conventional medical care and short, managed care office visits. Alternative medicine may also appeal to the need for consumers to have both their minds and bodies treated.

Medicine and the research establishment are responding. The National Institutes of Health have created the Office of Alternative Medicine, which has funded two full-scale research projects and given numerous study grants. Currently, more than 25 medical schools teach courses on alternative methods. Could there be a problem with this move toward alternatives such as homeopathy? Maybe. Herbal expert Varro Tyler and physician Stephen Barrett argue that homeopathy is a fraud. See "Researchers Question Validity of Homeopathy," *Nation's Health* (November 1997) and "Why Pharmacists Should Not Sell Homeopathic Remedies," *American Journal of Health-System Pharmacy* (May 1, 1995). Many of the studies supporting homeopathy appear to have methodological flaws. Despite this, many consumers seem to be drawn to unproven remedies.

Are there risks to homeopathy? Generally, it is assumed that the dosage is so diluted that there is little therapeutic effect or risk. The main concern is that patients will abandon conventional therapies in favor of the unproven. Readings that explore homeopathy and alternative medicine include "Homeopathy," *Prevention* (March 1998); "Are You Homeophobic?" *Village Voice* (February 3, 1998); "Flu Symptoms," *U.S. News and World Report* (February 17, 1997); "Homeopathy," *Harvard Women's Health* (January 1997); "Funding Alternative Medicine," *Popular Science* (January 1997); "Challenging the Mainstream," *Time* (Fall 1996); "Homeopathy: Real Medicine or Empty Promises?" *FDA Consumer* (December 1996); "Does Homeopathy Work?" *Healthline* (February 1996); and "Homeopathy," *Mayo Clinic Newsletter* (February 1996).

# CONTRIBUTORS
# TO THIS VOLUME

**EDITOR**

**EILEEN L. DANIEL,** a registered dietitian and licensed nutritionist, is an associate professor in and chair of the Department of Health Science at the State University of New York College at Brockport. She received a B.S. in nutrition and dietetics from the Rochester Institute of Technology in 1977, an M.S. in community health education from SUNY College at Brockport in 1978, and a Ph.D. in health education from the University of Oregon in 1986. A member of the Eta Sigma Gamma National Health Honor Society, the American Dietetics Association, the New York State Dietetics Society, and other professional and community organizations, she has published over 35 articles on issues of health, nutrition, and health education. Her publications have appeared in such professional journals as the *Journal of Nutrition Education,* the *Journal of School Health,* and the *Journal of Health Education.* She is the author of *Jumpstart With Weblinks: A Guidebook for Fitness/Wellness/Personal Health, 97/98* (Morton, 1997) and *A Guidebook for Nutrition* (Morton, 1998).

# AUTHORS

**ARTHUR ALLEN** is a freelance journalist based in Washington, D.C., who reports regularly on medical and scientific issues.

**BRUCE AMES,** a genetic toxicologist, is a professor of biochemistry and molecular biology and director of the National Institute of Environmental Health Sciences Center at the University of California, Berkeley, where he has been teaching since 1968. He is a member of the National Academy of Sciences and is the recipient of the most prestigious award for cancer research, the General Motors Cancer Research Foundation Prize (1983); the highest award in environmental achievement, the Tyler Prize (1985); and the Gold Medal Award of the American Institute of Chemists (1991). He has been elected to the Royal Swedish Academy of Sciences, Japan Cancer Association, and the Academy of Toxicological Sciences. He is the author or coauthor of 300 scientific publications.

**MARCIA ANGELL** is a physician, an author, and executive editor of the *New England Journal of Medicine.* She graduated from the Boston University School of Medicine and has done postgraduate work in internal medicine as well as in pathology. She frequently writes on ethical issues in medicine and biomedical research, and she is the author of *Science on Trial: The Clash of Medical Evidence and the Law in the Breast Implant Case* (W. W. Norton, 1996).

**GEORGE J. ANNAS** is the Edward R. Utley Professor of Law and Medicine at Boston University's Schools of Medicine and Public Health in Boston, Massachusetts. He is also director of Boston University's Law, Medicine, and Ethics Program and chair of the Department of Health Law. His publications include *Standard of Care: The Law of American Bioethics* (Oxford University Press, 1993) and *Some Choice: Law, Medicine, and the Market* (Oxford University Press, 1998).

**STEPHEN BARRETT** is a retired psychiatrist and a nationally renowned author, editor, and consumer health advocate. He is a board member of the National Council Against Health Fraud and a scientific and editorial adviser to the American Council on Science and Health. In 1986 he was awarded honorary life membership in the American Dietetic Association. He has written more than 36 books.

**HERBERT BENSON** is a physician and associate professor of medicine at Harvard Medical School and the Deaconess Hospital. He is also president and founder of their Mind/Body Institute.

**DENNIS BERNSTEIN** is an associate editor for *Pacific News Service* and a coproducer of KPFA's *Flashpoints* radio show.

**PATRICIA LANOIE BLANCHETTE** is a professor of medicine and public health in the John A. Burns School of Medicine at the University of Hawaii, Honolulu. She is also the director of their geriatric medicine program.

**NANCY BRUNING** is a founding member of Breast Cancer Action. A health and environment writer, she is the author or coauthor of 12 books, including *Breast Implant: Everything You Need to Know* (Hunter House, 1995) and, with Shari Lieberman, *The Real Vitamin and Mineral Book: Going Beyond the RDA for Optimum Health* (Avery, 1990).

**CHRISTOPHER CALDWELL** is a senior writer for *The Weekly Standard.*

**DANIEL CALLAHAN,** a philosopher, is cofounder and president of the Hastings Center in Briarcliff Manor, New York, where he is also director of International Programs. He received a Ph.D. in philosophy from Harvard University, and he is the author or editor of over 31 publications, including *The Troubled Dream of Life: In Search of Peaceful Death* (Simon & Schuster, 1993); *What Kind of Life: The Limits of Medical Progress* (Georgetown University Press, 1995); and *False Hopes: Why America's Quest for Perfect Health Is a Recipe for Failure* (Rutgers University Press, 1999).

**MICHAEL CASTLEMAN** is a health columnist and the author of *Nature's Cures* (St. Martin's Press, 1996) and *The Healing Herbs: The Ultimate Guide to the Curative Power of Nature's Medicines* (Rodale Press, 1991).

**SONJA L. CONNOR** is a lipid research dietitian at the Oregon Health Sciences University in Portland, Oregon. She is coauthor, with William E. Connor, of *The New American Diet Cookbook* (Simon & Schuster, 1997) and *The New American Diet System* (Simon & Schuster, 1991).

**WILLIAM E. CONNOR** is a professor of medicine and head of the Division of Endocrinology, Metabolism, and Clinical Nutrition in the Department of Medicine at Oregon Health Sciences University. He is the author of over 290 articles and three books on nutrition, coronary heart disease, and lipid metabolism. He is an internationally recognized researcher, and he has been chairman of the National Heart and Lung Institute and president of the American Society of Clinical Nutrition.

**JULIE FELNER** is a freelance editor and writer based in San Francisco, California.

**KATHLEEN M. FOLEY** is a physician in the department of neurology at the Memorial Sloan-Kettering Cancer Center in New York City. She is coeditor, with F. De Conno, of *Cancer Pain Relief: A Practical Manual* (Kluwer Academic Publications, 1995) and coauthor, with Richard Payne, of *Current Therapy of Pain* (B. C. Decker, 1988).

**MICHAEL FUMENTO,** a fellow with Consumer Alert in Washington, D.C., is a science and health journalist. He is a graduate of the University of Illinois College of Law and a former AIDS analyst and attorney for the U.S. Commission on Civil Rights. The author of numerous articles on AIDS for publications worldwide, he has written several books, including *The Myth of Heterosexual AIDS* (New Republic Books, 1990) and *Science Under Siege: Balancing Technology and the Environment* (William Morrow, 1993). He received the American Council on Science and Health's Distinguished Science Journalist of 1993 Award for *Science Under Siege.*

**ROSS GELBSPAN** was an editor and reporter at the *Philadelphia Bulletin,* the *Washington Post,* and the *Boston Globe* over a 30-year period. In 1984 he was a corecipient of the Pulitzer Prize for public service reporting.

**RONALD J. GLASSER** is a pediatrician in Minneapolis, Minnesota, and the author of *The Greatest Battle* (Random House, 1976) and *The Light in the Skull: An Odyssey of Medical Discovery* (Faber & Faber, 1997).

**SCOTT M. GRUNDY** is a professor of internal medicine and biochemistry in the

Center for Human Nutrition at the University of Texas Southwestern Medical Center in Dallas, Texas. He is the author of *Cholesterol and Artherosclerosis: Diagnosis and Treatment* (J. B. Lippincott, 1990) and *The American Heart Association Low-Fat, Low-Cholesterol Cookbook* (Thorndike Press, 1989).

**MARTHA HONEY,** a freelance journalist and author, is a research fellow at the Institute for Policy Studies in Washington, D.C. Among her publications are *Hostile Acts: U.S. Policy in Costa Rica in the 1980s* (University Press of Florida, 1994) and *Ecotourism and Sustainable Development: Who Owns Paradise?* (Island Press, 1999).

**DAVID JACOBSEN** is a surgeon with Harvard Pilgrim Health Care in Boston. He is coauthor, with Eric D. Jacobsen, of *Doctors Are Gods: Corruption and Unethical Practices in the Medical Profession* (Thunder's Mouth Press, 1994).

**ANDREW G. KADAR** is an attending physician at Cedars-Sinai Medical Center in Los Angeles, California, and a clinical instructor in the School of Medicine at the University of California, Los Angeles.

**WILLIAM B. KALIHER** is a disease intervention specialist in Orangeburg, South Carolina, who has 25 years of experience with communicable disease control.

**MARTIJN B. KATAN** is a professor of human nutrition at the Agricultural University in Wageningen, the Netherlands.

**DON B. KATES** is a civil liberties lawyer and criminologist based in San Francisco, California. He has authored or coauthored a number of books, including *Handgun Prohibition and the Original Meaning of the Second Amendment* (Second Amendment Foundation, 1984) and *The Great American Gun Debate: Essays on Firearms and Violence* (Pacific Research Institute for Public Policy, 1997).

**THEA KELLEY** is a freelance journalist based in San Francisco, California.

**LESLIE LAURENCE** is a health and medical reporter. She is coauthor, with Beth Weinhouse, of *Outrageous Practices: How Gender Bias Threatens Women's Health* (Rutgers University Press, 1997).

**WILLIAM B. LINDLEY** is an associate editor of *Truth Seeker* magazine.

**RICHARD MOSKOWITZ,** a homeopathic physician, is a former president of the National Institute of Homeopathy and a graduate of Harvard University. He is the author of *Homeopathic Medicines for Pregnancy and Childbirth* (North Atlantic Books, 1992).

**ETHAN A. NADELMANN** is director of the Lindesmith Center, a New York drug-policy research institute, and an assistant professor of politics and public affairs in the Woodrow Wilson School of Public and International Affairs at Princeton University in Princeton, New Jersey. He was the founding coordinator of the Harvard Study Group on Organized Crime, and he has been a consultant to the Department of State's Bureau of International Narcotics Matters. He is also an assistant editor of the *Journal of Drug Issues* and a contributing editor of the *International Journal on Drug Policy*.

**RICHARD W. POLLAY** is a marketing professor and curator of advertising archives at the University of British Columbia. He is editor and compiler of *Information Sources in Advertising History* (Greenwood Press, 1979).

**ERIC B. RIMM** received a doctorate in epidemiology from the Harvard School of Public Health in 1990 and has since been practicing there as a research associate. He also serves as project director of the Health Professionals Follow-up Study, a prospective epidemiological study designed to investigate the nutritional etiologies of chronic disease among over 50,000 men in the United States. He is coauthor of over 30 scientific publications, including articles examining associations between alcohol, coffee consumption, and dietary antioxidants (vitamins C and E and beta-carotene) and risk of cardiovascular disease.

**JOHN A. ROBERTSON** is a professor in and the Vinson and Elkins Chair of the University of Texas School of Law in Austin, Texas. He earned his B.A. from Dartmouth College in 1964 and his J.D. from Harvard University in 1968.

**ARTHUR B. ROBINSON** is a chemist at the Oregon Institute of Science and Medicine.

**ZACHARY W. ROBINSON** is a chemist at the Oregon Institute of Science and Medicine.

**GABRIEL ROTELLO** is a columnist and the author of *Sexual Ecology: AIDS and the Destiny of Gay Men* (Dutton, 1997).

**HENRY E. SCHAFFER** is a professor of genetics and biomathematics at North Carolina State University in Raleigh, North Carolina. He is coauthor, with Lawrence E. Mettler and Thomas G. Gregg, of *Population Genetics and Evolution* (Prentice Hall, 1988).

**DAVE SHIFLETT** is a writer living in Virginia. He is a regular contributor to *The American Spectator*, and his articles have

also appeared in such journals as *The New Democrat* and *The American Enterprise*.

**MEIR J. STAMPFER** is an associate professor of epidemiology at the Harvard University School of Public Health and holds an appointment at Brigham and Women's Hospital. His current research focuses on the influence of diet and exogenous hormones on health. He received a bachelor's degree at Columbia University, an M.D. from New York University School of Medicine, and a Ph.D. in epidemiology from Harvard University. He has published over 140 scientific papers and has a major interest in the influence of diet and exogenous hormones on health.

**MARG STARK** is a freelance journalist specializing in medical news and features and the author of *What No One Tells the Bride* (Hyperion, 1998).

**JOSH SUGARMANN** is the executive director of the Violence Policy Center, an educational foundation that researches firearm violence and advocates gun control. The former communications director of the National Coalition to Ban Handguns, he is the author of *National Rifle Association: Money, Firepower and Fear* (National Press Books, 1992) and coauthor, with Kristen Rand, of *Cease Fire: A Comprehensive Stategy to Reduce Firearms Violence* (Violence Policy Center, 1994).

**JACOB SULLUM** is a senior editor for *Reason* magazine. He writes on several public policy issues, including freedom of speech, criminal justice, and education. His work has appeared in the *Wall Street Journal*, the *New York Times*, and the *Los Angeles Times*. In 1988 he won the Keystone Award for investigative reporting. He has been a fellow of the Knight Center for Specialized Journalism.

**JOHN M. SWOMLEY** is a professor emeritus of social ethics at the St. Paul School of Theology. He has also team-taught biomedical ethics at Kansas University Medical Center summer seminars. He has published several books, including *Confronting Church and State: Memoirs of an Activist* (Humanist Press, 1997) and *The Case Against School Vouchers*, coauthored by Edd Doerr and Albert J. Menendez (Prometheus Books, 1996).

**ERIC A. VOTH** is chairman of the International Drug Strategy Institute and clinical assistant professor with the Department of Medicine at the University of Kansas School of Medicine. He is also the medical director of Chemical Dependency Services at St. Francis Hospital in Topeka, Kansas. He has testified for the Drug Enforcement Administration in opposition to legalizing marijuana, and he is recognized as an international authority on drug abuse.

**DIANA CHAPMAN WALSH** is a professor in the Department of Health and Social Behavior of the School of Public Health at Harvard University. She is the author of *Corporate Physicians: Between Medicine and Management* (Yale University Press, 1987) and coeditor, with

Richard H. Egdahl, of *Health Cost Management and Medical Practice Patterns* (Ballinger, 1985).

**JENNIFER WASHBURN** is a Brooklyn-based freelance writer.

**WILLIAM C. WATERS IV** practices medicine in Atlanta, Georgia.

**BETH WEINHOUSE** is a health and medical reporter. She is the author of *The Healthy Traveler: An Indispensable Guide to Staying Healthy Away from Home* (Pocket Books, 1987) and coauthor, with Leslie Laurence, of *Outrageous Practices: How Gender Bias Threatens Women's Health* (Rutgers University Press, 1997).

**ROBERT J. WHITE** is a professor and director of neurological surgery in the School of Medicine and MetroHealth Center at Case Western Reserve University in Cleveland, Ohio.

**WALTER C. WILLETT** is a professor of medicine at Harvard Medical School. He has also been a professor of epidemiology and nutrition at the Harvard School of Public Health. He earned his M.D. in medicine from Harvard Medical School in 1970 and a Ph.D. and an M.D. in public health from the Harvard School of Public Health.

# INDEX